James R. Evans
Editor

D1241819

Handbook
of Neurofeedback
Dynamics and Clinical
Applications

Pre-publication
REVIEWS,
COMMENTARIES,
EVALUATIONS . . .

"**T**his is a gem! The book will open and broaden the reader's knowledge base, whether you've been doing neurofeedback for years or are just thinking about using it. It gives the neurofeedback practitioner a window into the way some of our most experienced practitioners, engineers, and theoreticians think about neurofeedback. The very key issues of coherence, connectivity, and synchrony training are discussed at some length. The book includes chapters on audio-visual stimulation and on the combination of neurofeedback/entrainment, both from originators of these technologies.

The book has history, theory, fertile speculation, results of some group studies, and plenty of clinical case studies and anecdotes. Every chapter has a long and excellent reference section that allows the interested reader to go further into depth. The authors of the various chapters reveal the way they think about and conduct neurofeedback in ways I haven't seen in print before. It's more like sitting down with the authors over dinner and hearing what they really think is going on. Many of the chapters get very specific about what the author actually does in clinical practice, which I find very useful indeed. Whether the concepts challenge or reinforce the way you think about your own work with neurofeedback, you'll be stimulated and more connected with the field after reading this book."

John K. Nash, PhD, BCIA-EEG
Licensed Psychologist

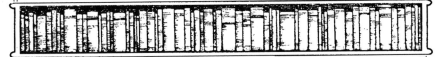

More pre-publication
REVIEWS, COMMENTARIES, EVALUATIONS . . .

"The field of neurofeedback has waited for a publication like Dr. James Evans' *Handbook of Neurofeedback: Dynamics and Clinical Applications*. With chapters written by some of the great pioneers and contributors to our field, it brilliantly solidifies in a single volume much of what is known about neurofeedback from a technical and clinical perspective. Whether you are a newcomer, technician, or advanced clinical practitioner, this is a reference work you want on the shelf of your library. This book will, undoubtedly, help advance the field of neurofeedback, and, by that, move it a step closer to earning its legitimate status as a meaningful, scientific, research-based procedure."

Robert E. McCarthy, PhD, LPC, BCIA-EEG
Executive Clinical Director,
McCarthy Counseling Associates, PA,
and the Center for Psychophysiological
Assessment and Treatment
Myrtle Beach, SC

The Haworth Medical Press®
An Imprint of The Haworth Press, Inc.
New York

Handbook
of Neurofeedback
Dynamics and Clinical Applications

THE HAWORTH MEDICAL PRESS®
Haworth Series in Neurotherapy
David L. Trudeau
Editor

Handbook of Neurofeedback: Dynamics and Clinical Applications
edited by James R. Evans

Titles of Related Interest:

Forensic Applications of QEEG and Neurotherapy
edited by James R. Evans

LENS: The Low Energy Neurofeedback System
edited by D. Corydon Hammond

New Developments in Blood Flow Hemoencephalography
edited by Tim Tinius

Quantitative Electroencephalographic Analysis (QEEG) Databases for Neurotherapy: Description, Validation, and Application
edited by Joel F. Lubar

Handbook
of Neurofeedback
Dynamics and Clinical Applications

James R. Evans
Editor

The Haworth Medical Press®
An Imprint of The Haworth Press, Inc.
New York

For more information on this book or to order, visit
http://www.haworthpress.com/store/product.asp?sku=5889

or call 1-800-HAWORTH (800-429-6784) in the United States and Canada
or (607) 722-5857 outside the United States and Canada

or contact orders@HaworthPress.com

Published by

The Haworth Medical Press®, an imprint of The Haworth Press, Inc., 10 Alice Street, Binghamton, NY 13904-1580.

PUBLISHER'S NOTE
The development, preparation, and publication of this work has been undertaken with great care. However, the Publisher, employees, editors, and agents of The Haworth Press are not responsible for any errors contained herein or for consequences that may ensue from use of materials or information contained in this work. The Haworth Press is committed to the dissemination of ideas and information according to the highest standards of intellectual freedom and the free exchange of ideas. Statements made and opinions expressed in this publication do not necessarily reflect the views of the Publisher, Directors, management, or staff of The Haworth Press, Inc., or an endorsement by them.

This book has been published solely for educational purposes and is not intended to substitute for the medical advice of a treating physician. Medicine is an ever-changing science. As new research and clinical experience broaden our knowledge, changes in treatment may be required. While many potential treatment options are made herein, some or all of the options may not be applicable to a particular individual. Therefore, the author, editor, and publisher do not accept responsibility in the event of negative consequences incurred as a result of the information presented in this book. We do not claim that this information is necessarily accurate by the rigid scientific and regulatory standards applied for medical treatment. **No warranty, expressed or implied, is furnished with respect to the material contained in this book. The reader is urged to consult with his/her personal physician with respect to the treatment of any medical condition.**

Identities and circumstances of patients and clients discussed in this book have been changed to protect confidentiality.

Library of Congress Cataloging-in-Publication Data

Handbook of neurofeedback : dynamics and clinical applications / James R. Evans, editor.
    p. ; cm.
  Includes bibliographical references and index.
  ISBN: 978-0-7890-3359-8 (hard : alk. paper)
  ISBN: 978-0-7890-3360-4 (soft : alk. paper)
  1. Biofeedback training—Handbooks, manuals, etc. I. Evans, James R.
  [DNLM: 1. Biofeedback (Psychology). 2. Electroencephalography. WM 425.5.B6 H236 2007]
RC489.B53H36 2007
615.8'51—dc22
                                                        2007000551

To the current generation of young practitioners
and researchers who, hopefully, will guide the field
of neurofeedback to its rightful position
as one of the dominant therapies
within the health care professions.

CONTENTS

SECTION III: GENERAL CLINICAL APPLICATIONS

SECTION IV: SPECIFIC CLINICAL APPLICATIONS

ABOUT THE EDITOR

James R. Evans, PhD, is Professor Emeritus at the University of South Carolina, where he taught for many years in the School Psychology Program of the Department of Psychology. He has more than thirty years experience as a school and clinical psychologist, providing psychotherapy and psychological evaluations in schools, prisons, mental health clinics, and psychiatric hospitals as well as in his own private practice. He is affiliated with the Sterlingworth Center of the Upstate in Greenville, South Carolina, where he conducts neuropsychological, psychoeducational, and quantitative EEG (QEEG) assessments and supervises neurotherapy sessions with a wide variety of clients. Dr. Evans has more than 40 publications in professional journals and is co-editor of three psychology-related books. He is co-editor of *Introduction to Quantitative EEG and Neurotherapy* and is a consulting editor to the *Journal of Neurotherapy*™ (Haworth).

Handbook of Neurofeedback
© 2007 by The Haworth Press, Inc. All rights reserved.
doi:10.1300/5889_a

CONTRIBUTORS

Helen K. Budzynski, PhD, Professor Emeritus, Psychosocial and Community Health, University of Washington, Department of Psychosocial and Community Health, Box 357263, Seattle, WA 98195-7263.

Thomas Budzynski, PhD, Affiliate Professor, Department of Psychosocial and Community Health, University of Washington, Box 357263, Seattle, WA 98195-7263.

Marco Congedo, PhD, Institute for Research in Informatics and Automatic, project i3d, Le Globe, 38410, Uriage, France.

Richard A. Crane, President, American BioTec Corporation and International MindFitness Foundation, 24 Browning Drive, Ossining, NY 10562.

Charles J. Davis, Chief Executive Officer, ROSHI Corp., 4806 10th Avenue # 4, Los Angeles, CA 90043.

Lester G. Fehmi, PhD, Director Emeritus, Princeton Biofeedback Centre 317 Mt. Lucas Road, Princeton, NJ 08540.

Joseph J. Horvat, PhD, Director of EEG and Neurofeedback at Mirasol, Mirosol, 10490 East Escalente St., Tucson, AZ 85730.

Victoria L. Ibric, PhD, Private Practice, Therapy and Prevention Center, Neurofeedback and Neurorehabilitation Institute, 65 N. Madison Ave., Suite 405, Pasadena, CA 91101.

Betty Jarusiewicz, PhD, Program Director, Atlantic Counseling Center, Inc., 27 Cypress Drive, Bayville, NJ 08721.

David Joffe, PhD, Lexicor Medical Technologies, 2840 Wilderness Place, Suite A, Boulder, CO 80301.

Handbook of Neurofeedback
© 2007 by The Haworth Press, Inc. All rights reserved.
doi:10.1300/5889_b

Lynda Kirk, MA, Executive Director, Austin Biofeedback Center, 3624 North Hills Drive, Suite B-205, Austin, TX 78731.

Gerald Kozlowski, PhD, Associate Professor, Department of Physiology, University of Texas Southwestern Medical Center at Dallas, 12870 Hillcrest Rd. #201, Dallas, TX 75230.

Robert Lawson, MS, Neurotherapy Center of Dallas, 12870 Hillcrest Rd., #201, Dallas, TX 75230.

Siegfried Othmer, PhD, Chief Scientist, EEG Institute, 22020 Clarendon St., Suite 305, Woodland Hills, CA 91367.

Susan F. Othmer, BA, Clinical Director, EEG Institute, 22020 Clarendon St., Suite 305, Woodland Hills, CA 91367.

Martha C. M. Rubi, MEd, Professor in School of Psychology, Graduate Studies, Universidad Nacional Autonoma de Mexico, UNAM. Nueva York #170, Col. Napoles, Mexico, DF 03810 Mexico.

David Siever, CET, Mind Alive, Inc., 9008-51 Avenue, Edmonton, Alberta T6E 5X4 Canada.

Hsin-Yi Tang, PhD, Assistant Professor, College of Nursing, Seattle University, 901 12th Ave., P.O. Box 222000, Seattle, WA 98122-1090.

Tim Tinius, PhD, Private Practice, 225 Benton Drive N. #104, Sauk Rapids, MN 56379.

Jonathan E. Walker, MD, Private Practice, Neuroscience Centers, Inc., 12870 Hillcrest Rd., Suite 201, Dallas, TX 75230.

Preface

By most peoples' reckoning, there is a major health crisis in the United States. Several reasons are commonly cited for this, including the high cost of healthcare, the high percentage of uninsured persons, increasingly impersonal treatment as managed care emphasizes profit over empathy, and the many negative side effects of often over-prescribed pharmacological treatments. Whatever the truth or relative importance of these factors, increasingly larger numbers of people are turning to alternative approaches to healthcare. Not without their own problems in terms of limited evidence of effectiveness, and in some cases, safety, these approaches generally are less expensive, involve personal contact with practitioners, and have few, if any, side effects. One problem faced by any individual seeking an alternative or complementary approach to healthcare is deciding which of these will be effective and safe for him or her. Should it be one with a long history, such as acupuncture, music therapy, chiropractic, or herbal treatment, or one of the newer ones? Should it be supported by both research and testimonials of former clients, or is the latter enough? Should it be one whose practitioners are certified or licensed, thus having demonstrated at least minimal competency in the field?

The approach, which is the topic of this book, neurofeedback, also known as neurotherapy and EEG biofeedback, is one of the newer and perhaps lesser-known ones. It did not really begin until the late 1960s, and has seen sustained, rapid development only in the last 15 to 20 years. It now is a field with rapidly growing research and clinical support and readily available lists of certified practitioners. Neurofeedback has been rather quietly gaining acceptance worldwide, with practitioners from diverse fields successfully applying it to ever widening numbers of disorders. The field has a professional journal, *Journal of Neurotherapy,* devoted exclusively to related research and clinical reports. In the United States, there are two certifying boards, the Biofeedback Certification Institute of America and the Neurotherapy and Biofeedback Certification Board as well as two professional societies composed largely of persons who practice neurotherapy on at least a part-time basis, the International Society for Neurofeedback and Research (ISNR) and the Association for Applied Psychophysiology and Biofeedback (AAPB). In addition, there are professional neurofeedback associations in Australia, Canada, the European Union, and Mexico. At least five books dealing primarily or exclusively with neurofeedback have been published in the past ten years. It seems safe to say that few, if any, of the other newer alternative approaches (and some of the older ones) can make all those claims.

Neurofeedback is a method that falls under the "umbrella" term, biofeedback. Both are characterized by use of electronic equipment to record and provide immediate feedback concerning ongoing psychophysiological processes such as skin temperature, muscle tension, heart rate, or in the case of neurofeedback, brain electrical activity (EEG). Feedback typically consists of tones changing in pitch or volume, "scores" visible on a computer monitor raising or lowering, and/or some graphic display continuing, diminishing, or vanishing depending on whether the goal of normalizing or modifying certain aspects of one or more psychophysiological processes is or is not being met. For example, feedback might reflect whether degree of EEG power within some frequency band, such as theta, is decreasing as desired. Without feedback, these processes would be extremely difficult or impossible to control. But with proper feedback, most persons can develop varying degrees of control. Such control may occur consciously through use of different strategies and/or unconsciously via passive association of the feedback signals with progress toward normalization. In any event, with continuing practice, processes usually normalize and this is associated with decreases in or remission of unwanted symptoms. Furthermore, at least in the case of neurofeedback such positive changes tend to be enduring.

Some skepticism of neurofeedback may be aroused by reports of neurofeedback successes with a very wide variety of disorders, for example, Attention Deficit/Hyperactivity Disorder, depression, obsessive-compulsive disorder, recovery from traumatic brain injury, addictive disorders, chronic fatigue syndrome, sleep disorders, anxiety disorders, chronic pain, tinnitus, and other disorders associated with central nervous system function. As a society, though, we have little doubt that pharmacological treatments can be effective with an even wider range of disorders through their effects on the central nervous system. When it is realized that neural function is electrochemical in nature, why should it be surprising that modifying the electrical activity of the central nervous system may be as effective as modifying neurochemistry through medications?

While dealing with medications the emphasis is on neurochemistry but a whole new realm is entered when dealing with the electrical aspects of neural function. Terms such as neurotransmitter are replaced by concepts such as frequency and amplitude of brain waves, phase relationships between waveforms, and entrainment of waves. Based on over 30 years of reports from neurofeedback practitioners, it seems that intervening in the electrical realm not only can be very effective, but also carries much less risk of adverse side effects than seen with pharmacological interventions.

The chapters of this book provide a comprehensive view of the field of neurofeedback and should be of interest both to experienced neurotherapists and those curious about or interested in entering the field. Most are written by pioneers in the field and reflect their many years of clinical experience with a variety of neurofeedback-related techniques. Readers will find a wealth of information regarding the history of the field in Section 1, speculation on the mechanisms by which neurofeedback yields positive results for clients in Section 2, and details concerning training protocols and combinations of protocols, which have been found especially effective for various conditions in Section 3. Attempts have been made to minimize use of technical terms and mathematical formulae. Thus, most of the material should be readily comprehended by readers with no more than minimal acquaintance with the concepts of biofeedback, EEG, and quantitative EEG (QEEG). Readers should keep in mind that in many cases chapter authors are expressing their own opinions and conclusions, and these may not be supported by research data or general consensus within the field of neurofeedback.

It is hoped that this text will provide further impetus to the rapid development of the field of clinical neurofeedback by stimulating theorizing and research on why and how neurofeedback is effective in a wide variety of applications and will provide practicing clinicians with valuable information on how to improve their skills, and provide a sort of historical "snapshot" of where this rapidly evolving field has been and is at this point in time. A further hope of the editor, and most likely of all contributors, is that publication of the text will stimulate wider recognition and acceptance of the field by healthcare professionals, neuroscientists, and the general public.

Acknowledgments

The editor wishes to thank various persons who contributed significantly to the completion and publication of this book. Dr. Shrikrishna Singh, Managing Editor, Science and Technology, The Haworth Press, and Dr. David Trudeau provided continuing encouragement throughout the editing process. I am very appreciative of the efforts of Ms. Jerlean Noble of the Department of Psychology at the University of South Carolina who managed details of manuscript organization and style. I also am indebted to associates who read and commented on early drafts of chapters, including Ms. Susan Ford, neurotherapist from Tryon, NC, and business associates Dr. Susan Hendley and Ms. Jane Price of the Sterlingworth Center of the Upstate in Greenville, SC. The advice and efforts of Ms. Tracy Sayles, production editor with The Haworth Press, and Ms. Vidhya Jayaprakash, head of the copyediting team from Newgen Imaging Systems, Ltd. are much appreciated. And, certainly, I thank my wife, Martha Young-Evans, for her patience during the many months when I was more or less an "absentee husband" as I edited the chapters of the book.

Handbook of Neurofeedback
© 2007 by The Haworth Press, Inc. All rights reserved.
doi:10.1300/5889_d

SECTION I:
HISTORICAL BACKGROUND

Chapter 1

Infinite Potential:
A Neurofeedback Pioneer
Looks Back and Ahead

Richard A. Crane

WHAT HAS BEEN

I thought, pioneers were those guys with arrows in their backs—
the ones whom the settlers stepped over as they took over the territory!
But since I have survived for 35 years, and even modestly prospered
in the neurofeedback business, I guess, that makes me a pioneer or
a settler of sorts.

I wonder how many others entered the neurofeedback business because of an epiphany—like experience. Probably quite a few. Mine
came in October 1970, after a day of meditation overlooking a quiet
lake behind our weekend house in Rhinebeck, New York. Dagne, my
wife, asked me to read a magazine article titled "Alpha, the Wave of
the Future," describing the company Gene Estribu had developed to
manufacture the Aquarius Alphaphone, which I believe was designed
by Tim Scully.

I was stunned and euphoric by the promise and beauty of a technology with such promise for enhancing self-knowledge. It has always
seemed to me that self-knowledge is the greatest of all challenges for
all of us. From childhood, I have been passionately interested in the
integration and interplay of mind, technology, science, and psychology, especially transpersonal psychology. I continued my retreat for
another three days and realized there was no choice but to sell my

Handbook of Neurofeedback
© 2007 by The Haworth Press, Inc. All rights reserved.
doi:10.1300/5889_01

business, and put all I had into making this technology (and the learning processes it serves) as understandable and affordable as I could. I did that, and 36 years flowed by like a summer afternoon.

At the November 1970 meeting of the Biofeedback Society of America (BSA) in New Orleans, I bought my first biofeedback instrument—an Aquarius Alphaphone. Those early BSA meetings were like heaven to me. There was so much to learn. There were scientists, educators, yogis, shamans, philosophers, business people, and health practitioners of virtually every discipline in attendance. It was a time of transformation amidst the company of renaissance men and women. The enthusiasm was palpable. Many were "on fire" with the promise of this great new scientific art form. Expectations ran high that biofeedback and what we now refer to as neurofeedback would quickly sweep the world.

Using the Alphaphone made me realize the enormous potential of brain wave training. I attempted to partner with its producer, Aquarius, but this did not work out. However, I did strike a deal with Buryl Payne of Psychophysics Labs, apparently the first biofeedback instrument company. We began marketing his equipment, which included a small battery-powered EEG monitor, which seemed to work better than the Alphaphone. Our collaboration ended in 1971.

In May 1971, I joined Hershel and Margerie Toomim of Los Angeles. They were producing a small, but effective neurofeedback device known as the Alpha Pacer, and it was selling well. We changed the name from Toomim Labs to Biofeedback Research Institute and tried to take it public. When the underwriting did not succeed, I resigned and cofounded Qtran (which developed the original "Mood Ring"), and a year later, established American BioTec with its own line of instruments. This included the A-3 EEG modeled after a fine little battery-powered instrument designed by Les Fehmi of Princeton, New Jersey. Production of these instruments continued for about 20 years.

About 1980, I met Sam Caldwell and we collaborated on development of the UniComp software series designed to work with practically all types of biofeedback instruments available. We multiplexed the raw EEG output of the A-3 EEG through five hardwired filters and produced the first computerized, commercial, multibandwidth neurofeedback system in 1982. During the 1970s and 1980s, there were several EEG biofeedback (neurofeedback) systems available. These ranged in price from a little rig made by Cyborg Corp. for about $125.00 to custom computerized systems put together by Chuck Stroebel and Jim Hardt, which cost millions. Stroebel's EEG synchrony research at the Institute for Living in Hartford required a $2,000,000 computer, and Dr. Hardt told me that his synchrony feedback system cost millions to develop. Elmer Green of the Menninger Foundation and his associate, Rex Hartsell of Topeka, had designed excellent systems for the times. The early ones involved large, hard-wired enclosures that could give feedback on four bandwidths, simultaneously. In 1973, these cost $9,000 each.

Hartsell improved the system, made it smaller, less expensive, and sold many. About 1979, the Biofeedback Research Institute developed the Apple II Plus compatible BioComp, which had EEG capability and sold for about $9,000. In my opinion, it was the best value in multimodality computerized systems for years. Cyborg's BioLab also originally ran on an Apple II, had EEG feedback capability, and sold for about $15,000. Autogenic Systems produced a large, battery-operated EEG biofeedback system, which sold in the $5,000 to $6,000 range, and the J&J Instrument Co. of Seattle made a quality stand-alone EEG instrument for a few years in the 1970s. Remember, we are talking in terms of 1979 to 1986 dollars.

Les Fehmi developed the first four-channel phase synchrony system. It was hardwired, battery-operated, sold for around $5,000, and is still in production. Tom Budzynski, in conjunction with Biofeedback Systems, developed the Twilight Learner designed to enhance the creative process using alpha/theta training. Dan Atlas built an EEG biofeedback system in Israel, and Len Ochs of Walnut Creek, California designed an early computer-based system.

By the late 1970s, neurofeedback equipment was being sidelined in favor of other modalities. Manufacturers continued to make EEG systems on a lower priority basis. Some of us, however, continued the quest for improved equipment and furtherance of EEG. In 1986, Chuck Stroebel inspired me to begin development of the CapScan. Sam Caldwell enlisted John "Pitch" Picchiottino, and we developed the CapScan Prism 5, which had four-amplifier synchrony capability and was years ahead of its time. Many still prefer the Prism 5 for synchrony feedback. Sam and "Pitch" built a remarkable system, which was as close to my "dream machine" as was possible at the time. Engineers advised us that it would be impossible to update a four-amplifier synchrony signal once per second. We eventually achieved ten updates per second. We began marketing in 1989. Both UniComp and CapScan were powerful for their time and included features that are still being replicated by others.

In the 1980s, David Joffe developed a neurofeedback/brainmapper system, which led to the birth of Lexicor Medical Technology, Inc., which became a major manufacturer of neurofeedback and quantitative EEG (QEEG) equipment during the 1990s. David told me that after we discussed Jim Lynch's best selling book, *The Language of the Heart* (Lynch, 1985), he looked up the Latin translation of Lynch's title, and so he chose Lexicor as his company name. There have been other neurofeedback systems developed in the United States and abroad, but space limitations prevent telling all of their stories.

Peniston's remarkable substance abuse study gave neurofeedback a second wind in the early 1990s, but counterintuitively, the attention deficit/hyperactivity disorder (ADHD) application became much bigger than substance abuse applications. Although that is still the case, I predict that substance abuse neurofeedback applications will eventually exceed attention disorder applications. Today, Thought Technology Ltd. produces the ProComp Infinity in Canada, and Tom Collura's Cleveland, Ohio-based company, Brain Master Technologies, Inc., produces the BrainMaster. We also are still very much in the game through Bio-Monitoring International Corporation (BMIC), which was formed to leverage the creative team originally assembled to produce the CapScan and UniComp systems. Using Internet development tools, we can utilize talents of hardware and software engineers, regardless of their physical locations. The focus of BMIC is cost-effective, breakthrough product development for the learning and performance enhancement and health science markets. Working with a major learning and performance enhancement company, we have jointly developed a unique and very successful peak performance product. We continue to work with the same company pursuing additional learning and performance enhancement products.

Readers new to the field of neurofeedback may be surprised to learn that, despite the early excitement, interest in the field decreased in the late 1970s and 1980s. Yet in the early 1990s, neurofeedback "took off." The evolution of our industry is a dramatic, often illogical, and even heroic saga. An extremely condensed personal perspective follows.

Collectively, we continue to make often-entertaining mistakes, and survive calamities (like massive decreases in third party compensation for mental health practitioners). However, the neurofeedback community as a whole keeps getting back up, brushing itself off, and charging (sometimes limping) enthusiastically onto the field of multiplying opportunities.

The "new" is often threatening to those economically rooted in the status quo. Paradigm shifts, such as those implied by neurofeedback and the "new psychology," have been viewed suspiciously by many who believed that the health care system was fine the way it was. Early on, it seemed obvious that biofeedback (and especially EEG biofeedback) could substantially reduce and/or augment numerous medications. In the early 1970s, I was told in true "Deep Throat" style by a government official that, in response to the medical and drug lobby, an effort to restrict the practice of biofeedback to persons with MD degrees was underway. It seems biofeedback was at that time a kind of banner for the alternative medical industry. Presumably, some misguided people believed that we were an economic threat. Restricting biofeedback to MD degree holders would have stopped or drastically slowed biofeedback's growth because there was less money to be made than by using more profitable (and often less effective) medical interventions. With a little help from Watergate, such restriction never materialized. However, the medical/industrial establishment continues to resist cost-reducing strategies such as biofeedback and other psychological interventions, and will probably continue to do so until the electorate becomes wiser.

My "Deep Throat" benefactor also told me that this effort was the reason that three underwriters had mysteriously abandoned our company's underwriting. At the time, some astute businessmen had expected our company to dominate the budding biofeedback business, but the collapse of our underwriting wiped us out financially. As it turned out, Autogenic Systems Inc. (ASI) came to dominate the industry, and then passed the baton to Cyborg Corp. I believe that ASI made a mistake in trying to develop its own computer instead of using an Apple. Cyborg later sold out to IBM, but IBM subsequently abandoned the biofeedback business. J&J (Jan Hoover) developed the powerful I330 System, and sprinted with the baton for about ten years before reluctantly handing it off to Thought Technology, Ltd., which now dominates the world professional biofeedback instrument market. While the U.S. government inhibits biofeedback manufacturers; the Canadian government assisted Thought Technology. Probably, the U.S. company that now has the best chance of leading the clinical neurofeedback field is BrainMaster Technologies, Inc.

One of the biggest problems our field has had to overcome is flawed research, which questioned the efficacy of biofeedback, including neurofeedback. Shellenberger and Green, in their book, *The Ghost in the Box* (1986), document twelve common methodological and conceptual errors researchers made in misguided studies, which indicated that biofeedback was ineffective, marginally effective, or too expensive. Such research hurt biofeedback badly. If any reader believes all these errors were made by accident, there is a bridge you may want to buy a piece of which links Manhattan and Brooklyn. These brutal pressures forced us individually and collectively to adapt or die.

The continuing works of those who love this field are transforming early curses into evolutionary blessings. We are a tougher, wiser breed now, and those who were not crushed can celebrate a bit before plunging into the challenges ahead. Clinical biofeedback as a field continues to spread. And a greater market seems to be emerging, namely, bringing the benefits of biofeedback-assisted self-knowledge learning to the general public. To quote Frank Lloyd Wright, "All that is done against the truth or for the truth, in the end, serves truth equally well."

Two reasons often given for biofeedback's relatively slow early growth, compared to some other less scientifically sound and effective clinical strategies, include the notions that it attracted too many "new age" people ("flakes" and "hippies") which tainted biofeedback's good name, and the lack of sufficient scientific research. It is true that some of those showing an early interest in the field believed that neurofeedback potentiates some psychoactive drugs (including some popular street drugs such as alcohol and marijuana), making less drug go farther. It appears they were right. In the author's opinion, however, both reasons basically are "straw men." The field has attracted all kinds of people, but I suggest that the weak rarely, if ever, survive. I've trained thousands, including some of the most successful, and have followed many of their careers. Being a successful biofeedback, and especially neurofeedback, practitioner is tough. It takes a lot of skill and integrity to make it an effective and profitable part of any practice.

The field has attracted some extraordinary minds. For example, I understand that Joe Kamiya (sometimes referred to as the "father of biofeedback"), once trained Abraham Maslow on a neurofeedback device. Dr. Maslow apparently was so impressed that he could not sleep for three nights because of his insight that neurofeedback could enhance the unfoldment of what he termed "Fourth Wave" psychology. During the course of training thousands of health care professionals, I have been impressed by the scientific acumen and humanity possessed by so many of them.

As for research, it is always politically correct to say there has not been enough. Certainly, we will always need more and better quality research. However, I assert, the research already published justifies biofeedback and neurofeedback being far more widely used and funded than it actually is. There is also the issue of the validity and appropriateness of much currently accepted research methodology. The late, great physicist David Bohm, a friend and mentor, told this author that he and other leading scientists feel the way scientific research is often done, with its emphasis on linear, reductionist fragmentation, is not adequate to meet the challenges facing science, and especially mind and body sciences. Also, the corrupting economic and political influences on research outcomes are leading to cynicism and somehow must be reduced. Great research often gets buried and bad research sometimes carries the day—at least for a while.

Still other factors add to the vulnerability of our field. Neurofeedback is labor intensive for both practitioner and client. Although there are a growing number of wealthy biofeedback professionals, it is likely that most would have become wealthier faster by applying their considerable talents to more lucrative forms of health care. Most practitioners agree that in order to get quality results the patient must undergo a true transformation of lifestyle. That appears to be why more intelligent, self-motivated clients usually have the best results. Those who believe that a pill or practitioner will fix a problem with little effort on the patient's part are not likely to pursue or continue in neurofeedback training.

Another vulnerability of biofeedback, and especially neurofeedback, is also one of its strengths. The author and others have observed that low frequency (alpha/theta) training sometimes leads to a peculiar kind of crisis causing some people to abandon training. The quieter the brain becomes, the more the deep recesses of the mind unfold, and a crisis of self-knowledge and self-image can occur. In these deep states, unconscious mental content may bubble to the surface, often dragging painful (trauma-related) material with it, providing therapeutic and deep insight opportunities. However, clients who sense that something uncomfortable may be coming, or that their self-image is incorrect, sometimes walk away from any process of self-discovery and necessary lifestyle changes. Similar phenomena can occur with meditation, as indicated by the Vedic saying, "In the beginning, meditation is roses, roses, but then it becomes thorns, thorns." I believe that this factor of fear phobia and identity challenge, whether conscious or unconscious, is responsible for slowing the growth of neurofeedback to a far greater degree than most practitioners realize—or will acknowledge.

Finally, the certification process has not worked as intended, which, I believe, has slowed our progress. Certification became too difficult, restrictive, and expensive, focusing too much on academic knowledge instead of practical, cost-effective, clinical training. Some of us fought for change within the system, and substantial change has been made. More improvement is needed. More than 50 percent of neurofeedback practitioners (including many neurofeedback research leaders) are not certified. Time will tell whether our certification processes can meet challenges and exert the unifying educational and quality control influences we need. Recently, New York instituted a licensing system which has driven some of the most experienced, respected BCIA certified practitioners out of business. If our national organization cannot better protect its own then, I believe, it will slow the healthy growth of our field. Hopefully, our introspection will pave the way to innovation and healthy growth. Alternatively, a case can be made that biofeedback and neurofeedback are probably progressing at about the rate than they actually are considering the magnitude of the therapeutic paradigm shifts implied and their real or imagined threat to the status quo.

WHAT IS NOW

I intended to begin this section with consensus statistics relating to total numbers of practitioners, revenue billed, equipment sales, fees, etc. However, discussions with colleagues, including some who run leading biofeedback equipment and training companies, yielded little new information. It seems, no one really knows how large the fields of biofeedback or neurofeedback are in the United States, much less in other countries. Perhaps, this is because the industry is not yet large enough to attract the expensive types of surveys needed to answer these questions. Another reason they are difficult to answer is that most, if not all, practitioners integrate neurofeedback with one or more other disciplines. Yet another reason may relate to the many ways biofeedback services are billed by practitioners. With no solid figures available, it will be necessary to venture some guesses here.

I estimate, there are between 10 and 20 thousand biofeedback practitioners in the United States, although, only a relatively few of their practices are limited to biofeedback. I estimate that there are between four and seven thousand practitioners who emphasize clinical neurofeedback. There are probably half the United States numbers in all other countries combined. As biofeedback and neurofeedback practices grow worldwide, a mass market in biofeedback, including neurofeedback instruments, is emerging. Indeed, there is evidence that this process is well underway.

I estimate that worldwide clinical biofeedback (including neurofeedback) equipment sales are between $15 million and $20 million annually. Worldwide patient/client billing is probably running between $250 million and $350 million annually. Biofeedback equipment packaged with accompanying DVD, CD, and/or software-training programs sold to the general public (mostly for performance enhancement and stress management training) is probably exceeding $15 million worldwide and growing. I estimate that neurofeedback equipment accounts for over 50 percent of that.

In the United States alone, my estimate for all types of clinical biofeedback billing would be between $150 million to $200 million, with less than 50 percent of that being through third party payment. Neurofeedback is probably at least a third of that and growing faster than other forms of biofeedback. I estimate that no more than 25 percent of neurofeedback is reimbursed by third party payers. These estimates seem reasonable. For example, just 5,000 practitioners billing $30,000 per year in services would amount to $150 million. Consider also that millions of dollars worth of increasingly efficient systems are sold every year in the United States; and many of the older units dating as far back as the 1970s are still in use. Some practitioners still use DOS based systems, which they like because of their speed, reliability, simplicity, and because their staff is trained on the software.

While exact figures are not available, it is obvious that neurofeedback is spreading throughout the world. Everyone known to the author who trains foreign practitioners comments that a substantial number of their trainees plan to take the practice back to their homelands. Over the years, seminars presented by our team have attracted people from every state, including Alaska and Hawaii, and from at least forty-nine countries. Thought Technology, Ltd. brochures claim clients in at least seventy countries. Quality equipment is being manufactured in several countries. I would wager that there is no country that does not have a practitioner trained in biofeedback in the United States.

The image of a powerful locomotive comes to mind in regard to the progress of neurofeedback. It is moving slowly along the tracks. Humans pushing on it from the back do not speed it up greatly; and others pushing against it from the front do not slow it down much. Of course, this does not prevent a number of us from harboring ambitions to "push the envelope" by ushering in breakthroughs and "killer applications." Most of us have wished more young people would choose biofeedback careers. However, it seems that especially neurofeedback is attracting young people, perhaps because of the combination of cutting edge science and the shining future of self-regulation and self-responsibility. As neurofeedback's usefulness as a tool for enhancing sensitivity, awareness, and consciousness (mindfulness) becomes more widely realized, ever more young people who are gifted will join us. And undoubtedly, some of them will provide the major breakthroughs needed.

In the author's opinion, one of the biggest stories now unfolding in the field is the application of neurofeedback to life and performance enhancement. We are contributing, through The International Mind-Fitness Foundation (IMF), to the growing field of life (job one) and performance (job two) enhancement. I have been inspired by psychologists like Seligman, Maslow, and others who claim that psychology and psychophysiology are evolving far beyond the traditional medical model into heuristic-type teaching of the science and art of increasing the quality of day-to-day consciousness. At IMF, we use neurofeedback (on an optional basis) as a super-learning tool in our coaching and training programs. We coined the term MindFitness® because it carries the implication that, like physical fitness, there is a relatively simple way to work—a process, whereby the mind can be strengthened, made more resilient and flexible, thus making it more capable of seizing the opportunities and avoiding the dangers that life continuously presents.

The learning applications for biofeedback and neurofeedback seem almost unlimited. We can begin as basic and relatively simple as using electromyograph (EMG) for relaxation and neuromuscular rehabilitation, and continue through hundreds of applications. However, there is a particular family of consciousness/life enhancement applications, which I feel is more challenging and has greater potential than the rest. Although this is difficult to articulate, I'd like to try. Biofeedback is a technology of self-knowledge. In my opinion, the ultimate application of such a technology is to directly enhance self-learning of the process of transforming the moment-to-moment, day-to-day quality of consciousness and awareness in real time. Of course, all biofeedback learning uses some such "mindfulness" principle to some degree. However, some of us feel we are taking the "consciousness of consciousness," awareness, and related principles to significantly more challenging and useful levels. I think it is fair to say that while most of what is done in the more common clinical biofeedback applications and in life and performance enhancement training is the same, there is a difference. This difference, I assert, is that self-learning skills have to be taken to a higher level in order to get satisfactory results in life and performance enhancement than is required to get clinically satisfactory results with more common applications. Various neurofeedback practitioners presently are doing their own versions of this "now power" (mindfulness) learning or something similar. The author's perspective in this area has been deeply influenced by numerous teachers and scientists, including the physicist David Bohm, J. Krishnamurti, and my wise, playful wife, Dagne. More detail on this perspective is available in the book titled, *Mindfitness Training: Neurofeedback and the Process* (Crane and Soutar, 2000), and at www.MindFitness.info, and I intend to go even more deeply into these principles and strategies in another book now in process. The Nobel Laureate, Francis Crick, and other leading scientists assert (as the ancient Greeks did) that better understanding of consciousness is the most critically important scientific challenge of any time. The importance of improving the quality of our own individual and collective consciousness cannot be overemphasized.

Our MindFitness Training is a synthesized, heuristic (self-discovery) process of understanding, applying, and integrating those principles and learning strategies, which, I believe, increase insight, self-knowledge, creativity, and energy. I assert there is a learnable process whereby, we become all we can be—whereby, we make the most of what we have—of what we are. Since everyone is unique, each person must discover his or her own individual process; hence the necessity for self-teaching and heuristic learning. The MindFitness Process intends to produce self-knowledge as quickly as possible. An important principle underlying this work is bringing order to the conditioned, "mechanical," computerlike aspects of the brain so there is easier access to higher, nonmechanical orders of intelligence, which can then manage the mechanical part efficiently and in line with highest, intrinsic, personal values. MindFitness Training is evolving, and tackles sometimes-difficult issues that affect quality of consciousness such as appropriate exercise and creating economic order. Implied is a lifelong heuristic learning process whereby the ordinary individual gains skill at discovering and continuously improving, renewing, and sustaining conscious and unconsciousness processes, including awareness, thinking, perception, attention, creativity, and health.

THE FUTURE

Biofeedback and neurofeedback as technologies of self-knowledge have a huge and complex future. Relative to this, Einstein said, "It will require a substantially different manner of thinking if humankind is to survive." Increasing self-knowledge, improving the clarity and coherence of thinking as well as sensitivity to orders of intelligence that lie beyond thinking must vastly improve all sciences and transform humanity's future. There is a crisis in the consciousness of mankind. The danger is obvious, yet opportunity lies before us. The unfolding of "a new manner of thinking," with greatly increased psychological freedom and enhanced consciousness, will surely lead to wiser, more compassionate electorates and societies.

Neurofeedback, in conjunction with the emerging science of consciousness is, I believe, already more useful than most now realize. I predict that neurofeedback is destined to become one of the most valuable, easy-to-apply consciousness-enhancing technologies in history. There is a hypothesis (and I assert a growing consensus) that enhancing the ability to observe thinking at the moment it is actually happening is critical to improving coherence of thought. If much, or most, of what is destructive in the world is due to incoherent individual and collective thinking, and neurofeedback can be substantially effective in increasing awareness and coherence of thought, then it seems to me that neurofeedback's potential stretches into infinity. Of course, much work is required to transform lofty words into practical, relatively easy to understand learning programs and strategies. The challenge lies in the execution, and execution is arduous and often expensive. The neurofeedback community includes wondrously creative individuals and teams. The economic tide is turning in our favor. We are on the right side of history.

The unfolding of neurofeedback's future will depend in large part on investment. Investment, in turn, will depend on the importance that society places on the nurturing of consciousness and self-regulation. For those of us who late middle aged, the question is, "How long will it take before neurofeedback attracts adequate capital to unleash its immense, pent up potential?" It would be much fun to live to see it and bask in its light. Presently, the U.S. health care system is in a liminal moment. Something old is dying and something new is being born. Futurists say our health care system must change immensely. It is savaging the working and middle classes as well as the small businesses that deliver most of the productivity critical to our prosperity.

Longevity experts believe that we are likely to double our life spans again in this century. It seems virtually certain to me that neurofeedback-assisted self-regulation must play a significant role in bringing another longevity evolution about. The mind-body principle (Green, 1977) implies that enhancing consciousness improves health and vice versa. I predict, therefore, that whatever new system emerges, biofeedback (especially neurofeedback) will flourish and attract much more scientific support and capital than it now does.

If my intuition is serving me well, biofeedback (including neurofeedback) could grow into a $20 billion or more industry within 20 years. Some may recoil from these numbers, because they seem too optimistic. But remember, we are talking worldwide, and almost all countries beginning to open up to biofeedback and neurofeedback are about where the United States was in the late 1970s. And some of those countries are more open to alternative, preventative and money saving strategies than we in the United States are. The Internet is spreading biofeedback information exponentially. The definition of what we think of as biofeedback is expanding. Some biofeedback systems are sold to complementary medicine practitioners, whose primary application is not biofeedback but as measurement tools to demonstrate effectiveness of their particular specialties. There is a huge mass-market potential that barely has been tapped.

I believe virtual reality (VR) feedback will ultimately deliver some of the most effective self-regulation learning systems ever seen. Internet applications will grow in terms of both training and diagnostics, including substantial growth in telemedicine. There will be decreases in size and cost, and the market will grow for portable, battery-operated, computerized instruments reminiscent of Palm Pilots. Four-amplifier neurofeedback/QEEG instruments will emerge just as four-channel evoked potential systems became common in neurological diagnostics. "MiniQ" (single and dual amplifier) neurofeedback systems already exist.

Clinical software has come a long way, but must evolve in order to catch up to hardware's capabilities. Programmers will develop software that is more intuitive and improve flexibility so that practitioners can more efficiently facilitate client learning, tailor reports to payers, and have more freedom to be creative. Normative databases have already been integrated with the top neurofeedback systems, and these databases will get better and easier to use. The technology, including software, is way ahead of creative applications.

Movies are arguably the most important art forms of our times, yet movie technology was in place years before artists, writers, directors, and actors emerged who knew how to use the technology in ways that delivered compelling stories and attracted the masses. I believe that improving consciousness will emerge as one of the greatest of scientific art forms as humanity plunges headlong into simultaneous technological, scientific, psychological, and physiological evolutionary leaps. Leading computerized biofeedback systems have capabilities crying out for creative practitioner/artists to more fully employ their existing potential.

The author joins those calling for a transformation of psychophysiological research so that it better deals with the mind and body as an interconnected system. There must be substantial reduction of the fragmentation and corruption existing in today's health care research establishment. Claire Cassidy (1994) does a brilliant job of both describing the problems and offering strategies for developing research methodology that better meets the challenges before us. All sciences including quantum physics, nonlinear dynamics, neuroscience, and neurophilosophy are under pressure to improve research methodologies and accountability. I predict that the maxim, "If it can't be counted, it doesn't count" will give way to "That which counts most can't be counted."

Many now believe that EEG synchrony and coherence training holds considerable promise. In fact, the first neurofeedback synchrony and coherence conference was held in New York in 2005. Synchrony and coherence training are more important than most realize, but it would require too much space to explain why in this chapter. I do, however, advocate for more development of synchrony training equipment that does as good or a better job than the CapScan Prism 5. Consensus is growing that such training can improve neurofeedback learning curves, facilitate breakthroughs, and prove invaluable with some difficult clients.

As more people realize the importance of self-knowledge, I predict that personal biofeedback instruments will become as ubiquitous as bathroom scales and mirrors, and beautiful instrumentation will be worn as clothing and jewelry. The original Mood Stone Ring developed by the Qtran Co. was a beautiful, durable, and effective personal temperature trainer. They cost about $150 and we sold about $30 million worth of them. Unfortunately, costume jewelry manufacturers found a way around our patents and flooded the world with cheap replicas that did not work. Although this destroyed Qtran, they sold about $500 million dollars worth of them.

These earlier personal instruments were trivial compared to what will emerge. Fashionable and useful instrumentation will be developed thus enabling individuals to increase awareness of both healthy and unhealthy internal and external influences such as stress, neuroimmune processes, air, radiation, etc. I believe that neurofeedback and heart rate variability (HRV) research, now underway, will lead to extraordinary instruments that feed back synchrony and coherence relationships between heart and brain. The neurophilosophical implications of integrating neurocardiology with neurofeedback (emotion and thought—autonomic and central nervous systems) have already aroused enormous interest among some neurofeedback practitioners. There is an ancient saying, "When the heart enters the brain, wisdom and compassion emerges."

Car seats and steering wheels can be modified to pick up physiological signals. Rear view mirrors can analyze eyes, and sensors can detect breath. Room temperature super conductors will allow the walls of houses to pick up most signals radiated by the body, including EEG, heart rate, breathing and muscle activity, making the whole house a biofeedback instrument. These things or something even more effective will happen.

In the book, *The Singularity Is Near,* Kurzweil (2005) makes a strong case that within about 30 years, a computer will pass the Turing Test, that is, artificial intelligence (AI) so sophisticated that a human cannot tell the difference between a computer thinking and a human thinking. It is rather scary at first blush, but I am betting that AI will bring more benefits than losses by extending and complementing human intelligence. Biofeedback already is a form of AI. Perhaps the most elegant definition of intelligence the author has heard is "Intelligence is sensitivity." Biofeedback instruments increase sensitivity like prostheses such as glasses, a hearing aid, a blind man's cane, etc. The continuing explosion of AI will mean almost unimaginable increases in effectiveness and ease of use of self-knowledge technology including biofeedback. I predict a way will be discovered to obtain real-time feedback on brain chemistry changes, enabling self-regulation strategies for modifying brain chemistry (which we already do indirectly).

Biofeedback, including neurofeedback, has much power to potentiate drugs. I predict that under enlightened medical supervision, practitioners will achieve results with drug and biofeedback combinations that will astonish skeptics and motivate politicians. Inspiring applications to neuroimmune disorders will unfold. As health care costs escalate, pharmaceutical companies will come to realize that making less drugs works better in their long (and maybe short) term interests. An extensive article in the New York Times (October 2, 2006) included the following: "Panel Urges Warning Labels for Stimulants" and "Stimulants like Ritalin could have dangerous effects on the heart, and federal drug regulators should require manufacturers to provide written guides to patients and place prominent warnings on drug labels describing the risks, a federal drug advisory panel voted." What a shame it will be, if it turns out that those children who have been on these medications for the last 15 years or so develop heart trouble unnecessarily as adults because they were discouraged from trying nonmedical alternatives such as neurofeedback.

The author is enthusiastic about the potential for conversion of physiological signals to musically corrected sound. I predict musicians will hold concerts in which they produce music and visual displays by manipulation of their physiology. Our group and some performance artists already have experimented with this type of conversion. But what we have done so far is crude compared to the art form envisioned—rather like playing a bowstring compared to an orchestra. When I first heard the sounds produced by our own crude experiments, I had an "aha" perception that much of jazz music is a supersensitive expression by the artist of signals coming from his own physiology. It is easy to speculate that being able to make our own mind/body music audible can increase our self-knowledge and ability to learn how to improve the moment-to-moment quality of consciousness. Imagine listening to "body music" coming from another, and being attracted or repelled by it much as we might be when listening to speech. In some ways, it could be more revealing than speech.

Signals of incredible subtlety will become detectable and incorporated into clinical and personal biofeedback instruments. The International Society for Subtle Energy and Energy Medicine (ISSEEM) was founded over 15 years ago. One of its goals is to encourage scientific research into energies that are recognized in Indian, Chinese, and other older medical sciences, but are not yet officially recognized in modern Western science. For example, many master acupuncturists, while acknowledging that acupuncture owes much of its effectiveness to modification of electrical energy in the meridians, assert that there is an additional kind of energy, which they also can manipulate. They usually assert that this other energy, which many call "chi," is more important than its electrical aspect. There are over 200 Ayurvedic medical texts that document treatment strategies for dealing with an energy called Kundalini. Perhaps, energies such as these will prove to be aspects of quanta fields. In any case, we will learn much more about these during this century. Subtle energies fed back and brought under conscious control could have incredible consequences. If these energies are as powerful as Buddhist, Ayurvedic, ancient Greek, and Chinese teachers suggest, we will need a lot of wisdom and balance to avoid the dangers and seize the opportunities.

How we decide who is qualified to be a neurofeedback practitioner is likely to change. Many prominent practitioners disagree with the current Biofeedback Certification Institute of America's (BCIA) certification process, and protest by allowing their certificates to lapse. I suggest that certification become as inclusive as possible. Today, many practitioners are uncertified. By allowing more people into the certification family, we are in a much better position to influence the field, and assist those who need skill upgrading. It also would be possible to offer levels of certification, for example, from technician to diplomate. There are at least two competing certification organizations, and there are rumors of two more organizations emerging with the backing of large professional societies. Recently New York has instituted a licensing process which has put some of the most experienced and respected BCIA certified biofeedback practitioners (including Senior Fellows) out of business. If our national organization cannot do a better job of protecting its own then that weakness will further delay the healthy evolution of bio and neurofeedback.

One of the strategies the author and his associates have undertaken in order to meet twenty-first century biofeedback and neurofeedback challenges is to reorganize our approach to the traditional clinical biofeedback business by creating a new corporation, Biofeedback Resources International (BRI). Our intentions for BRI include (1) bringing innovative strategies to performance enhancement and to the spectrum of biofeedback equipment and training needs, from clinical to mass market, (2) going beyond "motivational" training by focusing on what is actually required to maximize quality of life regardless of its commercial potential. Through BRI and the International Mind-Fitness Foundation, we intend to make our work available at lowest cost possible, yet prudent. Margaret Mead said, "Try to develop models which are not arbitrary and man-made, but organic and natural. The difference is in the intention. Arbitrary, man-made models have as their intention manipulation and control. Natural, organic models have as their intention resonance and reverence." We take her insight to heart.

To my mind, the most important factor in therapy, or in life and performance enhancement, is the creative process. Discovering and/or refining creative process strategies, including neurofeedback and other forms of feedback, should have high priority. Neurofeedback continues to attract creative people from many disciplines, thus bringing a fecund holism to our field.

I have come to believe that the field of neurofeedback probably is progressing about as fast as it can, considering the magnitude of the scientific revolution embedded in it. Implied is that self-knowledge technology, services, and education are a critically important part of our emerging future, and that true self-knowledge therapy and education will result in huge changes in the status quo. Thus, it is reasonable to believe that the 40 or so years it has taken us to get this far is about on track. The Old Testament says, "Your young shall see visions; your old will dream dreams." The combination of visionaries and dreamers in neurofeedback will continue to give birth to astounding developments. I joyfully "hide" and watch.

REFERENCES

Cassiday, C. (1994, Winter). Unraveling the ball of string: Reality, paradigms, and the study of alternative medicine. *Advances: The Journal of Mind-Body Health, 10*(1): 4-31.

Crane, R. A. & Soutar, R. (2000). *Mindfitness training: Neurofeedback and the process.* Lincoln, NY: Writers Club Press; San Jose, Shanghai.

Green, E. (1977). *Beyond biofeedback.* New York: Dell.

Kurzweil, R. (2005). *The singularity is near: When humans transcend biology.* New York: Viking; Member of the Penguin Group.

Lynch, J. J. (1985). *The language of the heart: The body's response to human dialogue.* Baltimore, MD: Bancroft Press.

Shellenberger, R. & Green, J. A. (1986). *From the ghost in the box to successful biofeedback training.* Greeley, CO: Health Psychology Publications.

SECTION II:
THEORETICAL CONCERNS

Chapter 2

Implications of Network Models for Neurofeedback

Siegfried Othmer

INTRODUCTION

The context for this chapter is provided by the strains developing within the dominant paradigm for the psychopathologies namely, their codification in terms of discrete disorders and their presumed traceability to underlying deficits in neurochemical functioning. The prevailing model fails to account for the prevalence of comorbidities and multiple diagnoses; it fails to address developmental aspects of disorders; it categorically fails to acknowledge the progressive time course of many disorders and the episodic nature of many others; and it cannot account for the interaction of psychodynamic and neurophysiological variables. In short, the idealized models fall considerably short of being able to describe real-world clinical complexity. Finally, the prominence of side effects in pharmacological remedies can be taken as evidence that the actual underlying deficits have not been well targeted.

Unfortunately, this unsatisfactory state of affairs is sustained in the clinical realm by the third-party reimbursement environment that is also based on the flawed codification scheme, and sustained by a drug delivery system that has successfully recruited the research and academic communities into dependency. In research, the paradigm enforces a continuing preoccupation with the fixed diagnostic categories, which sustains the paradigm past its dotage, and prevents any

Handbook of Neurofeedback
doi:10.1300/5889_02

engagement with the clinical complexities ordinarily encountered. Finally, the paradigm motivates a focus on genetic causation that cannot offer near-term relief even under the most optimistic assumptions. The genetic model cannot, in any event, account for the rapid increase in the ranking of mental disorders in the global burden of disease. If we disregard the childhood mortality attributable to poor hygiene in the Third World, depression already ranks at the top of the hierarchy in terms of disability adjusted life years, ahead of cancer and heart disease.

On the positive side, this chapter is motivated by the growing conviction that neurofeedback offers broad efficacy that cuts across diagnostic boundaries. By virtue of the fact that neurofeedback entails essentially no side effects, one is tempted to conclude that it is targeting the source of the problem. And in view of the fact that it tends to reduce requirements for psychoactive medications, it stands as a direct challenge to the conventional view that disorders are grounded in neurochemical disregulation. But even if these assertions are regarded as lacking strong evidentiary support in the literature to date, the fact that neurofeedback is effective at all for any condition is already sufficient reason to provoke inquiry into the mechanisms that may be at play.

If we regard the cumulative clinical evidence from anything other than a doctrinaire rejectionist frame of mind, then the following propositions can be taken as starting points for a discussion of mechanisms: (1) Remediation of various psychopathologies has been achieved with an increasing variety of neurofeedback techniques, based in turn on a variety of model assumptions. (2) Although some symptoms appear more intractable than others, the general clinical experience bespeaks a broad improvement in function that encompasses a wide variety of symptom categories that may have no obvious connection. (3) Remediation is observed not only with respect to the conditions commonly addressed with psychopharmacological agents but also with respect to classes of conditions that are clearly resistant to medical management: (a) specific learning disabilities; (b) traumatic brain injury and stroke; (c) the autistic spectrum; (d) Parkinson's; (e) the dementias; (f) chronic pain syndromes; and finally, (g) coma.

Significant insights are also furnished when we consider the time course of neurofeedback training. Curiously, the dimension of time is not typically under discussion when it comes to psychopharmacology. For most of the medications, no immediate impact on functionality is even anticipated. The clinical improvement is expected to accrue gradually. In the case of neurofeedback, the experience of state change is often prompt, occurring routinely in the first session and often in the first few minutes. The immediacy of the change, and its correlation with the contingencies of reward, makes it more likely that a bioelectrical description of state change should suffice. Any change in neuromodulator status should be secondary to such change in the timing and frequency domains. It cannot be the prime mover.

Most likely, the same is true when sudden state change is experienced in the clinical population. The excursion into seizure, into a migraine, into a panic attack, or into a sudden suicidal episode is likely to have been first triggered in the bioelectrical domain. This seems obvious when one considers the known triggers of migraines and seizures—rhythmic photic stimulation, for example. In the case of seizures, the presumption is also favored by observations of the EEG during transitional states. One can often discern the gradual and progressive development of seizure-like activity in the EEG prior to the onset of full-blown seizures. Further supporting this conjecture is the observation that neurofeedback is particularly effective for such transient excursions into dysfunction. That is to say, if one were to appraise the relative efficacy of neurofeedback and pharmacology for steady-state conditions (such as dysthymia and generalized anxiety) versus transient conditions (such as panic disorder or migraine), the relative superiority of neurofeedback for the transient conditions would be quite unambiguous. Hence, intervening in the timing and frequency domains of function appears to be preferentially efficacious for those conditions that exhibit a rapid time course. It would be straightforward to postulate that both the "immediate cause" as well as the remedy lie in the bioelectrical domain for such conditions.

The same argument is more difficult to sustain for the conditions that are more stable over the short term. Nevertheless, we shall invoke the kindling model to make the case. First applied to seizures, it was subsequently adduced by R. M. Post in application to the precursor phenomena seen in Bipolar Disorder (Post, 1986). Even though the diagnosis of Bipolar Disorder was often not made until maturity, a history of dysphoria could often be identified going all the way back to early childhood. A first observation of major depression sets the stage for a repetition. The period between occurrences of major depression becomes ever shorter. Episodes of mania may occur, ultimately eventuating in full-blown manic-depressive illness. Progressivity can be identified throughout the whole time course of the illness.

Other conditions have since been recognized as being progressive in character, to which the kindling model could similarly be applied: anxiety disorder, major depression, panic disorder, migraine, obsessive-compulsive disorder, Tourette syndrome, asthma, schizophrenia, posttraumatic stress disorder (PTSD), and finally chronic pain. The kindling model permits one to attempt a partitioning in these conditions between the psychodynamic and the neurophysiological realm. Whatever partitioning one may have assigned at the outset in a particular case, progressiveness of the condition gives evidence of the increasing role of physiological disregulation. Eventually the condition takes on a life of its own, with little mooring to life events. Since synaptic activity is the first nexus, or point of linkage, between the psychodynamic realm and that of state regulation, it is straightforward to propose that the disregulation may also be encoded as a neural network property.

This supposition is perhaps somewhat easier to accept when attention is restricted to posttraumatic stress disorder, borderline personality disorder, and dissociative identity disorder. All of these are deemed to be of traumatic origin, and all such traumas start with encoding in the bioelectrical realm. That is to say, the first representation of an event within the central nervous system (CNS)—traumatic or otherwise—is in terms of a distributed transient activation of particular neural networks. In the case of trauma potential, the particular pattern of activation is accorded such valence that it is likely to be encoded permanently for later recall. In PTSD in particular, we observe in flashbacks the intimate connection between historical memory and physiological state. It has been proposed to simply enlarge the concept of memory to assert that the body-mind records the trauma as a unitary event. The "content" memory becomes inseparable from the "state" memory. The traumatic memory becomes "state-stamped" more than "date-stamped." The starting point for such encoding must necessarily be the bioelectrical realm.

Finally, it must be said that no hard line is being drawn here between the bioelectrical and the neurochemical domains. If matters are discussed at the right level, then that simply facilitates a greater economy of ideas and simpler descriptions. Ultimately, what is claimed here must not be at war with what we have found to be valid in the pharmacological management of mental disorders. When we are done, however, it may be easier to understand pharmacological efficacy in terms of the bioelectrical or network model than by restricting the discussion to the neurochemical realm. Most likely, the two will largely remain different descriptions of the same phenomenology, appealing to different scientific constituencies with few points of contact.

What has shifted the author's perspective has been the need to bring the dimension of time into the picture. If we did not have to contend with the history of the neurochemical model, the case for the priority of bioelectrical models would be straightforward. After all, the brain must satisfy stability conditions just like any other feedback control system. There is no dispensation. The brain must organize its affairs on all behaviorally relevant timescales. Behavioral demands require the brain to organize the most rapid responses possible, and that "bandwidth" takes our brains to the edge of instability. Instability is a hazard in all control systems, and it can be treated in a manner that is universally applicable to all of them. More generally, the tight constraints on brain timing make it only too reasonable to suppose that functional deficits might be traceable to disregulations of various kinds in the timing or frequency domain. This may be particularly relevant to conditions of dysfunction that have little manifest organic or structural basis, such as minor traumatic brain injury, fibromyalgia, chronic fatigue syndrome, and premenstrual syndrome (PMS).

The fact that this shift in perspective happens to be difficult to bring about is likely to be attributable to the traditional preoccupation of medicine with structurally based models. The neurochemical models of neuroregulation still belong in the domain of structure, even when they are used to describe brain function and its deficits. The moment we move to a description in the bioelectrical realm, however, we are unambiguously in the functional domain. There is, unfortunately, no good incremental way to get there, and science tends, by and large, to move incrementally.

THE TRANSITION FROM STRUCTURAL
TO FUNCTIONAL MODELS

The conceptual chasm has been partly filled by the concept of brain plasticity, which used to be rare in the literature but is now commonplace. Brain plasticity is a useful transitional phrase that allows phenomena that used to be regarded as structurally immutable to move to being regarded as functionally malleable and adaptable. Where we are along that continuum of transition has once again to do with the dimension of time. The shorter the timescale of change, the more it is evident that we should apply a functional description, most likely out of a bioelectrical model. As an example, one may consider the finding that sensory receptive fields are not permanently fixed upon initial maturation but are adaptable following injury or even alteration in usage. Ultimately, it was found that such reallocation of cortical real estate could occur within mere seconds. Such a time rate of change surely stretches the traditional conception of brain plasticity, and motivates a reappraisal in terms of functional models. The term brain plasticity may ultimately have only a transient utility as concepts are conveyed, one by one, from a structural perspective to a functional description.

When it comes to functional models, we confront the daunting complexity of the central nervous system. It does not seem possible to get it all into view at the same time. We may have to content ourselves at one level with general principles, and at another, with drawing the most general conclusions we can from specific research findings. With nominally 10 billion cortical neurons, and an average number of some 10^4 synaptic connections to other neurons, and with an average firing-rate of between one and ten impulses per second, we are dealing with a density of between 10^{14} and 10^{15} action potentials being generated within cortex per second. How is this activity managed, and in particular, how is stability to be assured if the typical neuron propagates its activity with a gain of some 10^4? Why is there not a huge hazard of an information catastrophe, of an exponential runaway of activity, of a cortical Melissa virus?

First of all, it must be observed that even though excitatory synapses dominate in cortex, in the cerebrum as a whole there is a predominance of inhibitory connections. (The neurosurgeon Joe Bogen used to describe the brain, only somewhat tongue in cheek, as consisting of inhibitory systems inhibiting inhibitory systems which inhibited yet other inhibitory systems.) Second, the inhibitory postsynaptic potential excursions generated by such inhibitory boutons also have a longer duration, and hence much larger impact, than the excitatory postsynaptic potentials. This is illustrated in Figure 2.1. Together, these factors account in significant measure for the fact that excitatory signals incur considerable attrition through running the gauntlet of inhibition in their progression through cortex.

Also illustrated in Figure 2.1 is the generation of an action potential through an overlapping of excitatory postsynaptic potentials sufficient to meet threshold. A single excitatory postsynaptic potential excursion (EPSP) is insufficient to generate an action potential in the target neuron. At least one co-conspirator is required. Moreover, the timing sensitivity of this coalescence of events is the width of an EPSP, that is to say, on the order of 10 msec. This means that every action potential must be gated forward by at least one other facilitating excitatory transient. The extraordinary timing sensitivity of this coin-

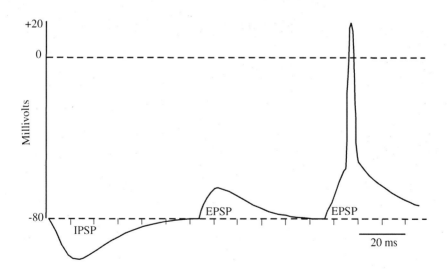

FIGURE 2.1. Illustration of the basic process of action potential generation as a threshold phenomenon. The generation of an action potential depends upon the coincidence of excitatory post-synaptic potential excursions (EPSP). The allowable time window is on the order of 10 msec.

cidence makes this the most significant impediment to the potential hazard of information runaway.

Stephen Wolfram, author of the software Mathematica, said in his recent book, *A New Kind of Science* that, ". . . all processes, whether they are produced by human effort or occur spontaneously in nature, can be viewed as computations" (Wolfram, 2002, p. 715). Further, he stated, as a general principle, that simple generating functions are capable of explaining a remarkable variety of behavior. That is to say, the essential computation may even be simple. The phenomenon under discussion may be a case in point. Whereas, the neuron can also be regarded as an analog computer of incredible complexity, in its role as a propagator of action potentials, we may be dealing with the utmost in simplicity: the neuron is acting as a coincidence detector. The simple generating function of behavior at the most basic level may be coincidence detection. This makes timing and its integrity within the network of the utmost importance, which in turn makes timing itself effectively the bearer of information. That allows us to view every neuron in the network as a mediator of timing, and as a propagator of timing information, effectively the signature of the event. Finally, it makes timing and its organization a prime suspect in mental disorders, and it makes the manipulation of timing and the restoration of timing integrity within the neural network the most obvious candidate for the mechanism of efficacy of neurofeedback.

Collectively, these considerations highlight the role of the individual neuron in bearing and propagating crucial timing information. That having been done, it is necessary to argue an apparent contradiction; namely, that the goings-on at the single-neuron level are ultimately of no import. As Sir John Eccles once said, the firing or non-firing of a single pyramidal neuron cannot be of any consequence to brain function. This is only a dramatic way of illustrating that information is embodied in ensembles—neuronal assemblies—rather than being the property of individual neurons. This has made it difficult to resolve the puzzle of the neural code, the question of how information is encoded in the neural signal stream. In one illustrative experiment, for example, some 100 neurons involved in gill movement in a marine animal were instrumented and firing rates monitored during subsequent events of spontaneous gill movement (Wu, Cohen, & Falk, 1994). There was often a gross similarity in firing patterns in particular neurons among successive ostensibly identical gill movements, but there was no microscopic reproducibility to be found in any neuron. If the ensemble firing is considered collectively, however, there was excellent tracking between events. The control of movement cannot be treated as other than an ensemble property. Below that level, synaptic events lose meaning.

Matters are similar on the sensory processing side. Neurofeedback pioneer Les Fehmi reported on an early experiment in which monkeys were trained in food reward to a visual cue appearing above one of two bins (Fehmi, Adkins, & Lindsley, 1965). After only a brief exposure to the visual cue, a bright blanking pulse was applied for purposes of perceptual masking. Progressively, the exposure time to the cue was shortened. Remarkably, the monkeys were able to perform the task correctly down to less than 50 msec exposure, and they were down to chance level only when exposure was reduced to less than 25 msec. This means that all of the information required for the choice was available to the brain in less than 50 msec. Visual processing had to take place in parallel. Sequential processing would not be fast enough or sufficiently discriminating, given limitations in cell firing rates.

Parallel processing of visual information means that the continuous visual input is packeted into ensembles that, from then on, must be treated by the brain as belonging together. This packeting occurs at a nominal rate of 40 Hz. The corresponding period is 25 msec. This digital representation of the image is then processed in various brain regions, each dealing with some feature or aspect of the visual field, yet we ultimately experience the event as one coherent image. This need to bring together disparate information into one percept is known as the binding problem. In fact, however, each of the constituent areas of visual processing also has a binding problem to solve.

An elegant solution that has been proposed is that "time does binding," that is, simultaneity defines belonging (von der Malsburg, 1981). As Wolf Singer, one of the early contributors to this model has put it, "what fires together wires together." This dictum was first applied to the Hebbian understanding of the gradual strengthening of synaptic junctions in accordance with their utilization. Now it was seen to apply at the network level as well, in the sense that what fires together belongs together functionally in the moment. Coincidence detection at the neuronal level is therefore to be seen as the irreducible binding event upon which the entire communication scheme of synaptic information transport is constructed. However, such binding only becomes meaningful to the brain when it manifests as a group property. Every neuron's axonal tree can be seen as propagating a timing signature, and the dispersal of every action potential in such a tree can be regarded in terms of its essential role in binding. Only if the context is favorable does this process bear fruit, and for present purposes the context is subsumed under the rubric of "state management."

ON THE UBIQUITY OF STATE MANAGEMENT

It may be helpful in this regard to distinguish formally between the information being conducted up the signal processing chain and the contextual inputs that either facilitate or disfacilitate this process. This is illustrated in block diagram fashion in Figure 2.2. Significantly, this process occurs at every neuron, and thus, every neuron can be thought of as an analog computer that brings together the realms of information transfer and of state management. The central nervous system (CNS) quite literally gets a vote at every synapse. This brings to mind the early work of John Basmajian, in which the electrical output of a single motor unit was displayed on an oscilloscope and the firing rate was brought under complete voluntary control with some reinforcement for success (Basmajian, 1963). In practice, control could be exercised in such exquisite detail that the experimenter could

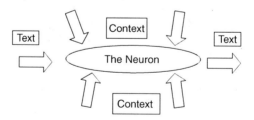

FIGURE 2.2. Synaptic transport of information can be seen as governed by a variety of synaptic modulations that jointly determine whether the context for the propagation of the signal is favorable. All such influences can be subsumed under the rubric of "state regulation." Hence, each and every neuron represents an interaction zone between the realm of information transfer and of state management.

beat out the rhythm of Yankee Doodle Dandy on the oscilloscope screen with the firing of his motor unit. Because the seriousness and sobriety of scientific work should never be called into question, however, this little fillip did not make it into the published paper. That is unfortunate because it illustrates that voluntary control could be exercised in this case from moment-to-moment. It was on/off control in real time rather than merely the consequence of a long learning process that ended up with a different set point of function for the motor unit. The question then comes to mind as to whether there is something unique about the motor unit that makes this possible. One suspects that there is not. Provided the relevant information can be made available, the CNS can no doubt be mobilized to influence the firing rate of any neuron in the system. The knowledge that the architecture to support such control is in place at every neuron is sufficient for present purposes.

One experiment in particular reveals for us the surprising degree to which the CNS exercises regulatory control. The experiment has to do with visual processing, and will be discussed below, after we establish the context. Our life experience eventually persuades us that our internal representation of the visual world matches up fairly well with what is actually out there. One may be forgiven for thinking that our visual system must map this outer world fairly directly. But we have learned from Edwin Land that full color vision may be discerned even from the projection of a black-and-white transparency (with only one reference color in addition to the full white spectrum), and Karl Pribram showed us that the visual system is actually a hybrid of topographical and frequency domain mapping (spatial frequencies in this case) (Pribram, 1991). Moreover, there are only about a million neurons in the optic nerve to convey the signals from over 100 million optical sensors in the eye. A lot of preprocessing must necessarily occur in the eyeball itself. The pipeline is not big enough to give us a full topographic representation of the actual image in real time and with full signal bandwidth. The visual complexity we experience must therefore be the endpoint of a process of reconstruction from very limited data, or from data that has been very efficiently encoded, or both. In addition, it is subject to considerable central regulation.

In the experiment at issue, the firing rate of a single motion-sensitive neuron in a cat's eye was monitored as a visual target was moved at a constant rate across a screen (de Ruyter van Steveninck, Lewen, Strong, Koberle, & Bialek, 1997). Surprisingly, the firing rate was highly nonuniform, as was confirmed with the repetitive transit of the same target. When the transit velocity was increased, the average firing rate of the neuron went up as expected, but the high variability was still present. When the variance was calculated for each value of the transit velocity, it was found to be even larger than would be the case if the neuron fired completely at random! (The results are shown in Figure 2.3a and b.) In a random process, the variance equals the average value (as in radioactive decay, for example). When the calculated variability is even greater, the noise must be correlated. This would be the case if the firing rate were being modulated by another function.

When the same neuron is exposed to a variable rate of movement across the field of vision, however, the firing rate tracks the signal much as expected, and the pattern repeats with great fidelity on repetition of the challenge (see Figure 2.3c). If the variability is calculated as a function of the ambient firing rate on this new signal, it is found to be much smaller, as shown in Figure 2.3d. In fact, the variability essentially matches the theoretical limit for such a grainy signal detection scheme, that is, for rate coding. Note the curve for random noise also entered on Figure 2.3d.

It is the level of interest in the signal which determines whether the neuron is engaged with the process or not, and of course, it is the central nervous system that specifies the level of interest. Hence, it is the CNS that is modulating the response somewhat carelessly in Figure 2.3b, whereas it is sharply linearizing the response in Figure 2.3d. The target neuron goes from being noisier than random noise to matching the theoretical detection limit given by information theory. It does so under control of the CNS. This shows that even our first cortical sentinels to the outside world are not responding in a totally representational fashion. On many levels, it is the CNS that allows us to observe what we see, and in particular, this is even true on our first cortical encounter with the information from the outside world.

There is one more remarkable aspect to this research that needs to be mentioned. The authors repeated the aforementioned experiment with a fly's eye. The results were identical to what was seen in the cat. One must conclude, therefore, that the basic principles of central modulation of sensory sensitivities as well as of behavioral responses must go back rather far in our evolutionary history, even so far back that the term central regulation is not well delineated. Every organism equipped with functioning action potentials had the capacity for the development of interacting networks engaged in mutual regulation. Action potentials gave us the first capability for rapid transport of in-

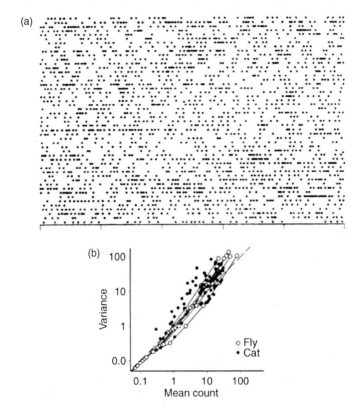

FIGURE 2.3. Spike trains observed in a single motion-sensitive neuron upon passage of targets of different velocity characteristics crossing the field of view repetitively. (a) Spike trains successively observed for a constant velocity target. (b) Variance of the signal in (a) determined for a range of target velocities for the visual system of a cat. The dashed line represents the condition of variance equal to mean velocity, a relationship that holds for a random process. Results are also shown for the visual system of a fly. (c) Successive spike trains for a modulated-velocity signal transiting the field of view. (d) Variance of the signal corresponding to (c). The dashed line represents the condition of variance equal to mean velocity, as in (b). *Source:* From de Ruyter van Steveninck et al., *Science,* 275: 1805-1808 (1997). Reprinted with permission from AAAS.

FIGURE 2.3 *(continued)*

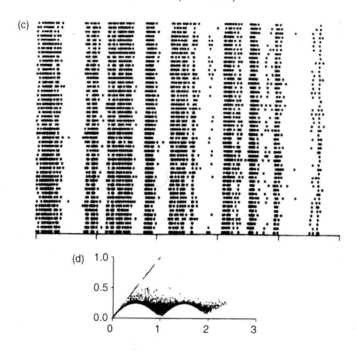

formation, presumably in the service of the prompt correlation of disparate sensory inputs, along with the rapid recruitment of behavioral responses on the output side. Undoubtedly, action potentials and network relations developed essentially contemporaneously, around the basic objective of organizing engagement and disengagement, activation and rest, that is, organismic arousal. (But, irrespective of precisely how we got here developmentally, it is not possible now to understand brain function without understanding networks.)

BRAIN ORGANIZATION IN THE TIMING AND FREQUENCY DOMAINS

The very next question then relates to how the brain actually modulates attention and engagement in the primary sensory systems. That question was addressed in another experiment that also touches on related matters of interest. The experiment was to monitor neuronal

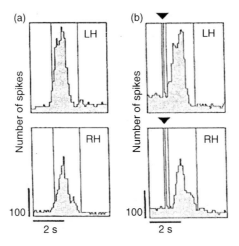

Figure 2.4. Firing rate of a neuron in striate cortex with the transit of a light bar, shown for a neuron in the right and in the left hemispheres. (a) Firing rate in baseline, without any specific measures to alert the animal. (b) Firing rate observed immediately subsequent to an alerting electrical stimulus to the mesencephalic reticular formation (locus coeruleus). *Source:* From Munk et al., *Science,* 272: 271-274 (1996). Reprinted with permission from AAAS.

firing rates in the primary visual, or striate cortex of a cat as a simple target was moved uniformly across the visual field. The experiment was done first in baseline, and again upon electrical stimulation of the mesencephalic reticular formation, in particular the locus coeruleus. The target was a light bar. Comparison was made between representative neurons in the left and right hemispheres (Munk et al., 1996).

The time course of the firing rate is shown in Figure 2.4a for both hemispheres. Figure 2.4a shows the response in baseline, whereas Figure 2.4b shows the response after the electrical stimulus. The stimulus artifact appears in Figure 2.4b just before the light bar comes into the field of view of the sampled neurons. Surprisingly, there is no difference outside of normal variability between the respective firing rates in Figure 2.4a and 2.4b, so the increased arousal level of the responding animal did not appear to have an impact. The mystery was resolved by looking in more detail at the actual signal trains and comparing them with high time resolution. By plotting the coincidence in events between the two hemispheres, a dependence on level of attention could be discerned. The determination was made as follows:

Given a bin width of 2 msec, a coincidence was identified for a particular bin if at the time one neuron fired the other one fired as well.

In the absence of stimulation, there was no observable event-related correlation between the two neurons. There was only a steady-state ripple traceable to the basic 40 Hz rhythm operative in visual processing, as discussed earlier. After the stimulus, however, the depth of modulation, or degree of correlation, was quite marked. When the light bar was subsequently replaced with two light bars moving in opposite directions, the neurons "illuminated" by one of the light bars in both hemispheres coordinated according to Figure 2.4b, whereas a cross comparison between the different light bars yielded the random pattern of Figure 2.4a. It is apparent that the heightened attention being given to the light bar was encoded via enhanced temporal correlation. One might also interpret this as the means for the encoding of figure/ground separation.

These results are puzzling for a number of reasons. First of all, they prompt the question of how inter-hemispheric timing is organized at the millisecond level, in view of the fact that there is no direct cortical connection between the hemispheres at visual cortex. All pathways that connect the two regions are plagued by significant transport delays, and are therefore unlikely candidates. The reticular formation in the brainstem only knows about activation/deactivation. It has no knowledge of one light bar versus two, or even any light bar at all. The thalamus does have a one-to-one topographical mapping of cortical regions, and the thalamocortical loop mediates timing between them. But the thalamus is also hemispherically organized, and coordination between the two does not seem to be a priority for the brain. The massa intermedia connects the two thalami, but alas, not every human being has that structure. It does not seem essential to our human existence. Whereas the thalamus would appear to be an excellent candidate for organizing intra-hemispheric timing in its regulatory dance with cortex, when it comes to inter-hemispheric coordination, it must remain largely passive.

It is impossible to ignore the corpus callosum in this discussion, given the fact that it contains nominally 4 percent of all cortical neurons (referenced to one hemisphere) for the purpose of communicating between the hemispheres. Transport delays have already been mentioned, but the fact is that two resonant systems can remain in some kind of resonance even if the coupling between them involves significant transport delays. However, it may be more difficult to understand multiple resonances at a variety of frequencies through such a mechanism. It may be possible to rule out an essential role for the corpus callosum by the arguments to follow.

When the corpus callosum is cut, as is sometimes done to abort medically intractable seizures, there is indeed a loss in the observed coordination of inter-hemispheric timing, as seen in terms of changes in cross-hemispheric EEG coherence. Nevertheless, the brains in such individuals are still able to solve the binding problem. There is not suddenly a problem of two visual images that are difficult to merge, for example, or any other gross problem in sensory integration. The person still has a unitary sense of self. Further, with a view toward what is to come when we bring neurofeedback into the discussion, it must be observed that cutting the corpus callosum also does not render a person subject to a host of psychopathologies. People don't suddenly become depressed or bipolar. In fact, specific cognitive testing may have to be done to demonstrate that the hemispheres have been severed. And in people with agenesis of the corpus callosum, the deficits can be difficult to detect in the absence of formal psychological assessment. Identified deficits tend to be complex and at a high level, in terms of subtle emotional judgment, for example, rather than in terms of more basic functionality (Brown & Paul, 2000).

The forty-Hertz rhythm that we see in striate cortex is not observed at the thalamus, nor is it observed in the brainstem. However, this does not rule out a role for either of those structures in establishing the basic timing—the phase—with which the 40-Hz rhythm plays out in cortex. What emerges here is a picture in which every "circuit element" in the network—cortex, thalamus, brainstem—plays a distinct role in the overall coordination of timing that is not shared by the other circuit elements.

When all the aforementioned is taken into consideration, the candidates for mediating temporal simultaneity between the hemispheres finally come down to one: the brainstem. In the nuclei sourcing the neuromodulators, we have neurons that project broadly to cortex and to the thalamus, and of course, they also impose their timing regimen everywhere. The brainstem is also the one structure among those discussed that is not lateralized. In addition to mediating cortical timing directly, brainstem nuclei may also mediate timing coincidence between the two thalami. We may have something here that gets close to the conductor's baton in terms of setting the basic timing scheme against which all of cortical activity plays out. But as with the conductor, whose role may be essential but nonetheless modest, the role of the brainstem may be essential but quite limited. The fuller picture is that each part of the network contributes its piece to the adaptation and unfolding of brain timing. We must consider brain timing to be a distributed network function in which each element both acts and is acted upon. Whereas a hierarchy of regulation can be identified, it is not a dictatorship. There is no autonomy. And to continue with the political metaphor, one can also identify a separation of powers and a system of checks and balances. The obvious implication for neurofeedback is that any disturbance of brain timing—either through reinforcement or through stimulation—is likely to have repercussions for the whole network involved in timing regulation.

In summary, then, the experimental result can be explained if the brainstem nucleus [LC] establishes a common timing reference for both hemispheres, presumably via thalamus, and that the thalamocortical circuits establish and maintain the timing of the neuronal pools involved in processing the light bar with respect to that presumptive timing reference. This involves establishing the phasing of the 40-Hz activity that is presumably largely cortically generated. Such phase-control could be effected with subharmonics of the 40-Hz rhythm, thus imposing the requirement of an ordering of the temporal relationships of high- and low-frequency activity. In the presence of an activating signal from the locus coeruleus, there is then an additional selection in favor of activity at the 40-Hz rhythm that is coincident across the hemispheric fissure, which shifts the rhythmic activity of these neuronal pools into greater synchrony.

The particulars may not be available to us from this experiment, but it suffices for present purposes to know that the control of timing cannot be lodged in one "circuit element" or another, but rather must be constituted out of the collaboration of a number of elements. If the control of timing is a function of distributed networks, then the expected effects of neurofeedback should be considered in the same way. On the other hand, there is a hierarchy of control, at the top of which is that circuit element which plays the most global role, that is, the brainstem. This means that the same "circuit elements" that play a pre-dominant role in the neurochemical model also play a dominant role in the bioelectrical model. Hence, psychopharmacology and neuro-feedback appeal largely to the same structures when it comes to the principal psychological and psychiatric conditions.

In addition to looking at timing coordination between the hemi-spheres, Munk and others tracked the distribution of EEG amplitudes with and without the application of a stimulus. The results are shown in Figure 2.5a with and without stimulation. Whereas a broad distribu-tion in EEG amplitudes is observed over the frequency domain in the steady state, after application of a stimulus there is a notable increase in EEG amplitudes in the 40-Hz region. At the same time, a decrease is observed in EEG amplitudes at lower and higher frequencies than 40 Hz (Figure 2.5b). The decrease at higher frequencies is not observed consistently, so we dismiss it from our considerations. The decrease at lower frequencies, on the other hand, is observed systematically.

The decrease is attributed quite simply to the whole-brain activat-ing effect of the pulse to the LC, with activation showing up as a segmentation of neuronal populations into subsets, each of which is

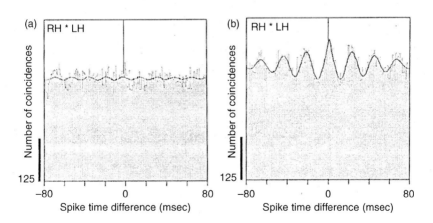

FIGURE 2.5. Correlogram of firing coincidences of the neurons in visual cortex of left and right hemispheres for the two conditions in Figure 2.4. (a) Absence of event-related correlations is seen over 180 msec window in baseline (see Figure 2.4a); (b) Event-related correlations are seen between the hemispheres subse-quent to the activating stimulus (see Figure 2.4b). *Soruce:* From Munk et al., *Science,* 272: 271-274 (1996). Reprinted with permission from AAAS.

characterized by its unique timing signature. Synchronous assemblies are thus dispersed into subassemblies that differentiate themselves slightly in the timing and frequency domains in order to subserve slightly different functions. They become desynchronized. Thus, paradoxically EEG amplitudes can be observed to decrease with an increase in activation, as overall synchrony is reduced. This is not in contradiction to the argument that specific neural events are contingent on the establishment of coincidence in the time domain, which equates to synchrony in the frequency domain. It is a question of scale. The need for differentiation in the time and frequency domain between the various neuronal pools appears on the larger scale as desynchronization.

The observation of reduced EEG amplitudes below the 40-Hz regime can be taken to define our principal region of interest in neurofeedback if our objective is the training of arousal regulation, and the modulation of activation/relaxation dynamics (Figure 2.6a and b). A general rule is applicable here that the more global regulatory functions must be organized at the lower frequencies, and the more specific, localized functions must be organized at the higher frequencies. Given our primary concern in neurofeedback with issues of state

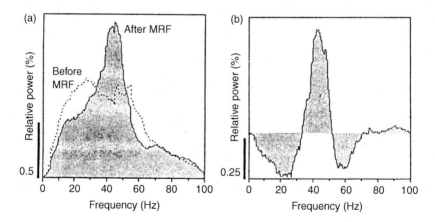

FIGURE 2.6. EEG Spectral amplitudes corresponding to the two conditions in Figures 2.4 and 2.5. The conventional distributions are shown in (a), and the difference between them is shown in (b). The null observed at zero frequency is attributable to the (standard) use of a high-pass filter. *Source:* From Munk et al., *Science*, 272: 271-274 (1996). Reprinted with permission from AAAS.

management, it is likely that our primary focus is going to be in this lower frequency region.

With respect to the coordination of inter-hemispheric timing, it has been argued earlier that subcortical processes must be determinative. The same question arises with regard to intra-hemispheric coordination. To shed light on this process, Steriade's group performed an experiment in which the cortical surface was surgically cut in order to disrupt the lateral communication pathways in cortex (Contreras, Destexhe, Sejnowski, & Steriade, 1996). The experimental configuration is shown in Figure 2.7a and b. Probes were placed at 1 mm intervals in order to monitor the spatial properties of coherence in spindle bursts. The spindle-burst waveforms are shown for both the intact cortex and the surgical preparation. There was a loss of EEG spindle-burst activity immediately adjacent to the cut, but beyond that, original patterns of temporal coordination were essentially preserved. Figure 2.8 illustrates just how well coherence relationships were preserved through this procedure. This means that the spindle-burst activity cannot be dependent upon cortical-cortical linkages for the organization of coherence. Rather, it must be constituted via nonlocal networks such as the thalamocortical loops.

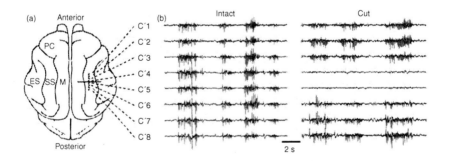

FIGURE 2.7. EEG spindle-burst activity is shown for eight sites spaced at 1mm intervals on the exposed cortex of a cat. (a) Sectioning the cortical tissue down to three millimeters did not disturb the coherence and synchrony of the spindles, except for the extinction of spindling adjacent to the cut. Hence, such coherence cannot depend upon intra-cortical connectivity. (b) Spatial dependence of coherence as influenced by cortical sectioning. *Source:* From Contreras et al., *Science*, 274: 771-777 (1996). Reprinted with permission from AAAS.

Figure 2.8 also illustrates the progressive dephasing that takes place as one migrates away from any cortical reference point. But the decline is not always monotonic. Between certain cortical locations, high coordination may prevail, particularly under brain challenge. And the coordination may well be non-zero everywhere. If this experiment had been done instead using a couple of microphones monitoring something like a waterfall, a monotonic decline in correlation would be found as the two microphones are moved apart, declining to zero correlation at some distance. The fact that this does not occur in the brain is proof that these relationships are under the active management of the CNS. The diffusion of phase information is not primarily a field effect, as in sound waves emanating from a waterfall. It is communicated via neuronal networks. By virtue of Figure 2.8, we know that even near-neighbor communications in cortex involve large-scale, nonlocalized networks. It is perhaps useful to take a network perspective on this whole issue of the organization of cerebral communication.

THE NETWORK MODEL

The theory of networks has received considerable impetus in the last few years, with more and more issues in biology being subjected

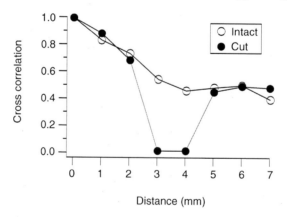

FIGURE 2.8. Trend of coherence as a function of distance from the reference point. Preservation of coherence relationships on both sides of the cut points to central mechanisms for their organization. Non-monotonic decline with distance argues for explicit management as opposed to passive mechanisms.

to network types of analysis. In these, one considers distributions of network nodes and their linkages to other nodes. An analysis starting from first principles would likely start with the assumption of a typical node of the network, with a characteristic number of linkages to other nodes, its connectivity. There would then be some distribution in connectivity around such typical characteristics, presumably a well defined, perhaps even a narrow spread. In the limit of large numbers, we would obtain the normal distribution. With nominally ten billion cortical neurons, most of which belong to a few morphologically similar types, this picture would appear to apply well to the neuronal networks at the level of complex characteristic of humans.

It is increasingly becoming apparent that most networks in nature do not follow this pattern. Instead of a narrow distribution in connectivity, we have very broad distributions. Typically, there is a high incidence of nodes that have a modest number of linkages to other nodes at one end of the distribution, and a small but important incidence of nodes that are much more highly interconnected than others are. The latter's highly connected nodes draw the whole assembly into more intimate connectedness, and this is referred to as the small-world model (Watts & Strogatz, 1998). The distributions for the two competing models are shown in Figure 2.9. The small-world model satisfies a power-law over some significant range of the variables. This has particular import in the tails of the distributions. Whereas the normal distribution falls off exponentially in the tails, the power law distribution falls off much more slowly at the upper end. Effectively the wings of the distribution dominate: at the low end in terms of incidence, and at the high end in terms of connectedness. There is no "characteristic value" as there is in the Poisson case. Hence, the small-world model is also referred to as the scale-free model (Barabási & Albert, 1999).

The human brain appears to exhibit salient characteristics of the small-world model, in view of its high degree of functional integration and internal network connectivity. This is documented later in the text. Yet, considerable homogeneity exists within the large populations of cortical neurons. If we did not know about the small-world model when looking at the overall distribution of neuronal connectivities, we would undoubtedly attempt to make a best fit to a normal distribution for our ten billion cortical neurons and that would have been that.

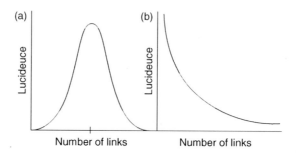

FIGURE 2.9. Distributions in connectivity are shown for two different types of networks. Nodal incidence is plotted vertically, and nodal connectivity is plotted horizontally. (a) Distribution in connectivity for a random network. The Poisson distribution approaches a normal distribution for large networks. Connectivity falls off exponentially in the tails of the distribution. (b) Distribution in connectivity for a small-world or scale-free model. Logarithmic compression on both axes yields a straight-line, or a power-law relationship. No characteristic node exists for such a power-law dependence. On the contrary, the distribution is dominated by minimally-connected nodes in terms of incidence, and by heavily-interconnected nodes in terms of network governance. Whereas the cerebral network organization exhibits features of both, developmental and evolutionary forces have driven the CNS toward the small-world model. *Source:* Following Watts & Strogatz, 1998, and Barabási & Albert, 1999.

Cortex might indeed resemble Figure 2.9a reasonably well, and we would then continue to treat cortex as an exemplar of a random network. The deviation from Gaussian behavior at some distance from the mean would not have raised any concern. Real-world systems are rarely Gaussian in the tails of the distribution. Case closed. But from the perspective of the small-world model, we must take explicit account of the tails of the distribution, and we find that even a small population of neurons there far exceeds the predicted incidence under the Gaussian model. Given the ubiquity of small-world networks in nature, such a development cannot be dismissed as an accident of nature but rather must be seen as the result of developmental and evolutionary "pressure." Whereas, the typical neuron has perhaps 10^4 synaptic connections to other neurons, some neurons interface with as many as 5×10^5 other neurons, some fifty times greater. These obviously carry a lot more weight. And so it is the tail that tells the tale.

Since connectivity is most directly determinative for the control of timing in the brain, the small-world model directs our attention to the neurons at the upper end of the distribution. The dominant nodes in small-world networks are referred to as hubs, and in the CNS, it is the highly interconnected neurons with broadly distributed axonal trees that define the hubs. They reside in the brainstem. So by this new chain of argument, we have once again arrived at the realization of the crucial role played by the nuclei that source the neuromodulators in the brainstem. They constitute the hubs both in the neurochemical and the bioelectrical perspective on neuromodulation. Consequently, neurofeedback for the common psychological and psychiatric conditions is largely seen as engaging with the hubs. Even though we maintain that neurofeedback addresses itself to the entire domain of cortical timing, in its distilled essence, much of neurofeedback likely reduces to the education of a modest number of neurons in our brainstem.

Secondary hubs include all of the other subcortical nuclei in which timing information is shared broadly, and that principally refers to the thalamus. Other subcortical nuclei must lie somewhat lower in the dominance hierarchy. The brainstem serves as the "capo di tutti capi," the hub of hubs, by virtue of its controlling role with respect to the subsidiary hubs. Unquestionably, a hierarchy exists, and this has bearing on how we must think about neurofeedback. The earlier argument would lead one to expect a considerable overlap of conditions addressed with pharmacotherapy and neurofeedback, by virtue of their convergence on the brainstem, and that is in fact the case. The centrality of hubs in the network model also means that neurofeedback is not necessarily targeting features that have an obvious cortical or, more particularly, a localized manifestation. The disregulation may be too diffuse to be readily observable in the EEG as it is conventionally measured. The conclusion one would like to draw is that any challenge to network timing impinges on the entire network. One simply has to tie into the network in some fashion in order to effect the reorganization.

It is also true, however, that neurofeedback is not limited to conditions affected by pharmacological agents. It can be helpful with disregulations of network timing in considerable generality, including in particular conditions where there is manifest injury in cortex, as in the case of stroke, or a localized seizure focus, or white matter injury as in MS or autism, or in case of deficits in certain functional networks, as, for example, in the case of specific learning disabilities.

At this point, it is still not clear to what extent the scale-free or small-world model should dominate our thinking with respect to timing organization in the human brain. It is helpful to look at evolutionary history in this regard. The long-suffering nematode *C. elegans* has only about 300 neurons, but if we ask the question about how many synaptic connections lie between any one arbitrary neuron and another, the answer is 14. Not much of a premium is placed on interconnectivity in such a nervous system. If we ask that same question about the human brain with our ten billion cortical neurons, we might expect the number of links to be somewhat greater than when only 300 neurons are talking to each other. As it happens, the average number of synaptic connections linking any cortical neuron with any other such neuron is approximately three. Of all the superlatives one might list regarding our exquisite nervous system, this fact may just be one of the most extraordinary. The human brain puts a great premium on interconnectivity.

In fact, the average number of links connecting arbitrary neurons could hardly be less than three, under any conceivable circumstances. Matters have gone just as far as they can go in that regard. As it is, nearly every pyramidal cell contributes an axon to the white matter. If one nevertheless posits an increment in white matter axons, there would not be a comparable decrease in the "three links between neurons." It will typically take at least one link in the local network to reach the white matter neuron that connects to the particular distal region, and typically, another short link at the other end to reach the final destination. Having more white matter neurons does not substantially alter that circumstance. Significantly, then, a limit in connectivity has effectively been reached within cortex. Evolutionary pressure has driven us to the most connected of networks possible, namely, the small-world model, together with the highest level of interconnectivity that is plausible, at nominally three links between any two nodes.

The practical import with respect to neurofeedback is that this extreme degree of connectivity shifts our perspective once again toward delocalization of the organization of brain timing. That is, we must think about timing as a property of distributed networks. Then it becomes reasonable to expect that any influence on the timing or phase of neuronal assemblies at any point in the network challenges the entire regulatory machinery. We may still be talking mainly to the hubs, but we can do so from anywhere on cortex.

THE CONSTRUCTION AND MAINTENANCE OF NEURONAL ASSEMBLIES

Teasing out the neural code, the means by which information is encoded in neuronal firing streams has been a long-term, somewhat unfruitful preoccupation. One immediate difficulty was the realization that the firing rate code, the mapping of information onto the firing rate of neurons, was wholly inadequate to represent the information that had to be managed by the brain. The brain has to organize itself for the embedding of information in parallel data streams. This has already been alluded to in connection with visual processing. The continuous signals arriving in visual cortex have to be grouped into packets, and going forward, each packet can be considered as a virtual "wave front" of action potentials that must be recognized by the brain as belonging to a common entity.

It is now increasingly believed that the criterion of belonging is simultaneity, a temporal window that has a width of two overlapping action potentials, or about 20 msec. As Christoph von der Malsburg has said presciently, "We are in the middle of scientific revolution, the result of which will be the establishment of [time] binding as a fundamental aspect of the neural code" (von der Malsburg, 1995). Time binding means that other neurons, firing concurrently with the arrival of the "packet," engage in a kind of pattern recognition process as they gate the signal forward. The signal is further shaped through inhibitory attrition, a process charmingly referred to as "inhibitory sculpting." The progressively refined signal carries its timing signature forward until the brain is done with it, or it eventuates in a motor act.

A burden of simultaneity is placed on all processes that must interact with the visual signal, in association cortex and elsewhere. This means that the timing signature of the packet is gradually diffused through cortex. However, movement of information through cortex involves transit time delays that may compromise the very simultaneity on which information integrity depends. How is the simultaneity criterion met in the face of such delays? One is struck by the fact that there is no stasis here. To stay alive, the signal must move, much a like a shark that must keep swimming. The action potential is a very perishable entity. In order for our brains to organize continuity of state, and hence continuity of our experience, the process must allow for refresh.

Hence, periodicity is built into the process, as patterns substantially repeat themselves, but also allow for slow evolution and refinement. The process of information transport must therefore be embedded in a context-setting network whose essential characteristic is periodicity. The periodic reference signals effectively serve as time base correctors that restore synchrony to the ensemble in the network with every cycle. Timing disparities therefore don't progressively accumulate. They are periodically set to zero. Thus, state management in the bio-electrical domain is expected to exhibit the feature of periodicity, and the underlying circuitry must be organized to produce and maintain rhythmicity. Thus, when rhythmicity or periodicity is observed in the EEG, we are directly observing the regulation of state.

The circuit architecture for these reference signals must be such that it is not itself compromised by transit time delays. One solution to this problem is to have the reference signals originate at the center of the brain, so that the transit time delays to the cortical surface are nearly identical everywhere and thus have minimal differential effects. Simultaneity at cortex is then maintained. It has been observed, for example, that distant pyramidal cells can fire within 3 msec of one another (Buzaki & Chrobak, 1995). This is a challenge for the brain to accomplish. One surmises that it must be important. Simultaneity of ensembles at this level points to a central source of timing. This brings us to the consideration of the thalamus.

The importance of the thalamus in organizing frequencies observed in the cortical EEG has been recognized for a long time. Primarily, the role of the thalamus has been seen in terms of the gating of sensory signals as the final way station to cortex. But in the words of Rodolfo Llinas, ". . . rather than a gate into the brain, the thalamus represents a hub from which any site in cortex can communicate with any other such site or sites" (Llinas et al., 1999). He asserts a much larger role for the thalamus in terms of organizing functional networks. Two features of the thalamocortical networks support this conjecture, according to Llinas: (1) the rich thalamocortical interconnectivity, and

(2) the reciprocal nature of the thalamocortical loop function. To this, we now add the consideration of central location in the brain.

Another key argument from evolution can be brought to bear. The CNS had to perform the functions of sensory integration and the co-ordination of sensory inputs with motor output long before evolution graced it with a large neocortex. These essential functions must have been originally provided for within the thalamus itself. It could be that many of the timing-critical communications occurred then and occur now in networks within the thalamus itself, where transit times are negligibly small because of the short distances involved. These networks would just have to be sufficient to communicate essential timing information between regions. Hence, they could be "thin" networks of small-world character. With subsequent evolution, the neo-cortex simply evolved to modulate and refine such activities. It does not displace them. Whatever role intra-thalamic networks played early on is probably largely conserved through the later developmental stages.

So the thalamus is another "hub" in our construction of the hierarchy of the control of timing. It is the only structure that contains sufficient complexity for one-to-one topographical mapping of the sensory cortices. It is the structure that provides the bulk of the circuitry to organize thalamocortical rhythms. It is the structure that, along with the hypothalamus, mediates the role of the brainstem in the activation and relaxation of cerebral networks. And it is the thalamus that mediates the interaction of neurofeedback with the brainstem nuclei. We therefore theorize that the most immediate and direct engagement of EEG neurofeedback is with thalamocortical networks (Sterman, 1984; Othmer, Othmer, & Kaiser, 1999). It is most propitious that Rodolfo Llinas has in recent years explored the role of disregulation in thalamocortical network relations as the basis of much of psychopathology.

THALAMOCORTICAL DYSRHYTHMIA

It was at the neurosciences meeting in Miami in 1999 that Rodolfo Llinas first presented the model of thalamocortical dysrhythmias, and press reports the following day around the nation testify to the fact that this presentation, among the many at the conference, struck a particular cord with the attendees. It was suddenly the right time for the role of brain organization in the timing and frequency domains to be seriously confronted, and its potential role in functional disorders recognized.

This line of thinking had actually found expression as far back as 1994 in the book, *Descartes' Error,* where Antonio Damasio suggested, "[A]ny malfunction of the timing mechanism would be likely to create spurious integration and disintegration. . . . This may indeed be what happens in states of confusion caused by head injury, or in some symptoms of schizophrenia and other diseases." Sometimes authors allow themselves speculations in the popular literature that do not rise yet to the level of publishable science. This might have been a gem of that nature. However, in conversations years later, Damasio did not recall his earlier thinking, and in fact, denied that he would ever have linked schizophrenia to such a model. Obviously, the idea of attributing such major disorders to something this ephemeral as disregulation in brain timing had been only a passing flirtation. It had not taken over his thinking.

Even further back in history, Oliver Sacks had conjectured in his 1970 edition of the book *Migraine* that the Sterman research on the control of seizures via EEG biofeedback might well have application to migraine. And even though Sterman's work was [mistakenly] considered a scientific dead end by the nineties, Sacks retained this conjecture in the 1992 edition of his book. It remained for Llinas to propose a testable model.

What started off this line of thinking was imaging data from magnetoencephalography (MEG) on several kinds of mental disorders. MEG can be thought of by analogy to EEG data with respect to signal bandwidth. That is, we can discern the same frequency spectrum that we see in the EEG. The difference is largely due to the use of magnetic detection that one is able to detect small currents below the cortical surface, whereas EEG data are obtained with voltage sensors that see only the voltage of the probe itself. With surface electrodes, subsurface events would have to be deduced. The use of MEG can be considered as simply historical in this case, not at all essential to the story.

Llinas refers to a comparison of four clinical cases with normals. There was one case of deep depression, one case of tinnitus, one case of Parkinson's, and one case of chronic (neuropathic) pain. In each of these cases, a bispectral analysis revealed an excess coupling or correlation between various frequencies, quite irrespective of whether they were harmonically related. Whenever one of these specific frequencies was large in amplitude, the other was also. They were, to an extent, time-locked. This occurred over a broad frequency range, but most surprisingly extended even to high frequencies, specifically into the gamma range (40 Hz). It seemed reasonable, then, that the inappropriate coupling could be responsible for spurious sensory experiences such as tinnitus or even the internal voices in schizophrenia, on the input processing side, as well as unmotivated motor acts in Parkinson's on the output side. Similarly, the sensation of chronic pain could be exaggerated beyond what can be explained on the basis of ordinary sensory inputs.

Llinas even proposed a specific model that invoked an inappropriate coupling between low- and high-frequency thalamocortical loops, and between content-related, specific thalamic nuclei and the context-sensitive, nonspecific medial thalamic nuclei.

Upon publication of these results in late 1999, David McCormick, who had also invested his career in studying the thalamocortical networks, gave tentative support to the new model under the title "Are thalamocortical rhythms the rosetta stone of a subset of neurological disorders?" Referring to the Llinas paper, he said:

> Recent evidence indicates that "dysrhythmias" cause alterations in the normal function of the thalamocortical loop and lead to various types of neurological disorders. Will decoding this rhythm help us to understand the basis for movement disorders, chronic pain, and even neuropsychological dysfunction? (McCormick, 1999)

It was still an open question, but now others were asking it. It is possible that the Llinas paper finally gave permission for the consideration of models in the bioelectrical domain, or the domain of brain timing and frequency, as a basis for a number of the psychopathologies. This emerging perspective was framed elegantly by Simon Farmer only two years later: "We are beginning to understand that brain rhythms, their synchronization and desynchronization, form an important and possibly fundamental part of the orchestration of perception, motor action, and conscious experience, and that disruption of oscillation and/or temporal synchronization may be a fundamental mechanism of neurological disease" (Farmer, 2002). If the Llinas model indeed explains so much of what we have stumbled upon in neurofeedback, and if this evidence is equivalently available in the EEG, why should it have taken this long to come up with this tentative model? The problem is simply that bispectral analysis is rarely done in our professional community, so the temporal relationship between different frequencies has not been an active subject for study. Most EEG analysis software does not even provide for this capability. This state of neglect is only gradually changing, and that has come about due to the gradual convergence of two lines of inquiry in the field of EEG: the evoked or event-related potential (ERP) and what is becoming known as event-related synchronization-desynchronization studies (ERS-ERD), which looks at event-related effects in a frequency-resolved manner. Klimesch has found that ERPs can be well modeled in terms of time-locking of key EEG frequencies, with the stimulus serving to time-lock the different frequencies. Such time-locking can only be observed over brief poststimulus intervals as the different frequencies will quickly diverge in phase (Klimesch, 1999).

This gives us further reason to think in terms of the specific intentional coordination of different EEG frequencies as necessary to good function. Anything that gives rise to inappropriate coupling among these frequencies could then similarly be responsible for dysfunction. One reason this particular hypothesis has not been entertained previously is that other explanations for neurofeedback efficacy were already at hand. Explanations have been offered in terms of training the resting frequencies of cortical networks, the alpha rhythm in the case of the visual system, the sensorimotor rhythm in the case of motor output, toward lower levels of excitability. Explanations have also been offered with regard to resolving observed EEG anomalies in the amplitude domain, as well as in the domain of intersite relationships (coherence and comodulation). As it turns out, the tactics of neurofeedback that have been devised to address these anomalies also address Llinas' "thalamocortical dysrhythmias." This follows from the use of broadband inhibits both in the high and low frequency region of the EEG, so that if elevation occur in either or both of these domains, the reward is inhibited and the behavior is gradually shaped toward more normal amplitude distributions.

The use of inhibits cues the brain broadly and nonspecifically with respect to any activity that correlates with the time interval over which the inhibit is engaged. It is therefore sufficient to detect the elevations in any band in order to address this particular mechanism in feedback. The cross-coupling is nonlinearly dependent on the amplitudes of both frequency constituents, and if these are both trained down in amplitude, the cross-coupling will diminish even more dramatically. By virtue of the cooccurrence of the cross-coupling with the amplitude elevations of the constituents, one does not have to target the cross-terms directly.

However, there may be a pathway here for devising better discriminants for an inhibit strategy in the future. At the moment, a common strategy is to inhibit the reward entirely whenever an inhibit threshold is crossed. Such a gross disruption of feedback is not well tolerated if it is applied too indiscriminately. Hence, in practice, it is always used sparingly, which means that only the most severe excursions into disregulation are called out. The use of more sophisticated discriminants may lead to a much more subtly prescriptive strategy for functional renormalization.

The prior models for neurofeedback efficacy have not been displaced by the new insights derived from the Llinas model. Rather they have been complemented. It is now possible to say that the objective of neurofeedback at the tactical level is to challenge the brain toward improved management of neuronal assemblies. This encompasses, first of all, the extent of a particular ensemble in time, in frequency, and in spatial dimension. Second, it encompasses its interaction with other cortical regions in space, and now with other regions in the frequency domain as well. Nonlocality of effects in physical space follows from the network model, and nonlocality of effects in the frequency domain is broached in the Llinas model.

The primary implication for neurofeedback is that there can be no narrow prescription for a proper protocol or strategy. The application of the small-world model allows us to conjecture that any cortical location, at any EEG frequency, and under any and all circumstances, is capable of yielding information with respect to the disregulation status of the brain, and thus of a strategy of renormalization of brain behavior. Any appeal to either the phase, frequency, or amplitude of rhythmic EEG activity, whether by stimulation or reinforcement through feedback, challenges directly the instrumentalities of state regulation, and sets up a response by the brain that is likely over time to restore more efficient regulation. It is merely required that such an appeal must be sufficiently small so as not to have adverse consequences for the system in its own right, and it may have to be selected somewhat judiciously so as not to destabilize or further disregulate a vulnerable brain. Significantly, the challenge does not have to target a known deficit. It is merely necessary to provoke a regulatory response by the system.

Since in practice all feedback occurs on short timescales, the detection of disregulation always amounts to detecting a transient deviation from ambient behavior. There remains considerable arbitrariness in the discrimination of disregulation from merely rare but normal excursions in brain behavior. Fortunately, the technique of operant conditioning in general, and of neurofeedback in particular, is tolerant to imperfections in a reinforcement strategy. Improvement on this score is to be found in resorting to multiple discriminants, so that various criteria of disregulation are available to corroborate each other. It is in facilitating and motivating such a strategy that the Llinas model may be most helpful to the practice of neurofeedback. We have difficulty corroborating specific models of neurofeedback because the implications of each lead to clinical success rather generally. But it would no doubt represent a step forward if we were to draw on all of them for the design of a multifaceted training strategy. We would have "inhibitory sculpting" at yet another level.

SUMMARY AND CONCLUSION

The present discussion is a beginning for a conception of neuro-regulation that is based entirely on bioelectrical and timing or frequency-based models. It has hopefully given a basis for understanding the generality of effects of neurofeedback across the range of psycho-pathologies and neurological deficits, and for the existence of a range of techniques that can be usefully deployed in a self-regulation strategy. To that end, it was important to abstract the discussion of both disregulation and of the compensatory self-regulation methodology from any particular mental disorder or deficit, and to construct the argument strictly on considerations of brain organization with respect to timing and frequency.

The hierarchical organization of cerebral networks argues for a key role for brain stem nuclei in mediating neurofeedback efficacy. This conception finds some empirical support in a companion chapter in this volume (Chapter 5) that addresses principally the reward strategy in neurofeedback. First, the centrality of arousal regulation in that clinical paradigm points to a key role for the reticular formation. And second, the universal utility of inter-hemispheric training implies a role for the brainstem nuclei as mediators of inter-hemispheric timing. In this regard, inter-hemispheric training at homotopic sites can be seen as a kind of triangulation strategy with brainstem function as a principal target. However, the small-world network model also highlights the integrated and distributed nature of timing regulation, which places bounds on any lumped analysis and on the localizability of neurofeedback efficacy. Formal empirical evaluation would be helpful to confirm the utility of such a generalized approach to the understanding and practice of neurofeedback.

REFERENCES

Barabási, A.-L., & Albert, R. (1999). Emergence of scaling in random networks. *Science, 286,* 509-512.

Basmajian, J.V. (1963). Conscious control of individual motor units. *Science, 141,* 440-441.

Brown, W.S., & Paul, L.K. (2000). Psychosocial deficits in agenesis of the corpus callosum with normal intelligence. *Cognitive Neuropsychiatry, 5,* 135-157.

Buzaki, G., & Chrobak, J.J. (1995). Temporal structure in spatially organized neuronal ensembles: A role for interneural networks. *Current Opinion in Neurobiology, 5,* 504-510.

Contreras, D., Destexhe, A., Sejnowski, T.J., & Steriade, M. (1996). Control of spatiotemporal coherence of a thalamic oscillation by corticothalamic feedback. *Science, 274,* 771-777.

De Ruyter van Steveninck, R.R., Lewen, G.D., Strong, S.P., Koberle, R., & Bialek, W. (1997). Reproducibility and variability in neural spike trains. *Science, 275,* 1805-1808.

Farmer, S. (June 2002). Neural rhythms in Parkinson's disease. *Brain Journal of Neurology, 125*(6), 1176-1176.

Fehmi, L.G., Adkins, J.W., & Lindsley, D.B. (1965). Electrophysiological correlates of visual perception in man and monkey. COM. 6 International Congress. *Electroenceph. Clin. Neurophysiol., 6,* 237-238.

Fehmi, L.G., Adkins, J.W., & Lindsley, D.B. (1969). Electrophysiological corre-lates of·visual perceptual masking in monkeys. *Experimental Brain Research, 7*(4), 299-316.

Klimesch, W. (1999). EEG alpha and theta oscillations reflect cognitive and mem-ory performance: A review and analysis, *Brain Research Reviews, 29,* 169-195.

Laughlin, S.B., & Sejnowski, T.J. (2003). Communication in neuronal networks, *Science, 301,* 1870-1874.

Llinas, R.R., Ribary, U., Jeanmonod, D., Kronberg, E., & Mitra, P.P. (1999). Thalamocortical dysrhythmia: A neurological and neuropsychiatric syndrome characterized by magnetoencephalography. *Proceedings of National Academy of Sciences, 96*(26), 15222-15227.

McCormick, D.A. (December 1999). Are thalamocortical rhythms the rosetta stone of a subset of neurological disorders? *Nature Medicine, 5*(12), 1349-1351.

Munk, M.H., Roelfsema, Pieter, R., Koenig, P., Engel, A.K., & Singer, W. Role of reticular activation in the modulation of intracortical synchronization, *Science, 272,* 271-274.

Othmer, S., Othmer, S.F., & Kaiser, D.A. (1999). EEG biofeedback: An emerging model for its global efficacy. In A. Abarbanel & J.R. Evans (Eds.), *Introduction to quantitative EEG and neurofeedback.* San Diego: Academic Press.

Post, R.M., Rubinow, D.R., & Ballinger, J.C. (1986). Conditioning and sensitization in the longitudinal course of affective illness. *British Journal of Psychiatry, 149,* 191-201.

Pribram, K.H. (1991). *Brain and Perception,* Hillsdale, NJ: Lawrence Erlbaum Association.

Sterman, M.B. (1984). *The role of sensorimotor rhythmic EEG activity in the etiol-ogy and treatment of generalized motor seizures.* In T. Elbert, B. Rockstroh, W. Lutzenberger, & N. Birbaumer, (Eds.), *Self-regulation of the brain and behavior.* Berlin: Springer.

Von der Malsburg, C. (1981). *Internal Report,* Max Planck Institute for Biophysical Chemistry, Goettingen, Germany.

Von der Malsburg, C. (1995). *Binding in Models of Perception and Brain Function, Current Opinion in Neurobiology, 5,* 520-526.

Watts, D.J., & Strogatz, S.H. (1998). Collective dynamics of small-world networks. *Nature, 393,* 440.

Wolfram, S.A. (2002). *New kind of science* (p. 715), Champaign, IL: Wolfram Media.

Wu, J.Y., Cohen, L.B., & Falk, C.X. (1994). Neuronal activity during different behaviors in aplysia: A distributed organization? *Science, 264,* 820-823.

Chapter 3

Ours Is to Reason Why and How

James R. Evans
Martha C. M. Rubi

INTRODUCTION

At this point in the short history of the field of neurotherapy (neuro-feedback), there is no doubt in the minds of most practitioners that the treatment has powerful effects. Many of us know this not only from results of published research and changes we see with clients, but also from actually using it with ourselves. However, many neurotherapists want to know why and how it is effective. Such knowledge not only could satisfy intellectual curiosity, but also should lead to more efficient and effective treatment. Perhaps, research in the field now needs to focus as much on why neurotherapy is effective as on whether and when it is effective. There are, of course, many directions and levels from which mechanisms of neurofeedback's efficacy could be approached. In this chapter, we take the approach of speculating on answers to two general questions (1) Why do nearly all neurotherapists, using a wide variety of treatment protocols, seem to achieve at least 60 percent success rates with clients? (2) Are there similar mechanisms underlying neurofeedback and other alternative/complementary medicine therapies, and, if so, is there anything about neurotherapy, which makes it a better treatment modality?

Newcomers to the field, as well as many veteran neurotherapists, must be very confused by the many claims at conference presentations, in books, and from other sources that certain approaches are

Handbook of Neurofeedback
© 2007 by The Haworth Press, Inc. All rights reserved.
doi:10.1300/5889_03

best. For example: "only QEEG-based treatment protocols consistently lead to positive treatment results"; "QEEG evaluation is a waste of time and money, which could be better spent for extra treatment using (speaker's/writer's favorite treatment protocol)"; "bipolar electrode placement is superior to monopolar"; "several short training sessions are superior to a few long ones"; "only equipment providing real-time, digital feedback enables optimal results"; "rewarding increases in power at certain frequencies is always preferable to inhibiting power"; "it is better (or worse) to train a frequency ratio than to inhibit or enhance one specific frequency"; "audio-visual or other type stimulation should (should not) be used to speed-up treatment results"; "my training protocol for disorder X is superior to all others"; etc. The authors, of course, are aware that a variety of views is to be expected, given the field's short history, and only many years of clinical experience and controlled research is likely to significantly decrease the confusion. We also believe that while some claims may have been motivated in part by desire for money or fame, many are true depending on great many factors, such as age, motivation, personality, and symptoms of individual clients. In the following paragraphs, we speculate on mechanisms through which a wide variety of nonspecific, treatment-specific, neurophysiological, and psychological factors may achieve positive results. We then discuss possible commonalities and differences between mechanisms of efficacy of neurotherapy and other treatment approaches often claiming equally impressive results. While certain of these speculations may be considered by some readers to be absurd and/or not amenable to scientific exploration, we believe that at this stage of our knowledge in this field, a very wide range of possibilities should be considered.

NONSPECIFIC VARIABLES

Several factors common to most, if not all, therapies undoubtedly account for much of the variance in treatment outcomes. Many of these have been studied extensively, especially in the field of psychotherapy, and demonstrated to influence treatment outcome regardless of the specific treatment theories and procedures involved.

Placebo and Expectancy

Probably the most common criticism of neurotherapy (as well as most alternative/complementary treatment approaches) is that "it is only a placebo effect." Some critics have even singled out neurotherapy as especially facilitative of such effects due to use of relatively expensive, computerized equipment, colorful "brain maps," use of impressive "intellectual" terms such as spectral analysis, etc. We have no doubt that client expectancy (placebo) effects are powerful, non-specific factors in neurotherapy, just as in all therapies, standard and alternative. In fact, it is now recognized as important enough to warrant funding by the U.S. National Institutes of Health for studying it as an independent variable in treatment. It has been said that no single medication has ever proven to have the approximately 35 percent to 40 percent success rate in alleviating symptoms of such a wide variety of disorders as the placebo effect, and if one ever is found, it probably will be hailed as a miracle drug. Successful neurotherapists undoubtedly capitalize on the placebo effect, some unwittingly and some deliberately through display of impressive equipment and other office surroundings, by emphasizing high success rates and never mentioning possible failure, etc. Some might argue that if this gets results, so be it. In our experience, however, it is the rare neurotherapist who believes that it is purely client expectancy that gets results; and most can cite experiences, which seem to prove there are other factors involved. Nevertheless, it likely will require several well-designed studies involving placebo controls and showing results favorable to neurotherapy to convince most skeptics that there is much more to the treatment than client expectancy of success.

Client Variables

Client motivation is a very obvious factor in the success of any treatment; especially those involving self-regulation (as opposed to "passive" treatment such as simply require only enough motivation to take medications at appropriate times). Neurotherapy can be quite demanding of clients in terms of the expenditure of mental energy involved in normalizing EEG patterns, persisting through almost inevitable learning plateaus, and, for some clients, just sitting still enough to prevent excessive artifacts. Although equipment manufacturers continuously strive to develop software for games and other type feedback, which may increase motivation, this remains an important variable in any neurofeedback situation. Client age, diagnosis, personality characteristics, and (especially in the case of children) family attitudes toward neurotherapy all relate to perseverance and compliance with treatment. In the authors' experiences, very young children and teenagers often show minimal motivation, while formerly high functioning adults attempting to recover from a head injury show strong levels of motivation. The demands of sitting still may be especially difficult for persons with attention deficit/hyperactivity disorder or autism; and the limited energy of many depressed persons could be expected to result in decreased motivation for training sessions of usual duration.

It seems predictable that persons with personality characteristics such as internal locus of control or "hardy personality" would be more highly motivated to learn self-regulation and persist through the required number of training sessions. Clients who are skeptical of neurofeedback's value may show sufficient motivation initially, but become much less motivated after the novelty wears off or they reach a learning plateau. Often, these are persons who have tried many other treatments without remission of symptoms. The same is true for some child clients when parents or other family members doubt the value of neurofeedback or have difficulty with its cost, and, consciously or unconsciously, "sabotage" the child's motivation and progress. Also, failure to complete a sufficient number of training sessions, or missing training for prolonged periods is typical when parents have a very busy life and do not find time to take their children for treatment.

Therapist Variables

Some neurotherapists, like some psychotherapists, have higher success rates than others. In addition to the possibility that they are the ones who develop client expectancy of success as discussed earlier, there are differences in relatively easily assessed variables of probable importance such as technical skills and years of experience, as well as intangible personality characteristics such as ability to empathize or show "loving concern." Surely, an empathic, encouraging, experienced clinician in most healing profession will be more apt to build motivation in clients to continue and succeed in treatment than an impersonal one, perceived by clients as a disinterested "cold fish." This is being recognized now in the field of medicine as more medical school curricula require training in appropriate "bedside manner."

Since preparing a client's scalp for placement of electrodes involves touching, the possibility that certain therapists exert a "healing touch" must be considered. There is a fairly large research literature on therapeutic touch, much of which supports its efficacy (Winstead-Fry & Kijek, 1999). The senior author once was told by a chiropractor with a very successful practice that he owed his success as much to his "healing hands" as to his skills with spinal manipulation. If so, could this be the "secret of success" of some neurotherapists? In addition, many neurotherapists are licensed mental health professionals. Undoubtedly, some of them consciously or unconsciously incorporate counseling and/or psychotherapy into their client training sessions. This, too, may constitute an often-overlooked nonspecific variable.

Finally, if factors specific to treatment protocols are important, the neurotherapist with skills to insure correct electrode placement, acceptable impedance levels, and appropriate reward/inhibit settings surely will have more success than one without the training, experience, ability, or ethical principles to do so. This, of course, relates to the often-contentious debates within the field regarding entry-level formal education, required number of supervised training hours, licensure, and certification.

Therapist/Client Interaction

The degree of rapport between a therapist and her or his clients is variable, even for the most empathic and experienced therapist. While picking the right "match" in choosing a neurotherapist may not be quite as important as in choosing a psychotherapist or counselor, certain matches are likely to lead to better client compliance with treatment and, hence, to more favorable results. A "good match" likely involves, and extends beyond, such factors as common education and socioeconomic levels, age ranges, and interests.

Of probable relevance here, is the concept of interaction rhythms or interpersonal synchrony (Davis, 1982). It may be what commonly is referred to as rapport, is a reflection of persons sharing common rhythm patterns in terms of movement tempo, voice intonations, etc. Perhaps, the more skilled therapists are those who entrain (set in motion) their own rhythm patterns in a variety of clients (or, conversely, are entrained by rhythms of clients) so that the two operate as a synchronous unit. A characteristic of such interpersonal synchrony may be that it exerts a healing influence. Perhaps, when a neurotherapist and client get "in sync" there is a simultaneous "getting together" (integration) within each, resulting in a healthier client (and a more satisfied, if not healthier, therapist). Such speculation on interpersonal rhythms seems especially appropriate in our field where, after all, we are dealing with frequencies and rhythms. The senior author years ago overheard a well-known EEG biofeedback research scientist mention being puzzled over his observation that certain research participants seemed more able to control their own brain rhythms in the presence of certain research assistants than in others. In private, he speculated on the possibility that some type of "subtle" energy from certain assistants had EEG entrainment power. For many of us, there is an intuitive sense that certain persons "are on the same wavelength." Whether this means having a therapist/client interpersonal synchrony reflected in harmony while speaking, shared thoughts, in-phase (coupled or coherent) EEG patterns, or some type sharing of "subtle" energy, it could be an important variable in success of neurotherapy.

Prayer By and/or For Client

Several neurotherapists known to the authors regularly pray for successful remediation of their clients' symptoms, during and/or between sessions, with or without a client's knowledge. In addition to the possible effect the knowledge of such activity itself could have on treatment outcome, some studies support the independent effectiveness of prayer. This is so with or without a client's knowledge and even at a distance, that is, distant healing or intercessory prayer (Ernst, 2003). In addition, as in many situations where some type of healing is needed, there may be prayer by a client's family members and friends, church groups, and the client himself or herself. This is a variable which would be nearly impossible (and unethical) to control, but may well be a factor in some cases of neurotherapy success.

Other Environmental Influences

As mentioned earlier, skepticism concerning neurotherapy by significant persons in a client's environment can have adverse effects on client motivation and perseverance over the course of treatment. However, other family environment factors may have equally strong impact. As noted by Lubar and Lubar (1999), neurotherapy progress can be impeded by various dysfunctional family variables. When such dysfunction is present, they routinely require family therapy prior to or concurrently with neurotherapy sessions with children. The senior author has noted a related situation, which may be of significance. This occurs especially in the families of some clients with ADHD where other family members have some of the same symptoms. Their abnormally fast tempos of moving and speaking and impulsive responding may be modeled on a daily basis by the client; or he or she may be entrained by these abnormal rhythms of siblings or parents. One or two hours per week of neurotherapy are not likely to completely counteract such environmental influences.

TREATMENT-SPECIFIC VARIABLES

Despite the likely influence of nonspecific variable such as those discussed earlier, much debate within the field of neurotherapy centers around treatment-specific variables such as appropriate electrode placement, duration of treatment, and equipment differences. Perhaps, such variables are especially important when there is some degree of commonality or standardization in the nonspecific factors. In other words, assuming a typical range of client motivations, reasonably empathic and adequately trained therapists, no strong client/therapist personality clashes and no major influence of other type treatment procedures, it seems almost certain that neurotherapy-specific variables are critical to high rates of success. In any event, their influences are likely to be more easily determined through controlled research. Some major treatment-specific variables will be discussed later.

Treatment Protocols

At this point in time, the most commonly used neurofeedback training protocols are designed to inhibit or increase EEG amplitude (power) within a frequency band or combination of bands. Probably the best-known example involves training to inhibit amplitude in a lower frequency band such as 4 to 8 Hz (theta) while simultaneously increasing amplitude in some higher frequency band such as 12 to

15 Hz or 14 to 18 Hz (beta). As all experienced neurotherapists know, this is a protocol commonly used with persons exhibiting symptoms of underarousal (as often seen with ADHD), and typically involves placement of electrodes at central and/or frontal sites. It has been used effectively for over 20 years, and continues to see wide usage. Another well-known example involves training increases in amplitude in some frequency band between about 6 and 12 Hz, usually at posterior scalp sites. This often is used to treat overarousal such as often seen in cases of anxiety disorder. Is it possible that any neurotherapist with average experience and skill, using only these two protocols, could have a 60 to 70 percent or higher success rate with clients exhibiting symptoms of underarousal or overarousal? It would seem so, judging from claims made by some therapists dating back to the early days of neurofeedback. If this is the case, and since it can be argued that the majority of neurotherapy clients suffer from either under- or overarousal, then it seems that other protocols and treatment-specific variables need to be considered only if it is assumed that success rates can be raised substantially by refining methodology and/or equipment.

Two of the pioneers in the field (Susan Othmer and Siegfried Othmer, this volume) discuss the evolution of their thinking as they and their associates refined their treatment procedures to achieve this goal of substantially raising success rates with a wide variety of clients. However, their conclusions do not always coincide with those of other experienced therapists who claim at conference presentations or in journal articles to have met the same goal. Such differences can be quite confusing, especially to those therapists who are new to the field, and can lead inquisitive people to ask, "Why and how can this be?" Presumably, the answer lies not only in variations in nonspecific variables such as those aforementioned, but also in differential emphasis on other treatment-specific variables such as presented in the next paragraph.

Over the years, neurotherapists have attributed unusually high rates of success to factors (or combinations of factors) such as the following:

1. Use of training protocols based on results of pretraining (or during training) QEEG data, considered in conjunction with a normative database such as Neuroguide Thatcher (2002);

2. Training using scalp electrode placements over localized cortical areas known to be heavily involved in mediating cognitive
   processes in which the client has impairment;
3. Adjusting training protocols based on minute-to-minute or day-
   to-day client reports of "satisfaction" or "comfort" with any
   given protocol;
4. Using so-called "canned" protocols widely reported to be effective for symptoms such as those reported by the client;
5. Directly training increases or decreases in frequency ratios
   (e.g., theta/beta) rather than individual bands;
6. Training a single frequency rather than a broader frequency
   band (usually based on QEEG results);
7. Doing cross-hemisphere training, usually involving homologous sites;
8. Using a "broadband inhibit" wherein abnormally high amplitude EEG is inhibited at all frequencies;
9. Using sequential (bipolar) electrode placements rather than
   monopolar (or vice versa);
10. Training decreases in EEG variability;
11. Providing "massed practice" by requiring daily or several times
    per day training rather than the usual two to three times per week;
12. Breaking training sessions into many small time segments or
    "runs," for example, 30, 60, 180 seconds, (or vice versa, requiring
    prolonged 30 to 60 minute sessions);
13. Requiring ten or more sessions after desired behavior change in
    order to "solidify" and insure permanency of change;
14. Concurrent use of adjunctive therapies such as audio-visual
    entrainment or disentrainment, hypnosis, cognitive-behavioral
    therapy, computer-based cognitive training activities, peripheral
    biofeedback (e.g., finger temperature), or hemoencephalography;
15. Using equipment that provides very rapid feedback, or real-time
    feedback (without the EEG signal first being subjected to Fourier
    transform); and
16. Using unique and inherently interesting forms of feedback, for
    example, virtual reality, music, etc.

While the aforementioned variables relate to frequency training,
most are also applicable to phase and/or coherence and comodulation

training, which some neurotherapists use in conjunction with, or independently of, frequency/amplitude training (see Horvath, this volume), and claim that it greatly increases effectiveness in many cases. Sometimes referred to as "connectivity training," it involves training increases or decreases in communication and neural timing between EEG signals from different sites.

Undoubtedly, there are other nonspecific and treatment-specific variables that are overlooked by the authors and touted by some neurotherapists as the ones primarily responsible for their treatment success rates approaching 100 percent. Certainly, there will be others as the field expands. As noted earlier, there are various levels regarding which one can question why and how neurofeedback "works." Two of these are the neurophysiological and psychological levels, as will be discussed in the next section.

UNDERLYING NEUROPHYSIOLOGICAL AND PSYCHOLOGICAL MECHANISMS

Several theorists in the field of neurotherapy have observed that neurofeedback itself, independently of nonspecific factors such as those discussed earlier, seems to be effective in the majority of cases using a wide range of training protocols, and have speculated on general mechanisms of efficacy.

Neurophysiological Mechanisms

Some theoretical explanations are quite broad and lack in detail. For example, there is the notion that a sort of natural "body wisdom" exists, so that when a normal or "healthful" frequency (or connectivity) pattern develops by chance during training, the brain "knows" it is helpful and tends to perpetuate the pattern. This seems to assume a brain separate from self-awareness or consciousness, and thus calls into question the self-regulation aspect of neurotherapy. However, the idea may be given some credence by the fact that many successfully trained clients say they have no conscious awareness of how they were able to maintain feedback during training. In what appears to the authors to be a somewhat related notion, it has been speculated that any change brought about by neurofeedback training in brain electrical activity (or perhaps other means such as electroshock or audio-visual entrainment) causes perturbation in the entire bioelectrical system. This, in turn, stimulates a generalized, natural, and reflexive normalizing reaction, leading to remission of symptoms.

Another general idea, which has been put forth elsewhere by the first author (Evans, 2002) involves the concept of EEG frequency imbalances. Since the majority of neurotherapy training protocols are designed to normalize abnormal frequency patterns at various electrode sites, it seems appropriate to invoke such a concept. The idea usually is understood and accepted by clients and other health practitioners, perhaps because they are used to thinking in terms of chemical imbalances and perceive an analogy to the latter. Since it is known that neural function is electrochemical in nature, it is reasonable to assume that electrical (EEG) imbalances and abnormalities are as likely as chemical imbalances to be associated with abnormal behavioral symptoms. And, it should follow from this concept that one should not be surprised by claims that neurotherapy is as useful as pharmacological treatment with a very wide variety of disorders.

Others have explored possible neurophysiological underpinnings of neurofeedback at much more basic levels. Abarbanel (1999) explored commonalities between pharmacological and neurofeedback phenomena, especially as they may relate to treatment of attention deficit/hyperactivity disorder (ADHD). He speculated that ADHD-related neural circuit systems are "adjustable" (have plasticity), and, through neurofeedback, clients learn to exert neuromodulatory control over these circuits. They appear to do this by modulating (adjusting) firing rate characteristics of individual postsynaptic neurons and group characteristics of entire neuronal circuits. He gives a related example from pharmacological research which indicated that the neurotransmitter dopamine is involved when a brain stem system responds to sensory cues arousing fear, and adjusts neural activity in higher brain centers, which then elicits motoric responses related to fight or flight. He speculates that similar neuromodulation also occurs in the bioelectric realm, but does so through oscillatory activity of individual neurons and groups of neurons. These oscillations of various frequencies open and close "gates" to affect neural information flow, and serve to switch states of brain centers or brain circuits. The mechanisms by which such rerouting of information in neural circuitry occur include frequency (oscillatory) entrainment of brain systems (e.g, limbic, thalamic), and facilitation/suppression of resonances between brain areas. In this view, neurofeedback permits adjustment of neural firing rates (oscillations), thus enabling "fine tuning" of aberrant, symptom-related brain centers.

Abarbanel further explains neurofeedback's efficacy by speculating that continuing the neuromodulation over a usual series of 20 to 40 or more training sessions result in long-term potentiation (LTP). The repetitive and apparently self-generated afferent signals involved in neurofeedback seem to stabilize and consolidate the client's enhanced neuromodulatory control, that is, the ability to regulate gating and state changes between brain centers. This apparently results in the enduring remission of symptoms so often noted.

In this view, imbalance in sets of neuronal circuits leads to psychopathology. Abarbanel notes, for example, that autonomous and exaggerated activity of prefrontal or subcortical neural circuits, which "code for" fixed behavioral or ideational circuits, may lead to symptoms of obsessive-compulsive disorder. Whether, by increasing one's general capacity for neuromodulation of imbalanced circuits over the course of training, and/or by continuing self-generated oscillatory entrainment of specific brain centers into desired (balanced) states, neurofeedback is seen as having wide ranging and lasting positive effects.

Siegfreid and Susan Othmer also theorize on the physiological mechanisms underlying neurofeedback's efficacy. Since their latest notions in this area are presented elsewhere in this volume, only a brief overview will be given here.

Their theories emphasize the inadequacies of neurochemical models for explaining such things as the origins and time courses of psychopathologies, while stressing the greater explanatory value of the bioelectrical domain. Pathology is viewed as due to disruptions of neural timing, with neurochemical imbalances being more a consequence than a cause. In this domain, concepts such as frequency, phase relationships, neural assemblies, neural networks, and time binding replace neurotransmitters, and function is emphasized over structure. Rhythmic firing of brain stem neurons is hypothesized to regulate firing of thalamic neural networks, which, in turn, regulate cortical networks (and vice versa). Dysrhythmias of thalamacortical function are associated with disintegration and disruption of regulatory functions of the brain. Transfer of neural information is seen as happening via "time binding," which involves neuronal events occurring simultaneously (even if in disparate brain locations); and integrity of timing between neural networks is critical to efficient information transfer. Coordinated coupling of different EEG frequencies and their harmonics, in addition to appropriate phase relationships within frequency bands, also is viewed as critical to efficient brain function.

In the Othmers' model, neurofeedback, acting through thalamacortical networks, affects brain stem mechanisms in a manner that enables the latter to then help restore timing integrity within all neural networks. In this regard, they note that any disturbance of brain timing, whether through the operant conditioning of neurofeedback or through other stimulation, elicits a brain response, which over time may restore normal rhythmicity, phase relationships, and timing integrity among neuronal assemblies, leading to more efficient information transfer and regulatory functioning. Since, such disturbance of brain timing can be by way of induced changes in frequency, amplitude, or phase relationships, it is suggested that many different neurofeedback training protocols derive their efficacy from this mechanism, that is, each challenges the existing neural timing, thus setting up a brain response that may result in improved management of timing relationships. This could help explain the high treatment success rates claimed by practitioners using many different training protocols.

Psychological Mechanisms

A notion that is occasionally discussed in neurotherapy circles assumes that traumatic or otherwise undesirable life circumstances cumulatively generate abnormally high EEG waveform amplitude. In other words, excessive amplitudes may be reflecting life's bad times. Presumably, lowering amplitude through neurofeedback can minimize negative effects of these past experiences. Those who advocate broadband inhibition of abnormally high amplitudes during training should appreciate this notion.

Another general and primarily psychological explanation of neurofeedback efficacy often espoused is that as a client learns to self-regulate EEG activity, a sense of empowerment develops with increased self-esteem and self-confidence, which generalizes to other life situations. He or she then more readily masters other life tasks, and many symptoms resolve. If this is the case, there is no apparent reason why neurotherapy should be any more effective than learning to self-regulate muscle tension, heart rate, or skill in sports. However, if the neurotherapy training specifically involved frontal lobe function, there may be enduring psychological and physiological effects wherein general executive control truly is improved, and accompanied by a conscious sense of greater self-efficacy.

Still another primarily psychological theory relates specifically to training increases in amplitude in slower frequencies. This often leads to client reports of experiencing deeply altered states of consciousness. A common example, usually referred to as alpha\theta training, reportedly is useful in treatment of posttraumatic stress disorder and dissociative identity disorder. Entering into an altered state of consciousness characterized by high-amplitude EEG in alpha or theta frequencies (typically 6 to 10 Hz), supposedly facilitates awareness of formerly unconscious memories of past trauma. Since such states usually also are accompanied by a sense of inner calmness, the client seems to be freed from psychological defenses, and therefore, able to confront and process the formerly repressed material in a manner which enables resolution of symptoms.

COMMONALITIES BETWEEN NEUROFEEDBACK AND VARIOUS ALTERNATIVE/COMPLEMENTARY MEDICINE APPROACHES

Although many reasons have been given for the often-reported low rate of acceptance of neurofeedback by the general public and mainstream medicine and education (see Crane, this volume), there is one that is rarely mentioned. It is the competition this field has with 150 or more alternative healing approaches offered by an array of practitioners who freely cite glowing client testimonials of their treatment value (Kastner & Burroughs, 1996). Many, if not most, members of the general public likely consider neurofeedback to be another alternative medicine. Even though very large numbers of persons are turning to these alternative approaches, if neurofeedback is to stand out among them, there is a need to demonstrate that it has unique value. To do this, it seems important to consider commonalities and differences among approaches. This not only could help determine neurofeedback's unique identity, but perhaps also shed more light on the why and how of its efficacy.

Oscillations and Rhythms

The Abarbanel and Othmer theories discussed earlier place heavy emphasis on concepts such as oscillations, frequency, resonance, entrainment, and rhythm. Many, if not most, alternative therapies do so as well. Therefore, this commonality will receive greatest attention in this chapter.

One of the most obvious applications of rhythmic stimulation to healing is seen in music therapy. Although some music therapists use music in a different manner, for example, employing opportunity to listen to favorite music as a reward for positive behavior change, for the most part, this type therapy can be conceived as involving entrainment via the pitch (sound frequencies) and rhythm pattern characteristics of music. While most details of the mechanisms through which music affects human physiology and behavior remain unknown or debatable, few would doubt that it has very strong impact at all ages and in all cultures. Neurotherapists and others who use audio-visual entrainment equipment are aware of the effects that exposure to relatively simple sound (and light) frequencies can have on EEG and other physiological measures as well as on consciousness (see chapter by Sevier, this volume). One might expect that even greater changes could be accomplished using more complex sound patterns that define music. The potential power of music to effect behavioral change is implied by parental fears that the music of each new generation of children will corrupt them, by the prohibition of listening to certain types of music by the governments of some countries, by the widespread interest in reports that listening to certain classical music can facilitate brain development of infants, and by reports of reversals (albeit usually temporary ones) of major symptoms of neurological disorders such as Parkinson's disease. Regarding the latter, a well known neurologist, Oliver Sachs (as cited in Comer, 2004, p. 577), reported case histories of several patients who could not walk, but could dance, could not speak, but could sing, or would not move until "activated" by music. In each case, he noted that the power of music was instantaneous, but effects lasted only while the music lasted. The parallels between music and EEG activity have been noted by many over the years, for example, both involve frequencies, harmonics, frequency patterns (rhythms), and resonance (as in harmony in music, and coherence and phase relationships in the EEG). This was implied in the title of one of the first published books on neurofeedback, *A Symphony in the Brain* (Robbins, 2000). A related recent development has been "brain music therapy" in which an individual's EEG patterns are converted into musical sounds and presented to him or her in two different forms, one relaxing and one activating. This reportedly promotes relaxation and activation in the individual. The extent to which this will develop and replace more commonly used entrainment procedures remains to be seen. However, the parallels between music and EEG are so great that it seems likely to the authors that technological developments eventually will enable creative persons to fully explore the relationships (Levin, 1988). This could yield greater insight into the mechanisms of neurofeedback, thus enabling development of equipment with power to effect greater, and more rapid, enduring changes in neurophysiological function than is possible with today's equipment. Perhaps, remissions from neurological diseases then will be permanent!

While music therapy is one of the oldest, best known, and most researched alternative healing method involving sound frequencies, it is not the only one. Chanting, as practiced extensively in some cultures reportedly induces alterations of consciousness, which may have healing effects. There have been reports of the healing effects of focusing high frequency sound waves on acupuncture points. And, the repetition of a mantra to induce meditative states may be an important factor in the frequently reported value of meditation in healing.

Rhythmic and repetitive stimulation is involved directly or indirectly in many other alternative healing approaches. Obvious examples include heart rate variability training, breathing exercises, dance therapy, poetry therapy, and rhythmic exercise such as walking and running. Rhythm and motoric timing are basic to the Interactive Metronome approach to working with attention deficit disorder, and the frequency of light flash stimuli (and perhaps the frequency of color of the lights) is considered important in the various approaches using auditory-visual entrainment. Less obvious may be the rhythmic or monotonous vocalizations (and sometime body movements) of the hypnotist during hypnotherapy, the rhythmic movements of massage therapists, and the color frequencies involved in color therapy or some types of art therapy.

Notions of disease being related to abnormal or imbalanced frequencies of body organs or disturbed "subtle energy" have existed for centuries. In "energy medicine" circles, the purported energies apparently are referred to as "subtle" because their exact nature remains unknown, and reliable measurement techniques have not yet been developed. A large number of complementary/alternative medicines purport to heal by manipulating these energies. The book *Vibrational Medicine* (Gerber, 1988) discusses many such applications, including acupuncture, healing with magnets, radionics, and homeopathy. In the latter approach, the fact that many homeopathic remedies have been diluted to the point that not a single molecule of the original substance remains has led to dismissal of claims of its value. However, some homeopathic practitioners claim that, "energy imprints" in the form of proper frequencies remain, and effect healing by interacting with disturbed body frequencies.

As with some theories of neurofeedback, the concepts of frequencies (vibrations or oscillations), resonance, and entrainment have been invoked by many practitioners of alternative healing to explain mechanisms of efficacy. However, even assuming the validity of such explanations, questions remain concerning how to best apply them. And it needs to be determined whether there is anything about neurofeedback that makes it more efficient, effective, economical, or enduring than these other approaches.

Relaxation

Many alternative healing methods involve a sense of (or actual) very deep physical and/or mental relaxation on the part of clients. This generally is true for peripheral biofeedback, such as that involving feedback of muscle activity [electromyography (EMG)] or skin temperature, meditation, breathing exercises, massage therapy, and some types of hypnotherapy. It also can be true for neurotherapy training, especially that involving enhancing power in lower frequencies.

It could be claimed that such deep relaxation itself is responsible for symptom removal. Perhaps, relaxation facilitates neural reintegration or improved function of one's immune system, or, via other pathways, frees the healing powers of one's "inner physician/psychologist." And, it needs to be determined whether a "good night's sleep" can be healing. Possibly, very deep relaxation can be even more so. Another possibility is that, when deeply relaxed, formerly anxiety-producing thoughts can occur without excessive arousal and a need for their suppression. Over time, such thoughts may become associated with relaxation rather than anxiety, and hence, lose their power to create symptoms such as those of anxiety and mood disorders. Even if deep relaxation is not the main reason for any treatment's efficacy, given its healing potential, it could be argued that it should be at least a part of any therapy. Again, however, one can question whether neurofeedback is a more efficient route to relaxation than other approaches.

Altered States of Consciousness

In several alternative approaches to healing, clients commonly report having experienced distinctly altered states of consciousness other than deep relaxation. This can be true regardless of whether or not there was a deliberate effort on the part of the practitioner to induce such states. Examples include hypnosis, meditation, auditory-visual entrainment, guided imagery, dream therapy, and some forms of biofeedback, including especially neurofeedback training of increases in lower alpha and theta frequency ranges. It could be argued that altered states occur even during training for increases in power of beta frequencies. For example, when a neurotherapy client with attention deficit disorder is focused, and thus meeting training criteria and receiving feedback, this focused state of consciousness presumably is altered from what is a "normal" state for him or her. As with deep relaxation, it could be speculated that altered states can be conducive to healing. Hypnotherapists, for example, often proceed on the assumption that a trance state enables access to formerly unconscious memories, enabling their entry into consciousness during subsequent therapy so that any negative impacts they might have had can be resolved and brought under self-control. "Alpha/theta" neurofeedback training dynamics may be similar; except that some claim the resolution can occur entirely in the altered state over a series of training sessions with little or no need for subsequent psychotherapy. The heightened suggestibility often noted in persons during some altered states could be another factor worth considering, especially if positive suggestions are given by therapists during treatment. As with the other variables considered in this chapter, it seems important to ask if and when an altered state of consciousness is important to treatment efficacy, and whether neurofeedback is the preferred way to induce it.

SUMMARY AND CONCLUSIONS

In this chapter, we have speculated widely (some might say wildly!) on various nonspecific, treatment-specific, neurophysiological, and psychological factors, which might explain why and how neurofeedback is effective in the treatment of wide variety of symptoms of disorders. Few, if any of the notions presented originated with the authors, but, rather, were gleaned from years of reading, attending workshops and conferences, talking with other therapists, and wondering about reasons this method should have such wide-ranging uses and effectiveness, and whether and when it is more effective than other treatment approaches. Surely, the nonspecific factors discussed are important to therapeutic success, but would be applicable to a great many healing approaches. The treatment-specific variables, singly or in combination, have been found valuable (or not valuable) by many experienced neurotherapists, and await further exploration through controlled research and accumulation of shared clinical experience. In all likelihood, value of each variable depends largely on factors such as symptoms being treated and skill in their applications. Some eventually may be found to be unimportant, and akin to "superstitious behaviors." Since neurotherapy deals primarily with brain electrical activity (the bioelectric domain), and since frequencies (oscillations, vibrations), resonances, phase relationships entrainment, and rhythms are concepts within that domain, related efficacy explanations seem especially promising. This is reinforced further by the large number of alternative healing methods, which include rhythmic/oscillatory features in their applications and/or theories of efficacy.

It seems fitting to conclude by speculating on why and how one might argue that neurofeedback is a preferred approach. In regard to this, we submit the following:

1. Neurofeedback (along with other biofeedback procedures such as EMG and hemoencephalography) requires clients to actively participate in treatment rather than be passive recipients waiting for a medication, homeopathic remedy, hypnotist's suggestion, massage, chiropractic manipulation, acupuncture procedure, auditory-visual entrainment stimuli, etc. to heal them. In theory at least, this has some advantage in that it facilitates emergence of (or strengthening of) a conscious sense of self-efficacy and inner control, and thus is likely to have more enduring effects.

2. Other than pharmacological treatment, only neurofeedback directly targets the electrochemical functioning of the central nervous system. Furthermore, only neurofeedback can directly address modification of specific frequencies, specific cortical areas (via electrode placement), and intracortical neural timing (via coherence/phase training). While other approaches undoubtedly modify central nervous system function, they do so more indirectly and in a more generalized fashion.

3. Neurofeedback deals with a recognized and reliably measurable energy (electromagnetic) as compared to the hypothetical "subtle" energies of many other approaches. This makes its claims more open to scientific study than is true of many other healing approaches.

4. Only neurofeedback can directly address the abnormal neural timing relationships and connectivity problems, which are believed by some to be basic causes of learning disabilities such as dyslexia.

5. Although it is also true of many other alternative procedures, neurofeedback has few, if any, negative and enduring side effects. Certainly, this gives it some advantage over many pharmacological treatments.

6. The field of neurofeedback is very supportive of scientific research, and rapidly growing numbers of studies generally validate its value.

7. Neurofeedback can be of special value for developing superior (peak) performance in normal (relatively symptom-free) persons.

For example, appropriate training protocols can increase one's timing sense in sports activities and increase ability to sustain attention in academic, avocational, and vocational settings.

By this point, some present-day readers may feel that trying to understand the mechanisms of efficacy of neurofeedback is a hopeless pursuit. They can be forgiven for this, considering the short history of the field and the fact that the exact dynamics of even such ancient healing approaches as acupuncture remain unknown. It is very likely that the nature of neurofeedback will still be debated long after we are gone. Nevertheless, inquisitive persons will continue to perform research, refine their clinical procedures, and help the field to evolve so that increasingly larger numbers of persons can be helped by this method—even if their therapists do not know for sure why or how.

REFERENCES

Abarbanel, A. A. (1999). The neural underpinnings of neurofeedback training. In J. R. Evans & A. A. Abarbanel (Eds.) *Introduction to quantitative EEG and neurofeedback*. San Diego: Academic Press.

Comer, R. J. (2004). *Abnormal psychology* (5th ed.). New York: Worth Publishers.

Davis, M. (1982). *Interaction rhythms*. New York: Human Sciences Press.

Ernst, E. (2003). Distant healing—An update of a systematic review. *Wiener Klinische Wochenschrift, 115*(7-8), 241-245.

Evans, J. R. (2002). Neurofeedback. In V. Ramachandran (Ed.) *Encyclopedia of the human brain*. San Diego: Academic Press.

Gerber, R. (1988). *Vibrational medicine*. Santa Fe, NM: Bear & Co.

Kastner, M. & Burroughs, H. (1996). *Alternative healing*. New York: Henry Holt and Co., Inc.

Levin, Y. (1998). "Brain music" in the treatment of patients with insomnia. *Neuroscience and Behavioral Physiology,* (28), 330-335.

Lubar, J. F. & Lubar, J. O. (1999). Neurofeedback Assessment and treatment for attention deficit/hyperactivity disorders. In J. R. Evans & Abarbanel (Eds.) *Introduction to quantitative EEG and neuro-feedback*. San Diego: Academic Press.

Robbins, J. (2000). *A symphony in the brain*. Boston: Atlantic Monthly Press.

Thatcher, R. (2002). *Neuroguide*. St. Petersburg, FL: Applied Neuroscience, Inc.

Winstead-Fry, P. & Kijek, J. (1999). An integrative review and meta-analysis of therapeutic touch research. *Alternative Therapies in Health and Medicine, 5*(6), 58-67.

SECTION III:
GENERAL CLINICAL
APPLICATIONS

Chapter 4

Multichannel Tomographic Neurofeedback: Wave of the Future?

Marco Congedo
David Joffe

INTRODUCTION

Electroencephalography (EEG) neurofeedback was conceived and introduced in the 1960s (Kamiya 1962; Engstrom, London, and Hart 1970; Travis, Kondo, and Knott 1974). Since then, it is our belief that other than the shift from analog to digital equipment, the overall methodology of neurofeedback has not evolved significantly. The general outline of what we will refer to as *traditional neurofeedback* in this chapter is shown in Figure 4.1. An electronic device records EEG activity at a particular scalp location and subjects it to signal processing. An electrophysiological feature is extracted and converted into visual and/or auditory representations, which dynamically covary with the target feature. The process is real-time, that is, the feedback modalities continuously represent brain activity with a minimum delay, which in modern equipment is on the order of a few tens of milliseconds. Typically, over 20 to 40 sessions of thirty minutes each, spaced two to three days apart, the participant acquires an enhanced awareness of the *causal relations* underlying the feedback process. As a consequence of neurofeedback training, it has been observed and documented that a certain ability to self-regulate overall brain functioning may be achieved (Lubar 1991). For example, sub-

Handbook of Neurofeedback
doi:10.1300/5889_04

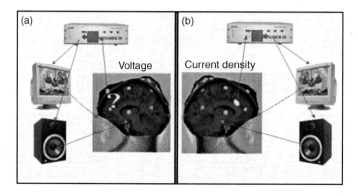

FIGURE 4.1. Schematic representation of traditional neurofeedback (a) and tomographic neurofeedback (b).

jects may learn how to increase the background power in the 8 to 10 Hz frequency range at a particular electrode location or to increase the coherence at one or more EEG frequencies measured between bipolar leads.

The amount of research accumulated in this area over the past 40 years is considerable, especially with respect to the clinical application of neurofeedback. However, many general aspects of the method are still largely ignored. Clearly, the neurofeedback loop is established by *association* of a spontaneous electromagnetic signal with the sensory information acquired through the feedback modality, but the manner in which the brain uses sensory information to drive physiological activity is unknown. There is also debate as to whether in humans, the learning associated with neurofeedback must be a volitional act or if it could be achieved against or outside the will by mere conditioning (Congedo 2003; Kotchoubey et al. 2002; Nowlis and Kamiya 1970; Sterman 1981).

In this chapter, we are interested in a more fundamental question regarding what can be considered the greatest limitation of traditional neurofeedback. The question mark illustrated just below the active electrode in Figure 4.1 signifies the *spatial-unspecificity* of the target brain feature, hereafter referred to as the target signal (TS). Otherwise stated, using only one active electrode (plus the reference and ground electrode), the spatial specificity and spatial resolution attainable are minimal. The electrical activity detected at the active site will reflect not only cortical activity directly underneath the electrode, but also electrical activity from other areas. This fact appears clearly, once we consider that the sum of *all* neuronal activity that is detectable by any given electrode (Nunez 1995; Nunez and Silberstein 2000). More specifically, the gray matter in the brain contributes to the scalp voltage according to the inverse of the square distance law, relative to the position of both active and reference electrodes. Thus, training a function of voltage at a single site results in training the whole brain. By choosing a particular active location, we merely assign larger "weights" to regions closer to it. See figure 1 in Kropotov et al. (2005) for an empirical verification of this phenomenon. Multiple EEG sources, noises, and artifacts, such as those contributed by electromyographic (EMG) and electro-ocular (EOG) activity, are all uncontrolled variables increasing the noncontingency of the self-regulating effort. That is, the participant is very likely to receive rewarding feedback due in part to electrical activity not related to the TS and to receive penalizing feedback even if the TS is in the desired state. It is important to recognize that the aforementioned limitations relating to the spatial specificity are serious and can be overcome only by using *multiple channels* and extracting the sources of the TS from all of them. Only in this case, it is possible to increase the spatial specificity. The idea is represented schematically in the right-hand part of Figure 4.1 and will be further elaborated upon from a *blind* perspective when we address issues concerning signal-artifact separation. As compared to traditional neurofeedback, the general functioning of such *tomographic neurofeedback* is unchanged. Only the electromagnetic origin of the TS differs (source) since we attempt to delimit its origin in brain space. The potential advantage of this approach is nevertheless considerable; the self-regulation of the electrical activity of interest may be easier and faster to achieve, making the neurofeedback training more effective and more practical. Training a specific anatomical region may engage target signals more closely related to the brain function of interest. And all this is possible using a noninvasive and relatively inexpensive method, which results in a form of EEG neurofeedback both affordable on a large scale and applicable to people of all ages.

In the next section, we describe relevant facts relating to brain physiology, and provide a foundation to the EEG/MEG (magnetoelectroencephalography) source localization problem as it is treated in linear physics, thus setting the stage for a discussion of the characteristics of standardized Low-Resolution Electromagnetic Tomography (sLORETA), which is one among number of related localization methods. The ensuing section describes our experimental study on tomographic neurofeedback. Next, we will suggest that by using multiple channels, it is possible to separate EEG activity from noise and artifacts, and possibly, to separate different EEG sources with the aim of training them selectively. In that context we will briefly introduce results from two modern signal processing techniques, namely, *blind source separation* and filtering by *beamforming,* and show how they could be used for our purposes. The chapter ends with a discussion, wherein we suggest possible paths for future research to establish new criteria for neurofeedback. We also briefly outline technical issues, which we believe must be addressed in order for multichannel tomographic neurofeedback to be introduced to the clinical setting in a responsible manner. It is worth mentioning that almost everything we discuss here with respect to EEG is also applicable to MEG, using suitable instrumentation.

This book is mainly addressed to the clinician. Consequently, in this chapter we restrict ourselves to a general discussion of those EEG/MEG neurofeedback improvements that can be obtained utilizing recent advances in digital signal processing methods pertaining to the biomagnetic source localization problem (Sarvas 1987), and to the question of why their application would be beneficial for neurofeedback. Our exposition will intentionally refrain from equations and other technical details to facilitate an intuitive understanding. Nevertheless, we provide a selection of relevant references where the reader interested in implementation can find all necessary details.

THE PHYSIOLOGY OF EEG
AND THE EEG INVERSE PROBLEM

Electrical fields, as measured on the scalp, are largely due to the postsynaptic potentials of neocortical cells (Nunez 1995), in particular, pyramidal cells (Figure 4.2). Within neocortical layers, pyramidal cells are organized in adjacent columns, normally oriented perpendicular to the tangent of the local neocortex surface (Figure 4.3). Because of their morphology and physiology, pyramidal cells act as clusters of

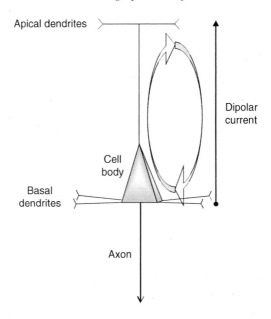

FIGURE 4.2. Schematic representation of a neocortical pyramidal cell. The thick arrow pointing toward the top of the figure shows the direction of the dipolar current (current flowing between two equal and opposite point charges). The moment of the dipole depends upon excitatory and inhibitory cortical and subcortical afferences in multiple layers of the cortex.

aligned, ionic dipoles, which rhythmically invert the polarity forming between the basal and apical portions. Now, considering a large enough volume of cortical tissue and admitting temporal independence of the columnar firing, we would not be able to record any rhythmic potential oscillation from the scalp. Instead, we would observe random noise. All these contradict our observations, according to which the spontaneous EEG signal, all over the cortex, oscillates according to the superposition* of both random and periodical components, as clearly indicated in periodograms and autocorrelation functions.[†] Thus, pyramidal cells over extended regions must not only fire simultaneously

---

*In the context of linear algebra, which applies here, *superposition* is synonymous with *weighted* summation.

[†] The periodogram (power spectrum) and autocorrelation function of random noise is flat, but this is not what we observe in spontaneous human EEG/MEG activity.

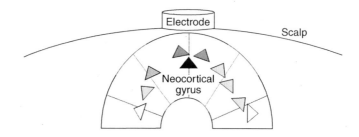

FIGURE 4.3. Schematic representation of a neocortical gyrus and an electrode upon it. Pyramidal cell bodies are organized in columns within the grey matter part of the gyrus. Their orientation is perpendicular to the tangent of the gyrus. In the figure, the "visibility" of pyramidal columns is color coded depending on their orientation with respect to the active electrode. Black represents maximal visibility and white represents minimal visibility. Dipoles perpendicular to the scalp (radial) are maximally visible, while dipoles parallel to the scalp (tangential) are invisible, i.e., their activity is not detected by the electrode [for MEG the visibility is somehow complementary, in that the radial component is either completely or almost completely silent (depending upon the head model employed), whereas maximal visibility belongs to tangential components].

but also synchronously (in phase). Given this state of affairs, the scalp potentials have been related proportionally to the number of cells acting synchronously and inversely proportional to the square root of the number of asynchronous cells (Nunez and Silberstein 2000). These considerations are intended to provide a direct organic interpretation of the physical intracranial measure of brain activity we next introduce.

Since scalp voltage results from intra-cortical current and since the head is a conductive medium, one may wish to characterize this current, that is to say, to know its *location, strength,* and *orientation* over *time.* For a given location and time instant (or time averaged Fourier frequency), electrical current can be expressed as a vector in three-dimensional (3-D) space (Figure 4.4). The *current density* can be represented by three components for orientation x, y, and z. The length of the vector is referred to as *source amplitude*, while its square is termed *source power* by analogy with the definition of power in the complex frequency domain. Typically, the TS will be chosen so as to be a function of one of these two quantities, which are basically analogous to absolute voltage amplitude and power. In summary, the observable

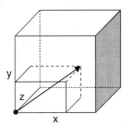

FIGURE 4.4. Representation of the current density as a vector spanning a three-dimensional orthogonal basis. This is the current space visualized by sLORETA. *Note:* Following Figure 4.4, whereas an orthogonal basis is represented by a cube, a non-orthogonal basis could be represented by a parallelepiped rectangle, one in which the angle between the faces is not necessarily 90° and in which the sides have not the same length. That is a way to visualize the fact that in a non-orthogonal space the three components are not all pair-wise independent from each other and/or there is no common unit among the three axes.

EEG is a mere effect of underlying source activity. By means of a source localization method, we try to characterize such *sources*. Said differently, a source localization method seeks the likely current source configuration engendering the EEG/MEG measurements.

The problem to be solved mathematically is called *inverse* and has no unique solution. Non-uniqueness is another way of saying that there are infinite combinations of current sources, which could generate the same exact scalp potential distribution. However, many of these hypothetical source configurations can be immediately eliminated on a physiological basis. Our choice in this paper is the minimum two-norm (least-square) solution of Hämäläinen and Ilmoniemi (1984) with standardization, as proposed by Pascual-Marqui (2002). This results in a distributed, discrete, linear, and instantaneous inverse solution known as sLORETA (standardized Low-Resolution Electromagnetic Tomography). In the aforementioned definition, *distributed* means that the current density is estimated all-at-once over the entire neocortical volume so that no assumption about the number of sources is required; *discrete* implies that the gray matter volume is divided into a certain number of cubic regions termed *voxels* (volume elements), for which the current density is estimated (this is just a matter of convenience); *linear* refers to the fact that mathematically, the inverse solution is obtained by seeking a solution to a linear equation; *instantaneous* indicates that sLORETA does not make use of second-order statistics of the sensor measurements, like variance-covariance matrix and similar statistics that need to be estimated using many data samples over time, thus, it is able to produce an image of current density for *every* time sample. Finally, *standardized* implies that the current space at each voxel is orthogonal (Figure 4.4).

sLORETA has been shown to have no localization error in exact measurements (noise-free) point spread function simulations (Pascual-Marqui 2002). In practice, this means, if the voltage vector measured on the scalp at a given instant of time is produced by a single source of current in the brain, than sLORETA allows the exact localization of the source, given noise-free scalp voltage measurement and an exact head model. This result holds even for a small number of measurement electrodes and has been proved theoretically (Greenblatt et al. 2005; Sekihara, Sahani, and Nagarajan 2005). The least-square solution is very smooth and sLORETA trades off spatial resolution to achieve excellent localization accuracy. By *low spatial resolution,* we refer to the spatial blurring of the sLORETA current density reconstruction. That is, even if the source is point-like (i.e., bounded within a single voxel), the reconstructed current density is approximately spherical with a maximum in the true location, which diminishes with increasing distance from that location. With real data, the actual blurring is found to be on the centimeter scale. The more the electrodes used, the better will be the spatial resolution, and with improved spatial resolution, the greater the chance that sLORETA will be able to separate two closely spaced sources. In conclusion, the major limitations of minimum norm inverse solutions are the low spatial resolution, the need for noise-free measurement, and the requirement for an appropriate head model. sLORETA is no exception, but it provides us with the very important localization accuracy feature, which can be considered the very essence of the inverse problem.

The proposals in this chapter relate to methods, which to a great extent may overcome the aforementioned limitations of minimum-norm instantaneous inverse solutions as applied to neurofeedback. We will examine recent methods designed to increase their spatial resolution and signal-to-noise ratio. These filtering techniques also address the multiple-source problem, and increase considerably the processing speed of EEG inversion algorithms. From a physiological perspective, the proposed advances should result in improvements of the spatial-specificity of the feedback, improvements of the feedback contingency, and decrease of feedback noncontingency. Furthermore, they should allow faster feedback and the possibility of training several regions simultaneously while minimizing the feedback delay. On the other hand, the problem of constructing adequate head models to enhance the accuracy of the correspondence between the ROI (region of interest) we train and the actual individual anatomical ROI we wish to train, is, for space limitations, left outside the scope of this work. Our proposals derive from the experience acquired with the first experimental study carried out on tomographic neurofeedback (Congedo, Lubar, and Joffe 2004). Hence, we begin by presenting this research.

TOMOGRAPHIC NEUROFEEDBACK: AN EXPERIMENTAL RESEARCH

In Congedo, Lubar, and Joffe (2004), we established a method for extracting and providing feedback on intra-cranial current density, and carried out an experimental study to ascertain the ability of the participants to drive their own EEG power in a desired direction by means of this tomographic neurofeedback. The fundamental question concerning the *efficacy* of such neurofeedback is related to whether spatial filters could be used to derive the TS. Moreover, in this research we set minimal standards for technical and statistical methods to be used in all steps of this kind of research. To derive current density within the brain volume, we used the low-resolution electromagnetic tomography (LORETA) (Pascual-Marqui, Michel, and Lehmann 1994), since at the time of the research the sLORETA method had not been widely examined.

Six undergraduate students (three males, three females in the age range of 19 to 22 years) underwent tomographic neurofeedback based on 19 electrodes placed according to the standard 10-20 placement (FP1, FP2, F3, F4, Fz , F7, F8, C3, C4, Cz, T3, T4, T5, T6, P3, P4, Pz, O1, and O2). Three participants underwent six sessions consisting of six three-minute trials, while the remaining three underwent 20 sessions of three 15-minute trials. The neurofeedback protocol was designed to enhance low-beta (16 to 20 Hz) and suppress low-alpha (8 to 10 Hz) current density amplitude in a region corresponding approximately to the Anterior Cingulate cognitive division (ACcd). Hereafter, we will refer to the protocol using the symbol $\alpha - |\beta +$. The region of interest is depicted in Figure 4.5.

The protocol was designed to improve the performance of the participants on the dimension of sustained attention, following convergent lines of research pointing to (1) the role of the ACcd in attentional processes (Bush et al. 1999; Devinsky, Morrell, and Vogt 1995), (2) the role of abnormally low frontal β/α power ratio in individuals affected by attention deficit disorder with hyperactivity (Barry, Clark, and Johnston 2003), and the beneficial effect for those individuals of a frontal low-beta enhancement protocol (Lubar 1991), and (3) the inverse relationship between low-alpha power and cognitive functions (Nunez, Wingeier, and Silberstein 2001), and between alpha power and metabolism (Leuchter et al. 1999). A merging of these lines of evidence resulted in our decision to suppress low alpha (α) and enhance low beta (β) power in the ACcd with the aim of facilitating attention processes. However, instead of using the typical β/α power ratio measure as a feedback signal, we employed a normalized function of the changes over time in α and β. We called this function Φ^1 and its description is outside the scope of this chapter. The reader is referred to the article for details on the precise nature of the feedback signal.

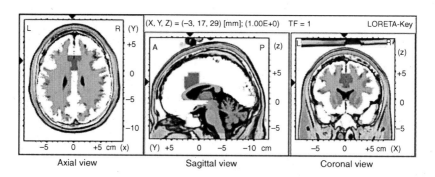

FIGURE 4.5. The Anterior Cingulate cognitive division (ACcd). The region of interest (ROI) used in LORETA modeling for training is shown with the LORETA-Key image viewer as a dark area. ROI extension = 38 voxels (area = 13.034 cm²). Axial view: left of picture is left of the brain. The slice is seen from the top of the brain. Sagittal view: left of picture is front of the brain. The slice is seen from the left of the brain. Coronal view: left of picture is left of the brain. The slice is seen from the back of the brain.

As already mentioned, least square inverse solutions, such as LORETA and sLORETA, are very sensitive to noise and artifacts, especially to episodic artifacts producing large potentials. In order to limit the influence of EMG and EOG artifacts, we implemented two inhibition filters, which constantly monitored the EMG and EOG activity during all neurofeedback sessions. Any time the EMG or EOG signal exceeded a threshold, the corresponding inhibit filters turned on and interrupted the feedback loop. The loop resumed one second subsequent to the inactivation of the inhibition filters. The status of each filter was communicated to the subject by means of flashing lights visible on the feedback screen together with a line plot of the Φ^1 signal constituting the feedback object. Thresholds for EMG and EOG were established and set in a pilot session for each individual separately. EMG activity was detected by computing the average LORETA current density in the ROI in the 35-55 Hz EEG filtered band (EMG channel). EOG activity was detected by measuring the maximum absolute voltage across frontal electrodes FP1, FP2, F7, F8, F4, and F3.

To test hypotheses regarding the modification of brain electrical activity as a result of the neurofeedback training in this research, we focused on two distinct types of learning associated with neurofeedback. The first, called *exercise learning* (EL), describes a monotonic trend of the TS over sessions. It shows that the relevant brain feature of the participant, as recorded during the sessions, tends to increase (or decrease, according to the direction he or she sought) as a function of the number of sessions. The second, called *volitional control* (VC), describes the acquired ability of the participant to shape his or her target brain activity in the desired direction at *will*.

Regarding the EL hypothesis, we analyzed five dependent variables. For each participant and for each neurofeedback session, we extracted measures of average amplitude of the current density in the ACcd in α and β band-pass regions, along with the β/α power ratio, the Φ^1 function, and the percent time spent in the reinforcement state. We also extracted average measures of the EMG and EOG artifacts. Those two variables were used as covariates. For the VC hypothesis, all participants underwent eight three-minute trials at the end of the experiment. In four of them, labeled as "A," the participants were instructed to obtain as much reinforcement as possible. In the remaining four trials ("B"), the participants were instructed to obtain as little reinforcement as possible. The participants underwent the trials according to the same protocol employed during the neurofeedback sessions. The order of A and B trials was randomized. The dependent variables analyzed were the same as those analyzed for the EL hypothesis. For both the EL and VC, all dependent variables were analyzed by means of an exact permutation-randomization OLS (ordinary least square) linear regression model (see Manly 1997). In both cases, EMG and EOG were treated as covariates in order to control for their confounding influence. The test procedure implemented in the program is the randomization-permutation equivalent of an analysis of covariance (ANCOVA), for which detailed explanations can be found in Cade and Richards (1999), Anderson and Legendre (1999) and Kennedy and Cade (1996). For the statistical analysis of data, instead of averaging the data from all individuals, we ran single-case statistical tests and then combined the p-values obtained across individuals. We used two combination functions, namely the *multiplicative* combining function ($P^{\times}$) due to Fisher and the *additive* combining function (P^{+}) of Edgington (Pesarin 2001). For details on these functions, the motivation for their use, and detailed results, the reader is referred to our original publication.

In summary, the results we obtained support both the hypotheses of exercise learning and of volitional control (Congedo, Lubar, and Joffe 2004); during adequate training, average current density β/α power in the ACcd could be increased (EL). Soon after the training, intention alone was sufficient to temporarily increase the β/α average power (VC). EL could be achieved through either motivation (self-regulation) or mere operant conditioning. On the other hand, the test on VC that we first introduced in the study, rules out any influence of unconscious processes. In a more general sense, the positive outcome of this experiment confirmed the intuitive hypothesis that it would be possible to train subjects using an arbitrarily weighted combination of electrode sites, or equivalently in this case, a more specific region of the brain. An interesting reciprocal relationship exists in that while the whole brain can be trained utilizing even one electrode site, training with spatial specificity requires a multiplicity of measurement sites.

BLIND SOURCE SEPARATION
FOR TOMOGRAPHIC NEUROFEEDBACK

EEG sensors (i.e., scalp electrodes) receive a multitude of signals, most of which do not represent neocortical activity. Figure 4.6 illustrates schematically a section of a simplified head model for the source localization scenario. The model is formed by concentric spherical shells. The EEG signal of interest, as seen, is produced mainly by pyramidal cells within the neocortical layer. EEG is known to be comprised of a considerable amount of *background noise* produced by summation of the electrical activity of a myriad of monopolar and dipolar neurons, the latter being oriented in all directions due to cortex convolution. The neocortex is also the origin of several intra-cranial artifacts such as cardiovascular pulse waves transmitted by brain vessels, which are not represented in Figure 4.6. Inside the neocortical

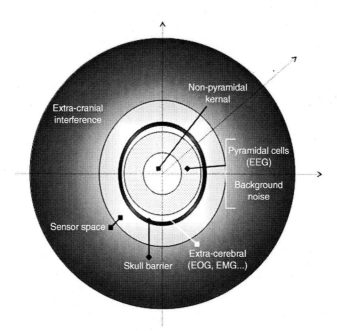

FIGURE 4.6. Schematic representation of a simplified head model indicating the spatial origin of several sources of electrical activity detectable along with (pyramidal cells) EEG and which constitute the main contributors to the source localization problem.

layer is the kernel formed by the white matter and all deep noncortical structures that it encapsulates. Despite the presence of many neurons in the noncortical brain, their contribution to the measurable EEG is considered to be negligible. On the outside of the cortical gray matter layer, we find, in the following order, layers for extra-cerebral arti-facts, the skull barrier, the sensor space, and extra-cranial interference. *Extra-cerebral artifacts* such as EOG, produced by all eye movements and EMG, produced by all facial, neck, and shoulder muscle tension, are probably the most energetic sources of confounding variables in the EEG recording, with their energy sometimes, for example, in the case of eye blinks, largely surpassing the contribution of the EEG neuronal signal itself. What we are calling as the *skull barrier* can actu-ally be decomposed into at least three layers, namely the cerebrospinal fluid, the cranium and facial bones, and the skin. Of the three, the most influential is the cranium itself, which acts as a frequency low-pass and spatial smearing filter with respect to the electromagnetic signal emanating from the brain and detected by scalp sensors. The *sensor space* represents the layer in which the sensors are located. This layer has been depicted intentionally large, so as to accommodate the actual location of either EEG sensors or MEG coils. Finally, in the *extra-cranial* interference layer, we group all external environmental elec-tromagnetic sources such as those produced by any electronic devices, power lines, etc.

A key characteristic of EEG measurements is that the observed signal is a *mixture* of all electrical sources so far described. This is shown in Figure 4.7. The left hemisphere is seen from inside. Suppose, we wish to select as TS—the ACcd, as in our research described ear-lier. This is represented by the larger white oval disk. The gray spheri-cal disks represent other active, but spatially separated EEG sources. The dotted oval disk represents EOG artifacts, for example, a lateral eye movement. In the figure, sensors (electrodes) are represented by small black disks. Each of these sources mixes with the others to pro-duce a signal at every measurement electrode, which is a uniquely weighted summation of their combined activity. *Blind source separa-tion* (BSS), sometimes confused with the more restricted, but essen-tially identical field of *independent component analysis* (ICA), groups an ensemble of well-known and widely used methods to decompose the sensor measurements into their sources (Cichocki and Amari

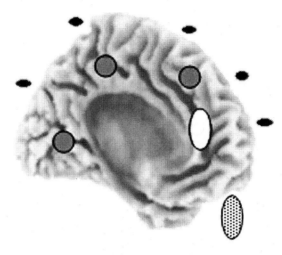

FIGURE 4.7. Schematic representation of multiple neocortical sources (gray disks) of which one is the ROI (white disk). The dotted disk represents an eye-generated artifactual source.

2002). To increase the efficiency of tomographic neurofeedback, one may use BSS to filter-out in real time the extra-cranial artifacts and other artifacts from the sensor measurements. The resulting current source density would be more accurate, in that the localization performance of inverse solutions such as sLORETA depends critically upon the purity of the source signal. In the research described in the previous section, we used detection filters to interrupt the feedback loop in the presence of EMG and EOG. Obviously, filtering-out those artifacts in real time would allow not only a better quality of source localization, but also an uninterrupted feedback modality. This may enhance the attention and concentration of the participant on the feedback and thus result in shorter training durations.

BSS estimates the waveform of the sources (temporal aspect) and also the corresponding spatial patterns in the sensor space. Therefore, by applying an inverse method to the BSS-estimated spatial scalp pattern, we may also be able to obtain an improved estimation of the source spatial location. Once *identified,* the non-EEG components of the signal (the EOG in our example) can be removed and the desired signal reconstructed ignoring their contribution. If the source separation is successful, the reconstructed signal will appear in a truly uncorrupted form as if the artifact sources had been physically removed from the head. The method is said to be "blind," since it does not assume *any* knowledge about the propagation channel (head) characteristics. This is in contrast to linear inverse solutions such as sLORETA, which explicitly require at least a formalization of the head model. Ideally, the knowledge of the participant's particular head anatomy should be incorporated. On the other hand, BSS makes use of statistical assumptions about the generation of the sources, namely, some aspect of the statistical *independence* of the sources (Hyvärinen, Karhunen, and Oja 2001). Therefore, any BSS method presupposes the estimation of some statistics, and its implementation in real-time calls for computationally intensive algorithms, which continuously and iteratively update such estimates and perform the decomposition. Still, the greatest difficulty with the implementation of BSS filters is the need for rapid and automatic systems for *detection* of artifactual sources. In other words, while BSS filters may be able to automatically separate signals from artifacts, they are not able to identify which is which. The important issue of correctly categorizing signal and noise is more properly a *classification* problem. Attempts to devise fully automated artifact detection systems have so far been fruitless. A reasonable solution appears to involve the use of supervised classification algorithms (Fukunaga 1990); in a preliminary stage, the algorithm would be instructed by an expert human. Once the algorithm had been trained, it could be allowed to accomplish the task alone, although its performance would always be monitored.

Attentive readers will have observed that BSS methods could be used to separate different EEG sources as well, thus to define entirely the target signal. This would be possible, given sufficient a-priori knowledge of the source signal, which is not always available. Note also how source localization and BSS differ in the way they define sources: instantaneous EEG inverse solutions focus on their spatial locations while BSS characterizes their statistical properties. Hence, rather than alternative, their contributions are complementary.

There already exist hundreds of algorithms for BSS and ICA with many new ones being developed each year. It is not easy to select the optimal version, which will perform best with EEG or MEG data under all conditions. In our experience, we have found algorithms exploiting second-order statistics, such as the SOBI algorithm of

Belouchrani, Abed-Meraim, and J. F. Cardoso (1997) or its variant, as proposed by Ziehe et al. (2004), quite efficient for the purposes of separating the most commonly encountered EEG/MEG artifacts. In general, these two algorithms successfully separate sources if they all have different power spectra, which also holds true for much artifactual activity as compared to the normal EEG background.

BEAMFORMING FOR TOMOGRAPHIC NEUROFEEDBACK

The spatial smearing of inverse solutions such as sLORETA implies that the measurements in the target ROI are influenced by activity in neighboring regions. More generally, the low-spatial resolution property, by definition, implies that by restricting the current density estimation to a particular ROI (e.g., the ACcD), we do not completely suppress the response of the sensors to activity outside the ROI. In practice, the influence of interfering sources can be considered important within a radius on the order of several centimeters. This is clearly another confounding variable jeopardizing the contingency of the feedback. Whenever a delimited ROI needs to be trained, it would be desirable to be able to enhance the response of the sensors to signals coming from the ROI, while suppressing signals arriving from the other sources. Source localization algorithms applied to such an enhanced signal would be more specific and accurate.

Virtually all sensor systems designed to receive spatially propagating signals encounter the problem of interference signals. In this section, we restrict the meaning of interference to noninteresting cortical activity, that is, to spontaneous brain activity produced *outside* the ROI as illustrated in Figure 4.6. The attenuation of these sources of electrical activity is addressed by *beamforming* methods as applied to the EEG/MEG source localization problem. "Forming beams" is an old term used in signal propagation for sensor arrays and antennas (Van Veen and Buckley 1988). When applied to *signal reception,* beamforming means constructing spatial filters for enhancing the reception of signal coming from a specified direction and suppressing the signal arriving from elsewhere. For example, the sensitivity of an antenna may be increased in the direction of a particular satellite, if the position of the latter is known. In fact, a variety of filters can be derived to target a desired aspect of the signal. Examples of filters designed to enhance the signal-to-noise ratio in the ROI can be found in Gross and Ioannides (1999) and in Sekihara et al. (2002). Filters to reduce the interference of nontarget ROIs have been described in Bolton et al. (1999) and in Rodríguez-Rivera et al. (2006). Beamforming is achieved by projecting the sensor measurements into a different space possessing the desired characteristics. Usually the beam space is of reduced dimension as compared to the original sensor space (exploiting the redundancy of the information contained in EEG). Hence, beamforming can accelerate the computation of inverse solutions, which may in turn result in faster feedback thus freeing up resources for other computer system functions. Beamforming filters may be constructed either in a data-independent fashion or based upon the statistics of the sensor data. Beamformers designed to take into account data statistics could be thought of as playing a kind of transitional role between purely spatial (sLORETA) and statistical (BSS) approaches. However, beamforming methods, which are strictly data-independent, are equally useful when combined with data-driven source localization methods such as described in Rodríguez-Rivera et al. (2006). An overview of beamforming filters used for EEG/MEG source localization can be found in Gross and Ioannides (1999). The combination of inverse solutions and spatial filters has been explored in Congedo (2006). An example application to the Brain Computer Interface problem can be found in Congedo et al. (2006). The interested reader is referred to the references for details.

SUMMARY AND CONCLUSIONS

In this chapter, we outlined physiological knowledge relevant to the EEG/MEG source localization problem. This knowledge created a framework within which to understand the relationship between traditional and tomographic neurofeedback. We listed and commented upon major advantages of tomographic neurofeedback as compared to the traditional form, namely, the spatial specificity with all its consequences. We summarized the methods and results of our experimental study on LORETA neurofeedback and we proposed the integration of inverse solution methods with blind source separation and beamforming filters. A supervised algorithm incorporating these three techniques simultaneously would offer a very powerful improvement over the current neurofeedback state-of-the-art. It is important to recognize that although sLORETA and other inverse current source solutions are capable of producing an image of current density at every time sample, and are therefore truly *high-temporal resolution* techniques, the actual application of these techniques often involves the use of fixed or moving averages. For example, evoked potential current source estimations are time-locked to a stimulus and averaged in the time domain. In neurofeedback, continuously recorded EEG is filtered or frequency transformed resulting in time domain delays or frequency domain averages. Furthermore, the TS is often subjected to an additional stage of moving average of a sufficient length in order to produce stability of the feedback signal. Selecting appropriate moving average lengths to guarantee a stable feedback signal, while at the same time minimizing feedback delay constitutes one of the most important tradeoffs and challenges involved in the use of both traditional and tomographic neurofeedback.

The sLORETA inverse solution, BSS, and beamforming algorithms have been presented in a linear sequence in earlier text for clarity of exposition. However, from a computational perspective, these individual components could be combined for the sake of efficiency. In some cases, such combinations would also yield a kind of hybrid vigor, in which redundancies in the separate algorithms could be eliminated so as to create more efficient and unified algorithms. But perhaps most importantly, the three combined classes of algorithms could be implemented in ways that would mutually constrain each other, or in other words, provide checks and balances on each other's operation to insure that each focused optimally on portions or subspaces of the space-time EEG/MEG data.

The clinical choices facing neurofeedback practitioners will dramatically increase when the next generation of multichannel spatial filtering systems becomes available. However, these new opportunities will be accompanied by new perils as well. In addition to the obvious sources of error, such as imprecise electrode placement or greater sensitivity to movement artifacts, more subtle confounding variables will also need to be taken into account. Multichannel spatial filtering EEG systems will have to be manufactured to more exacting tolerances than those required for current topographic mapping applications, since all three filtering methods discussed here are exquisitely sensitive to inter-channel amplification, phase, delay, and frequency response differences. Without a heightened appreciation for and attention to these details, it will be difficult to insure consistent results across the various platforms used for EEG data acquisition and analysis. It might surprise some that no universal standards presently exist regarding commercial EEG system amplitude, phase, delay, and frequency response. Device manufacturers often make independent design decisions resulting in performance inconsistencies between different brands of brain mapping or digital EEG equipment ranging from subtle to significant. This, coupled with the fact that the precise frequency response characteristics of the EEG systems used to acquire data referenced in most EEG research papers are seldom documented, introduces additional confounding variables, which may weaken meta-analyses and other forms of experimental study comparisons.

Although these considerations are strictly technical, those interested mainly in the clinical application of neurofeedback should be aware of the problems that could arise as a consequence of poor quality equipment. Prospective users of new equipment should be able to "look under the hood," since the instruments and techniques they use may have a significant impact on the clinical outcomes of their patients. More generally, "black box" approaches ("plug and play" for neurofeedback equipment) should not be encouraged.

As previously mentioned, the whole issue of signal, noise, and artifact detection and classification takes on an added importance when considered in the context of multichannel spatial filtering. The simple thresholding algorithms, accompanied by the temporary cessation of feedback in the presence of artifacts seem an unsatisfactory solution both for algorithmic and clinical reasons. Such data flow interruption is an additional problem to address for sophisticated hybrid inverse/BSS/beamforming algorithms. Future multichannel filtering "noise suppression" methods may consist of techniques whereby the various time/frequency subcomponents driving the ultimate feedback signal are individually tracked so that when significant deviations from their running averages are detected, particular components can be "shut down" or suppressed, while others continue, in order to insure continuity of overall feedback.

Finally, there is the issue of time delay to be addressed. The added computational burden of multichannel spatial filtering will inevitably impact the response time of the overall system. However, one of the key principles underlying classical feedback is that the time between a physiological change and the reporting of that change back to the subject must be as short as possible. Some combinations and implementations of the aforementioned algorithms may require the use of moving averages of varying lengths to generate stable estimates of different components of EEG or MEG activity. This in turn would result in nonsynchronous feedback of EEG components acquired at the same time. However, thanks to recent advance in microelectronics (64-bit high frequency dual-core multiple processing workstations), rather than constituting a liability, this is yet another fascinating challenge and opportunity for neurofeedback developers, researchers, and clinicians.

REFERENCES

Anderson, M. J., and P. Legendre (1999) An empirical comparison of permutation methods for tests of partial regression coefficients in a linear model, *Journal of Statistics Computation and Simulation*, 62: 271-303.

Barry, R. J., A. R. Clarke, and S. J. Johnston (2003) A review of electrophysiology in attention-deficit/hyperactivity disorder: I. Qualitative and quantitative electroencephalography, *Clinical Neurophysiology*, 114: 171-183.

Belouchrani, A., K. Abed-Meraim, and J. F. Cardoso (1997) A blind source separation technique using second-order statistics, *IEEE Transactions on Signal Processing*, 45(2): 434-444.

Bolton, J. P., J. Gross, L. C. Liu, and A. A. Ioannides (1999) SOFIA: Spatially optimal fast initial analysis of biomagnetic signals, *Physics in Medicine and Biology*, 44(1): 87-103.

Bush, G., J. A. Frazier, S. L. Rauch, L. J. Seidman, P. J. Whalen, M. A. Jenike, et al. (1999) Anterior cingulate cortex dysfunction in attention deficit/hyperactivity disorder revealed by fMRI and the counting stroop, *Biological Psychiatry*, 45(12): 1542-1552.

Cade, B. S., and J. D. Richards (1999) *User Manual for Blossom Statistical Software*. Fort Collins, CO. U.S. Geological Survey.

Cichocki, A., and S. I. Amari (2002) *Adaptive Blind Signal and Image Processing. Learning Algorithms and Applications*. New York: John Wiley & Sons.

Congedo, M. (2003) *Tomographic Neurofeedback: A New Technique for the Self-Regulation of Brain Electrical Activity*. PhD Dissertation. The University of Tennessee.

Congedo, M. (2006) Subspace projection filters for real-time brain electromagnetic imaging, *IEEE Transactions on Biomedical Engineering,* 53(8): 1624-1634.

Congedo, M., F. Lotte, and A. Lécuyer (2006) Classification of movement intention by spatially filtered electromagnetic inverse solutions, *Physics in Medicine and Biology,* 51: 1971-1989.

Congedo, M., J. F. Lubar, and D. Joffe (2004) Low-resolution electromagnetic tomography neurofeedback, *IEEE Trans. on Neuronal Systems & Rehabilitation Engineering,* 12(4): 387-397.

Devinsky, O., M. J. Morrell, and B. A. Vogt (1995) Contributions of anterior cingulate to behavior, *Brain,* 118: 279-306.

Engstrom, D. R., P. London, and J. T. Hart (1970) Hypnotic susceptibility increased by EEG alpha training, *Nature,* 227: 1261-1262.

Fukunaga, K. (1990) *Introduction to Statistical Pattern Recognition* (2nd ed.), New York: Academic Press.

Greenblatt, R. E., A. Ossadtchi, and M. E. Pflieger (2005) Local linear estimators for the bioelectromagnetic inverse problem, *IEEE Transactions on Significant Proceedings,* 53(9): 3403-3412.

Gross, J., and A. A. Ioannides (1999) Linear transformation of data space in MEG, *Physics in Medicine and Biology,* 44(1): 87-103.

Hämäläinen, M. S., and R. J. Ilmoniemi (1984) Interpreting measured magnetic fields of the brain: Estimates of current distributions, *Technical Report TKK-F-A559,* Helsinky University of Technology, Espoo, 1984.

Hyvärinen, A., J. Karhunen, and E. Oja (2001) *Independent Component Analysis,* New York: John Wiley & Sons.

Kamiya, J. (1962) *Conditioned Discrimination of the EEG Alpha Rhythm in Humans.* Paper presented at the Western Psychological Association, San Francisco.

Kennedy, P. E., and B. S. Cade (1996) Randomization tests for multiple regression, *Communications in Statistics-Simulation and Computation,* 25: 923-936.

Kotchoubey, B., A. Kubler, U. Strehl, H. Flor, and N. Birbaumer (Mar. 2002) Can humans perceive their brain states? *Consciousness and Cognition,* 11(1): 98-113.

Kübler, A., B. Kotchoubey, J. Kaiser, J. R. Wolpaw, and N. Birbaumer (2001) Brain-computer communication: Unlocking the locked in, *Psychological Bulletin,* 127(3): 358-375.

Kropotov, J. D., V. A. Grin-Yatsenko, V. A. Ponomarev, L. S. Chutko, E. A. Yakovenko, and I. S. Nikishena (2005) ERPs correlates of EEG relative beta training in ADHD children, *International Journal of Psychophysiology,* 55(1): 23-34.

Leuchter, A. F., S. H. J. Uijtdehaage, I. A. Cook, R. O'Hara, and M. Mandelkern, (1999) Relationship between brain electrical activity and cortical perfusion in normal subjects, *Psychiatric Research: Neuroimaging Section,* 90: 125-140.

Lubar, J. F. (1991) Discourse on the development of EEG diagnostics and biofeedback for attention-deficit/hyperactivity disorders, *Biofeedback and Self-Regulation,* 16(3): 201-225.

Manly, B. F. J. (1997) *Randomization, Bootstrap and Monte Carlo Methods in Biology* (2nd ed.), London: Chapman & Hall.

Nowlis, D. P., and J. Kamiya (1970) The control of electroencephalographic alpha rhythms through auditory feedback and the associated mental activity, *Psychophysiology,* 6(4): 476-484.

Nunez, P. L. (1995) *Neocortical Dynamics and Human EEG Rhythms,* Oxford University Press.

Nunez, P. L., B. M. Wingeier, and R. B. Silberstein (2001) Spatial-temporal structures of human alpha rhythms: Theory, microcurrent sources, multiscale measurements, and global binding of local networks, *Human Brain Mapping,* 13(3): 125-164.

Nunez, P. L., and R. B. Silberstein (2000) On the relationship of synaptic activity to macroscopic measurements: Does co-registration of EEG with fMRI make sense? *Brain Topography,* 13(2): 79-96.

Pascual-Marqui, R. D. (2002) Standardized low resolution brain electromagnetic Tomography (sLORETA): Technical details, *Methods and Findings in Experimental & Clinical Pharmacology,* 24D: 5-12.

Pascual-Marqui, R. D., C. M. Michel, and D. Lehmann (1994) Low resolution electromagnetic tomography: A new method for localizing electrical activity in the brain. *International Journal of Psychophysiology,* 18: 49-65.

Pesarin, F. (2001) *Multivariate Permutation Tests.* New York: John Wiley & Sons.

Rodríguez-Rivera, A., B. Baryshikov, and B. D. Van Veen (2006) MEG and EEG Source Localization in Beamspace, *IEEE Transactions on Neuronal Systems & Rehabilitation Engineering,* 53(3): 430-441.

Sarvas, J. (1987) Basic mathematical and electromagnetic concepts of the biomagnetic inverse problem, *Physics in Medicine and Biology,* 32(1): 11-22.

Sekihara, K., S. S. Nagarajan, D. Poeppel, A. Marantz, and Y. Miyashita (2002) Application of an MEG eigenspace beamformer to reconstructing spatio-temporal activities of neuronal sources, *Human Brain Mapping,* 15(4): 199-215.

Sekihara, K., M. Sahani, and S. S. Nagarajan (2005) Localization Bias and Spatial Resolution of Adaptive and non-Adaptive Spatial Filters for MEG Source Reconstruction, *Neuroimage,* 25(4): 1056-1067.

Sterman, M. B. (1981) EEG biofeedback: Physiological behavior modification, *Neuroscience and Biobehavioral Reviews,* 5: 405-412.

Travis, T. A., C. Y. Kondo, and J. R. Knott (1974) Alpha conditioning; a controlled study, *The Journal of Nervous and Mental Disease,* 158: 163-173.

Van Veen, B. D. and M. Buckley (1988) Beamforming: A versatile approach to spatial filtering, *IEEE ASSP Magazine,* 5: 4-24.

Ziehe, A., P. Laskov, G. Nolte, and R. K. Müller (2004) A fast algorithm for joint diagonalization with non-orthogonal transformations and its application to blind source separation, *Journal of Machine Learning Research,* 5: 777-800.

Chapter 5

Interhemispheric EEG Training: Clinical Experience and Conceptual Models

Susan F. Othmer
Siegfried Othmer

INTRODUCTION

There are presently two major thrusts within the field of neurofeedback. The first consists of neurofeedback training to improve physiological self-regulation and the second consists of the promotion of lower EEG frequencies for largely experiential, exploratory, and integrative purposes. The first of these has commonly been referred to as "SMR/beta" training, where SMR refers to the (nominally 12-15 Hz) sensorimotor rhythm. The second is usually referred to as Alpha/Theta training. This chapter concerns itself entirely with SMR/beta, the training directed toward functional normalization and optimization. Additional introductory material on SMR/beta training is available elsewhere (Othmer, Othmer, & Kaiser, 1999).

Whereas Alpha/Theta training has remained largely invariant in clinical approach over the years, SMR/beta training has multiplied into a host of specific clinical approaches tailored for different applications. These approaches can be grouped under three guiding philosophies (1) mechanisms-based, protocol-driven, or symptom-responsive training; (2) EEG normalization approaches based on stationary QEEG-measures; and (3) generalized approaches to neuroregulation based on

Handbook of Neurofeedback
doi:10.1300/5889_05

top-level insights derived from the theory of nonlinear dynamical systems. These three basic approaches were discussed recently (Othmer, 2002a,b).

This chapter addresses a particular evolution of the basic protocol-driven approach. This approach has set standards for treatment within the neurofeedback field since its inception. Its breadth of efficacy compels a reappraisal of the mechanisms that account for the utility of the method, which is also attempted here.

HISTORICAL DEVELOPMENT

The early clinical experience with beta/SMR neurofeedback protocols primarily involved training on the central, or sensorimotor, strip. This followed from the Sterman model in which the goal of training was to enhance the amplitude of the resting rhythm of the motor system in order to move the brain to a lower level of motor excitability. Such a lower set point of steady-state motor activation would then lead to a decrease in motor symptoms, including in particular motor seizures (see Sterman, 2000 for a review).

Training was predominantly done within the sensorimotor rhythm (SMR) band centered at 13.5 Hz, the peak frequency typically seen in sleep spindles in Stage II sleep. The sleep spindle can be viewed as the human homologue of the SMR spindles first observed in cat sensorimotor cortex. With a typical bandwidth of 3 Hz, 12-15 Hz came to be regarded as the standard SMR band in neurofeedback. Training was also done at 15-18 Hz during one early study, although Sterman decided that this yielded nothing beyond what could be achieved with 12-15 Hz reinforcement (Sterman, Macdonald, & Stone, 1974). Thereafter, Sterman concentrated his work exclusively on 12-15 Hz training, at least until such time as QEEG-based training altered the landscape.

Our initial EEG training beginning in 1988 followed the work of Ayers, Sterman, Lubar, and Tansey (Ayers, 1987; Lubar, 1995; Tansey and Bruner, 1983) by rewarding either SMR (nominally 12-15 Hz) or beta (nominally 15-18 Hz). Our early efforts focused on the central strip using bipolar montages, with training typically done at C3-T3 or C1-C5, as identified by the International 10/20 System of electrode placement (Jasper, 1958). Sterman employed C3-T3 or sometimes

C1-C5 (Sterman, personal communication). Tansey used a large electrode running both forward and aft of Cz on the midline, in a referential placement. Lubar initially followed Sterman in training the left hemisphere with bipolar placements, but then adopted midline placements, apparently following Tansey. With the increasing adoption of QEEG measures in the field, there came a general shift toward referential placement, and our placement changed accordingly to C3-A1, C4-A2, and Cz-A1.

While Sterman and Lubar settled on 12-15 Hz as the standard band, Tansey moved toward a more narrow focus on 14 Hz, derived from one-Hertz bins in a fast Fourier Transform (FFT). Ayers found that reinforcement at the higher frequency of 15-18 Hz was especially helpful in the remediation of minor traumatic brain injury (Ayers, 1987), although she also occasionally employed reinforcement at 12-15 Hz as well.

All of these protocols exemplify reward-based training: that is, the trainee receives a cue in the form of auditory or visual feedback designed to encourage EEG activity within the defined band. In addition, all the aforementioned protocols included an inhibit band. Excess amplitudes are detected within that band, and the rewards are inhibited for the duration that the inhibit threshold is exceeded. Sterman introduced the inhibit band of 4-7 Hz because of his interest in seizure reduction (Sterman and Friar, 1974), and that soon became standard in the field. The principal rationale for the 4-7 Hz inhibit was to make sure that the person was not given false rewards. (The appearance of a paroxysmal event in the EEG would be likely to trigger the SMR reward through its higher harmonics.) Since rewards were always meted out sparingly in early clinical work, there was a premium on assuring that the person was not inappropriately rewarded for paroxysmal bursts. Sterman also introduced a high frequency inhibit in order to intercept EMG (electromyographic) bursts that could inadvertently elicit rewards during EEG training.

In Sterman's implementation, the role of inhibits was indirect. They were intended to suppress contamination of what was essentially a reward strategy on SMR amplitudes. This was a particularly appropriate strategy for seizure control, in that the adverse theta activity was typically paroxysmal or episodic. It could usually be readily distinguished from the background activity. Of course, any rewards would have to be suppressed during such epochs. It was Tansey and Lubar who first utilized inhibits as an integral part of neurofeedback. That is to say, inhibits represented a clinical objective in their own right in cueing the brain toward improved regulation. Since, such improved regulation would be indexed by reduction in theta amplitudes, such inhibit-based training came to be referred to as a normalization strategy. This was appropriate for working with ADHD in particular, where the theta amplitudes were elevated nearly all the time, with an amplitude distribution that was more continuous than usually is found with seizures. For Lubar, this strategy involved only a conceptual shift in how the role of inhibits was understood, and not an alteration of the electronics required for the training. In Tansey's approach, however, the trainee received verbal rather than electronic cues whenever the low-frequency EEG amplitudes were elevated. Thus, Tansey himself became part of an active feedback loop to the client with respect to inhibits, and instrumental feedback was reserved for the 14 Hz component of the EEG.

Sterman's reward strategy was based upon his prior research with cats (Sterman, LoPresti, & Fairchild, 1969). Sterman's goal in that research was to reward cats for SMR spindle bursts. In cats, such spindle-bursts stood out clearly from the baseline in narrow-band filtered data, and therefore could readily be discriminated with a simple thresholding function. The bursts were brief and episodic, occurring no more than several times a minute. Hence, the training consisted in essence of a binary reward that required nothing more than unambiguous event detection. Matters were distinctly different when research shifted to human subjects. Since discrete rhythmic SMR spindles that stood out from the ambient EEG background could not be routinely observed in the normal waking human EEG, the target in human training became the highest-amplitude SMR spindles that could be observed within the individual record. That is to say, the rewards were restricted to the upper tail of a presumptively Gaussian distribution in SMR amplitudes. Consistent with the objective of emulating the cat research as much as possible, rewards were sparse so as to limit rewards to the largest amplitude excursions. In turn, this meant that the brain did not receive very many cues during training—a strategy that we view as relatively inefficient today with the benefit of hindsight.

Sterman's instrumentation also yielded analog information on the amplitude in the SMR-band, and human participants could be instructed to attend to the analog signal. With such instruction, the reward strategy moved from being a discrete, binary, go/no-go discriminant to having a significant "analog" component even though the instrumentation was unaltered. Recommending attention to the smooth variation in signal amplitude had the effect of increasing the level of engagement with the process at the conscious level. It may also have increased the capacity for pattern recognition by the brain at the subconscious level.

Yet another factor may have been at play. Clinicians may have been "shaped" by their clinical experience with difficult and unresponsive clients to move the reward incidence gradually upward to improve task compliance. This was done with the simple expedient of easing up on the reward threshold. As the reward incidence increased to a nominal 70 percent or as much as 85 percent, what started out as being a rare event in Sterman's original design became an expectation. The Sterman instrumentation provided for a maximum repetition rate of the discrete reward of $2\times$ per second. As a result, discrete rewards (tones) came with complete periodicity most of the time; the cadence would settle in, and the oddball event became the dropout of the sounds. With the rewards becoming periodic, their contingency on immediately preceding events was lost. This focused even more attention on the analog signal as a focus for engagement of the client, and the occasional dropout of the rewards effectively functioned as inhibit. Concomitantly, the training had shifted from being one of rewarding an extremum in state space to one of modulating state regulation near ambient levels. The state variable most immediately impacted was that of central arousal. With this simple alteration in the experimental contingencies, neurofeedback became relevant to a broad range of conditions of disregulation.

Arousal

Arousal refers here to an encompassing appraisal of the general state of activation of the central nervous system, and it involves the specific activations of a number of subsystems. Thus, a central constituent of arousal is the set point of excitability of the voluntary motor system. Another is the status of activation of the sympathetic and parasympathetic nervous systems, and of the balance between them. Finally, arousal involves the excitability of sensory systems, of cognition, and of the system of interoception.

The reliance on 15-18 Hz reinforcement by Ayers and in our own early work found its rationale in the arousal model. Many of the sequelae of minor traumatic brain injury were seen as depressive in character. Moreover, application to children with attention deficit/ hyperactivity disorder could find support in Satterfield's original underarousal model (Satterfield & Dawson, 1971). Moreover, profound positive effects were observed clinically in depressive syndromes of various descriptions with 15-18 Hz training, later known as "beta" training, on the left hemisphere.

As soon as we incorporated SMR-training on the midline (Cz) as an adjunct to beta training on the left hemisphere (following Tansey and Lubar), our clinical reach expanded considerably, and the arousal model received additional support. The beta training was seen as activating, and the SMR training was seen as calming. Eventually, the midline placement migrated to C4 (right side), and clinically it became a matter of discerning whether a person mainly needed to be moved to higher or lower arousal levels. Over time, we developed the approach of balancing left-side beta and right-side SMR training for each individual in every session.

It was clear throughout that left-side training was more effective and more comfortable with a slightly higher frequency reward than that for right-side training. There emerged an identification of left-sided deficits with underactivation and right-sided deficits with overarousal. Since there was also an arousal shift for the entire physiology as we rewarded higher (beta) or lower (SMR) frequencies, we found that we needed to balance left-side activation with right side calming for each individual according to arousal level, symptoms, and sensitivity to training.

Our extensive experience with training left and right hemispheres separately with different reward frequencies actually led us to resist interhemispheric training initially. Even though we were aware of the work of Douglas Quirk and George Von Hilsheimer with C3-C4 SMR, we couldn't see how two hemispheres that needed to train at different frequencies could be trained together effectively with one reward frequency (Quirk, 1995). The term reward frequency here refers to the center frequency of the filter transfer function of the reward band.

Interhemispheric training, as the term is used herein, consists of single-channel training using bipolar placement at homologous sites. The primary montage is T3-T4, but other site pairs play subsidiary roles. The principal montages are shown in Figure 5.1.

Instability

The arousal model, in which we conceptualized symptoms as arising in the context of some combination of left-hemisphere underactivation and right-hemisphere overarousal, enabled us to resolve a variety of clinical symptoms. The strategy received some theoretical support from the bihemispheric model of ADHD of Malone, Kershner, and Swanson (1994). In practice, we sometimes struggled with the more sensitive and unstable nervous systems. People with traumatic brain injury were sometimes so sensitive to training that we would find ourselves shifting back and forth within a 30-minute session so as not to take them too far into over- or underarousal. Clients with

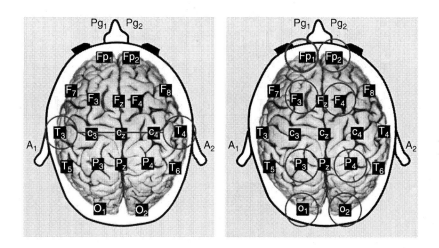

FIGURE 5.1. The principal interhemispheric montages employed in training are illustrated. Other pairings, however, are used as well for specific purposes, in addition to lateralized bipolar placements.

migraines or bipolar disorder could also be difficult to keep within a comfortable zone in terms of arousal level. Our earliest experience with interhemispheric training arose while working with migraines. Left-side training would often eliminate a left-side headache while allowing it to pop up on the right side. Training on the right would just cause the migraine to reappear on the left. We found ourselves chasing the migraine around the head. In frustration, we trained both sides together at one point and the migraines vanished, typically within the session.

EXPLORING INTERHEMISPHERIC TRAINING

Over the course of several years we gradually explored interhemispheric training for what we define as instabilities. Here the primary problem is conceptualized as instability of state leading to episodic symptoms such as migraines, panic attacks, mood swings, vertigo, hot flashes, seizures, and other episodic or paroxysmal events or sudden state transitions. Once we began to think in terms of instabilities as a core issue and began to use interhemispheric training as a means of improving stability long-term, this became an increasingly important part of our work. Interhemispheric training became a standard approach for us in this timeframe, but it brought some surprises and some changes in our understanding of how the brain responds to the challenge of EEG training.

It rapidly became clear that interhemispheric training is both more powerful and more specific in its effects than targeting the hemispheres individually. By separating the issues of electrode site placement and reward frequency, it allowed a more direct path to stability, but it also required more specific attention to the reward frequency. Our initial uncertainty was related to *which* reward frequency to use when training both hemispheres together as one difference signal. Our previous experience was that we could usually train left-side beta and right-side SMR (i.e., using standard bands) with satisfactory results for most people. When combining the two with C3-C4 or T3-T4 placement, we discovered that the optimum reward frequency could well lie outside of that range. In fact, it could be anywhere from zero to 30 Hz. And it was surprisingly specific for each individual. A one-half Hz shift in reward frequency could, in sensitive individuals, lead to an immediate and significant change in symptoms and state of arousal.

We began interhemispheric training with the temporal lobes (T3-T4) because many instabilities we targeted responded most strongly to temporal lobe training, and because the temporal lobes are the most likely to exhibit instabilities such as seizures. Shifts in reward frequency resulted in corresponding shifts in arousal level. We learned to move the reward frequency up or down even within a session from a typical starting frequency of 12-15 Hz while monitoring symptoms through client self-report of arousal level. It is useful to think in terms of finding the top of the individual's arousal curve—in the Yerkes-Dodson Law sense; namely, that optimal state in which the client reports being maximally alert and attentive without a feeling of tension or sedation. Too high a reward frequency may result in symptoms of overarousal such as agitation or increased muscle tension. Training too low can result in symptoms of underarousal, as if the person had been overly sedated. Symptoms of instability can arise strongly and suddenly with training either too high or too low. Hence, instabilities are manifestly correlated with arousal level, but they are still understandable as separate entities.

In practice, we look for the optimal reward frequency at which the person reports feeling relaxed, calm, alert, attentive, and euthymic. Interhemispheric training is an efficient path to training stability, but at the same time, it requires the most attention to the immediate effects of training within and between sessions. We think of the interhemispheric training process as exploring the "state space" of each individual. We can move anyone up or down in arousal level, but what symptoms arise at what frequencies is specific for each individual. The majority of people can feel and report these arousal shifts during the first session. For those who are unable to discern or describe the changes, we can work on the basis of reported changes session to session. Highly sensitive people with symptoms like migraine or fibromyalgia often require some continuing shifts in reward frequency over time as the person gradually assimilates the training.

What began as a method of training specifically for those symptoms arising from instability of state over time became a standard starting point for us. Interhemispheric training has the clinical effect of improving the function of both hemispheres as well as the communication and coordination between them. Even in a situation where a dysfunction is known to exist specifically in one hemisphere, training the two hemispheres together appears to offer an effective approach to reducing specific symptoms and improving overall brain function. And even when no symptoms of instability are present, we have found that there is still benefit to be derived from interhemispheric challenge.

In the emerging picture, in which the nervous system is viewed largely in terms of its obligations as a control system, there is, in addition to the requirement for fundamental stability, also the need for maintenance of dynamic homeostasis with respect to a variety of control functions. It is in this latter role that interhemispheric training has also shown itself as competent, even though the consequences may not be as dramatic as they are in the case of the instabilities.

Site-Specific Training

Initial work with interhemispheric training protocols concentrated on understanding T3-T4. Indeed, we observed that T3-T4 training was effective for stabilizing the brain against migraines, mood swings, panic attacks, and temporal lobe seizures. But eventually we moved to interhemispheric training at other sites in order to address symptoms that were not as responsive to temporal lobe training.

Our first move was frontal to address problems of attention and impulse control. We found specific and very different effects in training frontal (F3-F4 and F7-F8) versus prefrontal (Fp1-Fp2) sites. Interhemispheric frontal training is quite energizing. It gets people moving, thinking, and talking. It specifically impacts the initiation and sequencing of various output functions, and it can lessen depression. It can also be too activating for some people, leading to agitation and aggression—not unlike the effect of Selective Serabnin reuptake inhibitors (SSRIs) on some people with bipolar susceptibility. Although generally T3-T4 is an effective approach for stabilizing mood, F3-F4 appears to have a direct antidepressant effect of lifting mood. Interhemispheric prefrontal training has a very different and more calming effect. Fp1-Fp2 training improves executive function, which allows improved planning and organization as well as appropriate inhibition of impulsive and compulsive behaviors. It has an interesting settling effect, which reduces restless behaviors such as fidgeting or eating in an effort to calm the nervous system.

We train Fp1-Fp2 routinely with people who respond well to stimulants. Here we suspect that we access the prefrontal dopamine circuits that are targeted by stimulant medications. The objective with prefrontal training is not to increase arousal level, but to improve attention and impulse control. Appropriate reward frequency is a separate issue and is considered in the following text. Fp1-Fp2 training is also important for addressing symptoms that arise from behavioral disinhibition. Some people, for example, respond to sedatives, fatigue, or hypoglycemia by spinning out of control. Prefrontal training seems to strengthen the top-down inhibitory control of such inappropriate disinhibited behaviors.

The major surprise with interhemispheric training frontally or prefrontally was that a reliable relationship emerged between the optimal reward frequencies at those sites compared to T3-T4 (or C3-C4). After finding the most effective reward frequency at T3-T4 for a given individual, we simply subtract two Hz to yield the most appropriate frequency for training the frontal sites. In most cases, the two-Hertz shift works well. There are times when we need to adjust these frequencies independently, but a two-Hertz decrement is usually close to optimal. It is quite surprising that this two-Hertz rule should apply across the whole range of frequencies that we reward, and across a whole host of different conditions that we address.

It took us somewhat longer to move successfully to training the posterior cortex. We had often trained parietal sites when training the left or right hemisphere separately, but in our early attempts at interhemispheric parietal training, people often reported feeling uncomfortable. Eventually, we found that lower reward frequencies allowed effective training at P3-P4 and O1-O2. Again, the surprising finding was that interhemispheric parietal or occipital training required subtracting 4 Hz from the optimal reward at T3-T4 to obtain the best training frequency at these posterior sites.

P3-P4 training generally improves body and spatial awareness. It is physically relaxing and it opens people up to more emotional and social awareness. This is very important training for bipolar disorder, reactive attachment disorder, and the autism spectrum. More recently, we trained O1-O2 with success for visual sensitivity and visual processing deficits. We also find it emotionally calming and soothing for people with a trauma history. Our most recent work has targeted posterior temporal lobe training (T5-T6). The question was whether this would fall into the temporal lobe or posterior cortex domain in terms of reward frequency. The answer is that T5-T6 clearly trains at a reward frequency similar to more anterior temporal lobe training (T3-T4), and not like the parietal or occipital areas.

After emphasizing temporal lobe training rather than central in our clinical work because of its greater impact on emotional and pain symptoms, we finally returned to training C3-C4 in some cases. We find that C3-C4 can be useful for specifically addressing somatosensory or motor deficits such as those found in Parkinson's disease.

A Standard Approach

Some interhemispheric sites have emerged as more generally useful with a wide variety of individuals. In the majority of cases, we find our way to training some combination of parietal, prefrontal, and temporal sites within each session. We might explain this to a peak performance client as firstly a means to increase physical calmness and the brain's attention to and management of the body with P3-P4. Then Fp1-Fp2 training improves executive function—the ability to plan, organize, and reason, to act rather than react to life situations. T3-T4 training then improves emotional and physiological stability and resilience. The aforementioned is a combination of training sites that can improve function in most individuals, from the severely impaired to the peak performer. The other interhemispheric sites that we have explored are very useful in specific situations in which they can impact specific symptoms not addressed by the more standard training. But we employ them much less often.

Our general approach is to start a training program with T3-T4 when there are any presenting emotional or pain symptoms. This is the vast majority of cases in our practice. There are some situations with no headaches, no anxiety or depression, no panic attacks, and no rages, but still showing significant physical symptoms. In these latter cases, C3-C4 would be our starting point. Typically, we begin by training T3-T4 (or C3-C4) alone, long enough to optimize the reward frequency and to assess how symptoms are changing with this training. Then, we add other sites as needed to address other symptoms, with training of the posterior and frontal sites being of approximately equal duration for balance. A thirty-minute training session usually begins with some amount of posterior training, then frontal (including prefrontal), and concludes with T3-T4. The most stabilizing training is generally used at the end of each session. Specific sites are included for different amounts of time according to the desired training effect.

Inhibit Frequencies

We began our work with low- and high-frequency inhibit bands based on the earlier works of Sterman and others. Four to seven Hertz was chosen to inhibit inappropriate theta activity that might represent cortical inactivation related to attention deficits or abnormal activity related to seizures or brain injury. Over time, we found that targeting more specific abnormal brain wave activity was clinically useful. Frequent choices were delta-theta inhibits of 2-7 Hz for people with delta activity resulting from neurological injury or associated with developmental delay, or an alpha inhibit of 8-11 Hz for people with excess alpha activity possibly related to migraines, fibromyalgia, or depression.

More recently, we moved to the use of wide-band inhibits, which effectively inhibit high amplitude activity from zero to 30 Hz. We use a low frequency band of 2-13 Hz and a high frequency inhibit of 14-30 Hz. The separate bands allow us to set separate thresholds that are appropriate for the different amplitudes that typically occur at lower and higher frequencies. Because of soft roll-offs, the two bands effectively overlap so that all frequencies are within one or both inhibit bands. With inhibits covering the entire range of interest, we are faced with overlapping reward and inhibit bands. A slight iteration on this approach is the use of multiple inhibit bands distributed across the entire range of EEG frequencies.

The superimposition of the rewards on the wide-band inhibit requires that we consider the fundamental difference in the roles of the reward and inhibits in EEG training. We view the inhibit bands as detecting episodically elevated EEG activity at any frequency, with the reward then withheld for the duration. The inhibit thresholds serve as event detectors, which cue the brain when it wanders off track or when various artifacts intrude on the signal. We use these inhibits rather sparingly so as not to frustrate the client. Thresholds are typically set to inhibit excess low-frequency activity 10-15 percent of the time, and high frequency activity about 5 percent of the time. When no inhibits are exceeded, our goal is to reward increases in the amplitude of the reward signal, one which always reflects a narrow (3-Hz-wide) band around the indicated reward frequency. We understand this as a brain exercise in shifting and maintaining activation and arousal. Here we use the normal regulatory rhythms and their normal variations in amplitude over time to alter the overall levels of EEG activity. We reward slight EEG increases within the reward band, but also discourage larger amplitude bursts within that same band by virtue of our wide inhibits. We want the brain to exercise appropriate shifts in state, not abnormal bursts of activity.

Considering Amplitude and Phase

In the past, beta and SMR training could be reasonably explained as rewarding appropriately activated brainwave frequencies while inhibiting inappropriate higher and lower frequency activity. With interhemispheric training, we found ourselves rewarding high and low frequencies that did not fit this explanatory model. How could we explain a reward frequency of 1-4 Hz? Did we really want to take people to delta frequencies in the awake state? How can we explain that some people report feeling more awake and alert when we migrate to reward frequencies as low as 1-4 Hz? Interhemispheric training has forced us to reevaluate our explanations of the mechanisms that underlie neurofeedback generally.

With interhemispheric training, our EEG signal represents a difference measure between two signals of comparable amplitude. This applies, of course, to other bipolar placements as well. In essence, the issue is this: what does it mean to reward increases in the size or amplitude of this difference signal? Increases in the difference can result from amplitude changes in one or both of the constituent EEG signals or from shifts in phase between the two signals. Whenever the activity within the reward band at the two sites moves into phase, that is, toward synchronous activity, the difference signal will decrease— and vice versa. So in addition to rewarding amplitude shifts, we are generally rewarding shifts toward out-of-phase activity as well. It might even be easier for the brain to achieve rewards by shifting the phase relationship of these signals between the sites rather than the amplitudes at each site directly. One can also argue mathematically that spindle-burst amplitude is sensitively dependent on the phase distribution within the neuronal assembly. So it is quite possible that phase is the operative variable (both physiologically and mathematically) not only in the relationship between the two sites, but also with respect to the amplitude that we observe at each site.

When we perturb the system by rewarding shifts away from the instantaneous state of dynamic equilibrium, the brain might quickly respond locally to the challenge in first instance, and then also observe more globally that its own state has changed. In an attempt to maintain its state, it may then resist the change and to shift back toward the *status quo ante*. After all, the brain cannot allow its state to be changed arbitrarily. This repetitive push-pull exercise might be an effective mechanism for strengthening the brain's ability to coordinate its own activity over the cortex.

There remains a clear relationship between arousal level and appropriate reward frequency. People with very high arousal symptoms such as anxiety, agitation, and physical tension generally need to train with a lower reward frequency. Our experience shows that rewarding increases in the difference signal recorded during interhemispheric training at frequencies near the lower end of our 0-30 Hz range typically allow such persons to feel calmer. We have come to view reward frequencies not as a destination but rather as a direction of change. To achieve lower arousal levels with interhemispheric training generally involves training lower than 12-15 Hz, and to achieve higher arousal levels generally means training higher than 12-15 Hz. The more extreme the arousal level, the more extreme the reward frequency.

Thus, interhemispheric training has compelled us to stretch the arousal model to consider a larger range of EEG frequencies than when we worked exclusively in the SMR/beta domain. The arousal model cannot, however, provide an explanation of the high specificity of reward frequency that seems to be mandated by client self-reports. One must separate the issues of the essential stability of the nervous system from that of set points of functioning, including arousal. People can move into unstable states at any arousal level, and rapid movement in the arousal dimension can even precipitate an excursion into unstable states. Since neurofeedback can elicit abrupt changes in arousal level, this all by itself can constitute a precipitating event for instability. That observation should not be taken as an indictment of the neurofeedback process itself. It simply imposes constraints on how the exercise of neurofeedback must be performed. The training must take place within the existing zone of stability of the person, under circumstances where the induced changes of physiological state are of bounded variation. The tactical approach, therefore, is to seek out that part of state space in which the person feels most calm, alert, and euthymic. The person's self-appraisal in that regard includes awareness of arousal state, but must also take into account other self-reported symptomatology as well.

Although the proposition is speculative, the most probable direct impact of the interhemispheric training is on instantaneous phase relationships between the two electrode sites. It is therefore likely that interhemispheric training at the optimum frequency elicits changes in phase where the neurofeedback exercise is most benign, and is least likely to precipitate the symptoms of instability. Hence, the training can also be thought of as building upon strength (i.e., nervous system stability) wherever we find it in a particular system.

The idea that reward-based training would consistently result in persistent increases in the average amplitude of the reward band never really corresponded with our experience. While abnormal low– or high-frequency EEG activity might decrease with training, reward band amplitudes rarely changed substantially according to the direction of training. There might be observable shifts during a session, but not typically from session to session. So it seems more appropriate to think of these reward band changes as an exercise in self-regulation rather than as normalizing the EEG in the reward band. It is also true that quantitative EEG results might usefully inform our choice of inhibit frequencies, but they do not help us predict an appropriate reward frequency. There is no manifest EEG deficit that needs to be "filled" by the choice of specific reward frequency we have been able to detect.

The interhemispheric exercise in shifting brain state, while asking that a client maintain a calm and alert state, is quite different from the dynamic of alpha-theta training. With alpha-theta, we deliberately evoke alpha- and theta-dominant states. And we expect to see significant changes in the EEG associated with those state shifts. With beta/SMR training, we are running in place—more like a treadmill.

We now need a better name for what we have been calling beta/SMR training. Our reward frequencies are often far from standard beta or SMR frequency bands. And we really are not trying to take people to beta or SMR states and certainly not to theta or delta states. So it seems more sensible to name the various training bands by their frequency ranges and set aside the historical names for specific EEG rhythms. And we still need a better descriptive name for this process. Perhaps it would be less confusing to call these two processes "awake-state" EEG training and "deep-state" EEG training.

Clinical Validation

The clinical environment is not conducive to the conduct of formal comparative studies, but in significant respects, the clinical setting offers unique opportunities for hypothesis testing. The issue in this case is whether interhemispheric training offers systematic advantages over earlier protocols. The generality of such a claim is readily evaluated in a clinical environment where a large variety of clinical challenges are routinely encountered. A second consideration is that, in testing for specificity of the approach, one would wish to hold all variables constant except for the one under investigation. This can be accomplished by making comparisons within the same client and in the same time frame. These conditions are well met with A/B designs done on the same client, either in the same session or in immediately contiguous sessions.

Whereas group data in psychological research is often handicapped by significant population heterogeneity, single-subject data largely takes this issue off the table. Since nearly all clients are trained with more than one protocol, they are all capable of yielding data of interest to research through A/B comparisons. The clinician is always using his or her best judgment, but at the same time, the results are faithfully documented. This process of "local optimization" of protocols is qualitatively no different from what a psychiatrist does in refining a medication strategy with multiple medications involved. As a practical matter, it is very similar to the process of A/B comparison employed by the optometrist to refine a correction of refraction. It is this process of intrasubject comparison that led us over a period of years to adopt interhemispheric training as a mainline approach for an increasing range of symptom presentations. It remains to discern the circumstances under which the prior lateralized protocols continue to hold an advantage, to be drawn upon as an alternative or as a complement. This question, too, can be resolved through continuation of the A/B within-subject comparisons as real-world clinical challenges continue to be confronted.

At any point in this process, one can take stock and inquire as to whether the final outcome has been improved. Has the training process merely been made more efficient (a worthy goal in itself), or is the outcome also more assured and perhaps qualitatively better? In such an outcome evaluation, the heterogeneity of the clinical population is a disadvantage. But we have found that attentional deficits are ubiquitous in clinical populations, and can therefore serve as a common measure for all. For more than a decade, we have used a continuous performance test, the test of variables of attention (TOVA), to track clinical progress among clients (Greenberg, 1988). This extended choice reaction time task furnishes measures of impulsivity and sustained attention, along with reaction time and its variability. These measures usually respond to neurofeedback training, and we have found them useful as a change measure in the general case.

The result for a subset of clients (male and female, ranging in age from 7 to 62 years) with indications of attentional deficits are shown in Figures 5.2 and 5.3 for the inattention and impulsivity measures using the TOVA (Putman et al., 2005). These outcomes are more consistently favorable than those obtained years ago with standard left-side/right-side training, and they more consistently reach "saturation." That is to say, clients more consistently reach zero errors of omission, and hence saturate at the maximum possible standard score for attention. (For earlier data, see Kaiser & Othmer, 2000.) We do attribute the improvement largely to the change in protocols, both with respect to the switch to interhemispheric training and the inclusion of more training sites. However, over the years, there has also been an improvement in clinical skills and in the software arena (mainly with respect to presentation of the information to the client through better video media).

Theoretical Modeling

The fact that interhemispheric training with bipolar placement did not behave like conventional "up-training" with referential placement

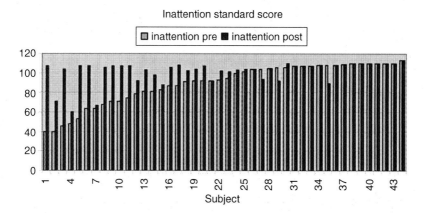

FIGURE 5.2. Inattention scores obtained from the TOVA test are shown for inter-hemispheric training. Observe the limiting score of nominally 108, referring to the maximum score possible in the event of zero omission errors. Note also that those starting out scoring above norms tend to maintain their scores.

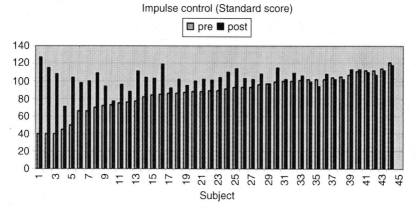

FIGURE 5.3. Impulsivity data obtained with the TOVA test for inter-hemispheric training. Gains are observed rather consistently, along with an absence of significant declines in scores.

compelled a reappraisal of what was being accomplished. The crucial element in interhemispheric training probably lies in the dependence of the reward signal on the relative phase of the EEG at the two sites. The reinforcement in a bipolar montage might not impinge so much on EEG amplitudes directly, but instead may serve primarily as a transducer of relative phase into amplitude information. Continuous reinforcement on the short-term integrated amplitude within the reward band then constitutes "pressure" on the ambient phase relationships to discourage synchronous or in-phase activity between sites.

It is easy to show the import of phase theoretically, using some simplifying assumptions to generate a set of surrogate data. If we assume a random distribution of amplitudes at each of the two sites (Gaussian-distributed), as well as random relative phase (uniformly distributed), a statistical sampling of outcomes can be modeled using a Monte Carlo procedure. That is, random choices of each of the three variables (i.e., two typically homologous amplitude measures, plus one phase measure) are combined to yield net amplitude, which would be seen in a bipolar measurement. The results are shown in Figure 5.4. A threshold criterion is then applied such that 70 percent of the resulting data points fall above the threshold, which reflects actual practice. In the event, this threshold is found to be nominally 40 degrees. Then we observe the distribution in phase of the resulting "data points" that meet threshold criterion. The results are shown in Figure 5.5, which confirms that the reward strongly discourages common phase: only 3 percent of the rewards fall within forty degrees in relative phase.

Admittedly, the modeling results presented in Figure 5.5 are not realistic in their assumption of randomness. It is known that there are significant amplitude correlations between sites, as discerned from determinations of spectral comodulation. But in this regard, the calculation has only been conservative. Any amplitude correlation between sites only serves to sharpen up the phase dependence as illustrated in Figure 5.4 to make the exclusion of synchrony even more complete.

In this view, then, bipolar placement should perhaps be seen more in terms of discouraging synchronous activity than in terms of a particular reward. That is, success in feedback is meted out broadly so long as the activity is not synchronous. There is no narrow target for success in phase terms. This is illustrated in the polar plot of Figure 5.6, which shows the net amplitude for two signals of equal amplitude as a function of relative phase. In effect, then, the reward serves as a "soft" inhibit on synchronous activity. Success can equally be had with appropriate amplitude shifts at the two sites. So the most general statement that can be made is that interhemispheric training broadly promotes differentiation between the two sites, however that may

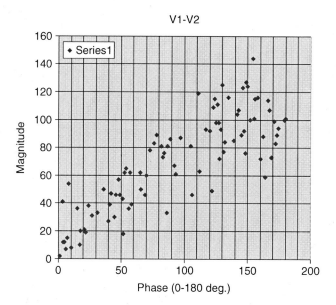

FIGURE 5.4. Results for a Monte Carlo calculation for the net signal amplitude for Gaussian-distributed amplitudes and random phase. With a reward threshold set for 70% success, the threshold in this case would be set at a magnitude of nominally 40.

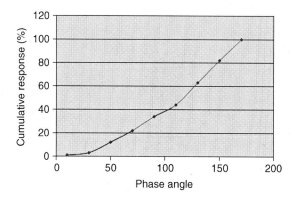

FIGURE 5.5. The cumulative reward incidence as a function of phase angle for the data of Figure 5.4 is shown. Note that only three percent of the rewards fall within the first 40 degrees of phase angle.

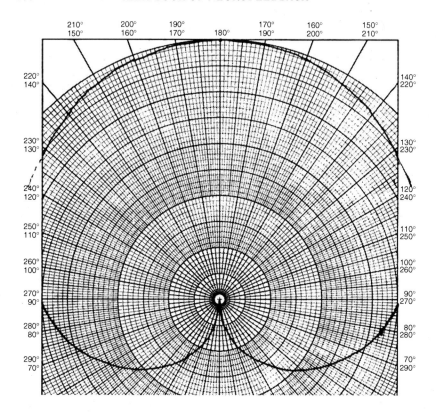

FIGURE 5.6. Polar plot of net signal amplitude as a function of relative phase for two signals, each of magnitude 100. Observe the strong dependence on phase angle near zero degrees. For other phase angles, the phase dependence is small.

manifest. The question remains about how the brain actually accommodates to the reinforcement.

Although empirical data are needed to resolve the issue, the foregoing speculations provide strong clues to the apparent breadth of efficacy of interhemispheric training. Specifically, altering phase relationships may represent the most efficient adaptive response by the brain. Challenging connectivity through altering phase relations between sites might be our most clinically effective option. Three circumstances may exist (1) there may be an excess in network connectivity between the training sites, as indexed by EEG synchrony;

(2) there may be a deficiency; and (3) a "normal" relationship may in fact prevail. If the protocol is to be considered universal in terms of its utility to enhance the quality of brain regulation for the purpose of improving the individual's function, then it must offer a net benefit in all three of these situations.

In the first of these categories, manifested through hypersynchrony, interhemispheric training would likely induce phase differentiation that would serve to reduce EEG synchrony to some degree. Specifically with reference to Figure 5.6, phase measurements over time would pile up near zero degrees in relative phase, and rewards would be garnered only for that activity which fell outside of that narrow phase range. In the second extreme case, sometimes referred to as a "disconnect syndrome," any effect at all of interhemispheric training would depend upon communication between the two sites, but it too is likely to be accomplished through phase changes. Enhancing such communication takes us in the right direction of improved connectivity, hence helping to resolve disconnect. And in the third case, that of enhancing normal function, it might be that any subtle challenge to the regulatory networks induced by interhemispheric training exerts a favorable influence in the quality of regulation. In other words, universality follows from the fact that the training is inherently bi-directional, involving both a movement away from the prevailing state, and mobilizing a restoration. The challenge to brain function is not contingent on the existence of any apparent deviation, or even on the proper targeting of an existing deviation.

The obvious shortcoming of this exercise model is that it cannot explain the sensitivity to choice of reward frequency. For any single individual, some frequency within the 0-30 Hz range is likely to lead to a favorable outcome, but for each individual most of the band could be contra-indicated. To explain this, one must consider not only the effects on regulatory mechanisms but also on the immediate status of the individual. In those who respond sensitively to this training, the tolerance to prolonged training at any arbitrary frequency may be low. One can think of this in terms of overdosing. The exercise model itself may be largely agnostic with respect to reward frequency. One might presume that training at any and all frequencies could be potentially beneficial in terms of regulatory response. As a practical matter, however, the person may have lower tolerance for the experience at some frequencies versus others. Fortunately, in most individuals a frequency can be identified where the training is not only benign but also favorable in terms of subjective states.

Remarkably, a frequency can typically be identified where adverse symptoms appear to be minimized (e.g., agitation, inattention, and somnolence) on the one hand, and positive attributes maximized on the other (e.g., alertness, vigilance, euthymia). It is tempting to propose that we are dealing here with a "saddle point" in phase space, where along one dimension we are operating at a local minimum with respect to adverse features, and along another axis we are operating at a local maximum with respect to positive attributes. This is illustrated in Figure 5.7, where the dependence of both a positive and a negative feature are shown as a function of frequency around the neighborhood of the optimum operating point. Small deviations around that point remain within the zone of stability. The training gradually alters the behavior surface in such a way that the zone of stability increases.

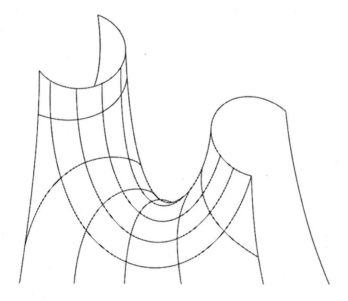

FIGURE 5.7. The behavior surface (for a range of EEG reward frequencies) shows one attribute whose values are to be maximized, and one variable whose values are to be minimized. A saddle point can usually be found that represents the optimum training frequency taking into account both criteria.

Mathematically, this would be reflected in a reduction of the curvature of the behavior surface at the saddle point.

The term saddle point follows directly from the fact that a real-world saddle exhibits the salient characteristics of both a positive and a negative curvature along two axes, with the respective maximum and minimum meeting at a single point. In the case of a saddle, both dimensions serve to push the rider back to the saddle point. In the present case of feedback, this must be accomplished through placing the therapist in the feedback loop in order to make the adjustment of operating point.

Figure 5.7 is limited to illustrating this concept with only a single dimension committed to an adverse feature, and a single dimension committed to a positive attribute. Remarkably, the curve would be much the same even if different behavioral variables were to be plotted. The saddle point identifies the optimum training locus in frequency for a variety of regulatory functions. The existence of such a saddle point has been implicit in our utilization of standard reward frequencies throughout the history of the field. It was simply assumed all along that this attribute was characteristic solely of certain special frequencies like the alpha resting frequency and the sleep spindle frequency. The modern challenge is to understand the large individual variation that appears to exist when this process is allowed to be particularized to the individual.

SUMMARY AND CONCLUSIONS

Even before our transition to interhemispheric training, we had begun to move beyond standard beta and SMR reward bands to achieve sufficient calming or activation, as needed. This was particularly important for high arousal conditions like autism and reactive attachment disorder. Yet, much of our clinical work continued with standard left-side 15-18 Hz and right-side 12-15 Hz. Interhemispheric training has shown us over the past several years the power of optimizing the reward frequency for each individual and each training site. Applying that lesson now when returning to target the hemispheres individually, we can significantly improve our efficacy by optimizing the reward frequencies in each individual case, as opposed to using the standard left beta and right SMR trainings.

We can also reconsider some of the specific problems we encountered when trying to train all sites on the left or right hemisphere with the same standard reward band. In particular, right prefrontal training had been contraindicated with a standard SMR reward. With interhemispheric training Fp1-Fp2 is quite manageable and useful. So we would expect Fp2 training to be possible in other configurations as well. We now find that right prefrontal training (Fp2-T4 or Fp2-A2) is well tolerated with a reward frequency that has been optimized for right-hemisphere training. A general relationship prevails that more potent the subjective effect on the client, the more crucial the choice of reward frequency. Right prefrontal training is a case in point. Because of the strong effect of training right prefrontal placements, there is a premium on the selection of the appropriate reward frequency.

Interhemispheric training has shown us the power of training with bipolar placements at homologous sites. Although the field started with bipolar training following the conventions of clinical EEG, most practitioners in time adopted referential placements due to the increased influence of quantitative EEG. We have now returned to bipolar training, even when we are training one hemisphere. For example, we consider C3-T3 to be preferable to C3-A1 generally. It is our impression that there is an additional benefit from challenging the brain to coordinate the activity between two sites as opposed to the simple activation of one site at a time. Whether this occurs via inter- or via intrahemispheric placements, we want to challenge the brain to improve its management of the phase relationship of the regulatory rhythms across the cortex. With such bipolar training, we reward increases in a difference measure, which is the difference derived from the two EEG sites. As noted earlier, this protocol most likely rewards the brain for phase shifts. We find that rewarding the sum of two signals, which rewards in-phase activity, is not as stabilizing. It may be that the brain is more at risk from inappropriately coherent activity in the awake state, and under the baseline conditions where training takes place. This may hold particular relevance for near-neighbor sites, as these may become too tightly coupled.

Our clinical experience and theoretical models are leading us to a particular approach to two-channel training wherein we reward the difference (within a narrow reward band), while inhibiting the sum of two signals. This rewards slight shifts toward an out-of-phase condition in the reward band, while also inhibiting larger abnormal bursts of in-phase activity. Broadband or multiple inhibits remain installed on the difference signal as well, as is presently done. Hence, the brain will be constrained with respect to large-amplitude excursions irrespective of the relative phase. We have some limited clinical experience that inhibiting on both the sum and the difference, along with a narrowly targeted reward on the difference of two channels, is clinically useful.

Perhaps the most important lesson from our work with interhemispheric training is that there are many more surprises and important lessons yet to be learned from our clinical experience with neurofeedback. The major objections to interhemispheric training arose because questions about mechanisms have remained unanswered. Theoretical models and the research necessary to clarify them nearly always come after the clinical results. That is likely to be particularly true in a field as clinically driven as neurofeedback. As clinicians, we need to remain open to new possibilities and let the theoretical models come with their explanations in our wake. Empirical research is needed to address the fundamental mechanisms that regulate neurofeedback generally, and interhemispheric training in particular.

Neurofeedback is a powerful tool that allows us to ask very specific questions in the real world of clinical practice. Every day, we have the opportunity to observe the specific results of different EEG training approaches with a variety of individuals. By being good observers and making our best clinical decisions day-by-day, we also help to move the field forward.

REFERENCES

Ayers, M.E. (1987). Electroencephalographic neurofeedback and closed head injury of 250 individuals. In *National head injury syllabus*, Washington, DC, Head Injury Foundation, 380-392.

Greenberg, L.M. (1988-2000). *TOVA: Test of variables of attention—Professional Guide*. Los Alamitos, CA: Universal Attention Disorders Inc.

Jasper, H. (1958). The ten-twenty system of the international federation. *EEG and Clinical Neurophysiology, 10,* 371-375.

Kaiser, D.A., & Othmer, S. (2000). Effect of neurofeedback on variables of attention in a large multicenter trial. *Journal of Neurotherapy, 4*(1), 5-15.

Lubar, J.F. (1995). Neurofeedback for the management of attention/hyperactivity disorders. In M. S. Schwartz & Associates (Eds.), *Biofeedback: A practitioner's guide* (pp. 493-522). New York: Guilford Press.

Malone, M.A., Kershner, J.R., & Swanson, J.M. (1994). Hemispheric processing and methylphenidate effects in attention deficit hyperactivity disorder. *Journal of Child Neurology, 9*(2), 181-189.

Nash, J.K. (2000). Treatment of attention deficit hyperactivity disorder with neuro-therapy. *Clinical Encephalography, 31*(1), 30-37.

Othmer, S. (2002a). Emerging trends in neurofeedback: I. On the status and future of mechanisms-based training. *Biofeedback, 30*(2), 21-23.

Othmer, S. (2002b). Emerging trends in neurofeedback: II. The challenge of QEEG-based and NLD-based neurofeedback protocols. *Biofeedback, 30*(3), 43-45.

Othmer, S., Othmer, S.F., & Kaiser, D.A., (1999). EEG biofeedback: An emerging model for its global efficacy. In J.R. Evans & A. Arbanel (Eds.), *Introduction to quantitative EEG and neurofeedback* (pp. 243-310). San Diego: Academic Press.

Putman, J.A., Othmer, S.F., Othmer, S., & Pollock, V.E. (2005). TOVA results following inter-hemispheric bipolar EEG training. *Journal of Neurotherapy, 9*(1), 37-52

Putman, J.A., & Othmer, S., Phase sensitivity of bipolar EEG training protocols. *Journal of Neurotherapy*, in press.

Quirk, D.A. (1995). Composite biofeedback conditioning and dangerous offenders, III. *Journal of Neurotherapy, 1*(2), 44-54.

Satterfield, J.H., & Dawson, M.E. (1971). Electrodermal correlates of hyperactivity in children. *Psychophysiology, 8,* 191-197.

Sterman, M.B. (2000). Basic concepts and clinical findings in the treatment of seizure disorders with EEG operant conditioning, *Clinical Electroencephalography, 31*(1), 45-55.

Sterman, M.B., & Friar, L. (1972). Suppression of seizures in epileptics following sensorimotor EEG feedback training. *Electroencephalogr. Clin. Neurophys., 33,* 89-95.

Sterman, M.B., LoPresti, R.W., & Fairchild, M.D. (1969). *Electroencephalographic and behavioral studies of monomethylhydrazine toxicity in the cat.* Tech Report AMRL-TR-69-3, Aerospace Medical Research Laboratory, Wright-Patterson Air Force Base, Ohio.

Sterman, M.B., Macdonald, L.R., & Stone, R.K. (1974). Biofeedback training of the sensorimotor electroencephalogram rhythm in man: Effects on epilepsy. *Epilepsia, 15*(3), 395-416.

Tansey, M.A., & Bruner, R.L. (1983). EMG and EEG biofeedback training in the treatment of a 10-year-old hyperactive boy with a developmental reading disorder. *Biofeedback and Self-Regulation, 8,* 25-37.

Chapter 6

The Combination
of Cognitive Training Exercises
and Neurofeedback

Tim Tinius

INTRODUCTION

The combination of cognitive exercises and neurofeedback as a treatment model to change or modify cognitive, emotional, and physiological processes in clients gives the trainer or clinician greater flexibility with a large variety of techniques that are easy to implement and interesting to most clients. This model is based upon a premise that education, teaching, and learning in a classroom situation is very important, but does not equal rehabilitation or necessarily result in quick responses on boring tasks. Education teaches and challenges students to learn because the more we know, the more we can know (Neath & Surprenant, 2003); and although there is a significant general effect of education on cognitive, emotional, and physical development, it may not specifically facilitate skills like attention, memory, and information processing in a developing brain.

If a student struggles with learning in a classroom setting, there are options that teachers or instructors have to facilitate learning or performance. The first option is simply to give more practice, for example, a student with trouble learning math concepts will benefit from the practice or repetition to complete a math problem over and over again. The second option is to reduce the number of problems so the student can finish in the same amount of time as other students. The

Handbook of Neurofeedback
doi:10.1300/5889_06

third option is to give a student more time to finish a task such as a test. The fourth option is a resource room with a low student-to-teacher ratio. The fifth option is one-to-one tutoring (as by a paraprofessional) in a classroom to maintain the attention or focus of the student. The sixth option is to decrease environmental distractions by placing the student in the front of the room. Finally, a teacher can use a variety of techniques such as using a schedule book, writing assignments on the board, or hands-on exercises. Each method is an environmental change in an attempt to facilitate the flow of information into the brain so that the student can learn information that other students may learn faster, easier, or more efficiently. While all of these methods assist a student to learn, they lack the capability to provide immediate (less than one second) feedback about changes in basic cognitive skills such as attention, impulse control, and variability of processing speed. Such cognitive functions are important to classroom learning, and are facilitated in cognitive training exercises combined with neurofeedback. This type of training can easily be implemented in an office or classroom.

The treatment model proposed in this chapter has four components to facilitate changes in brain information processing and subsequent changes in cognition and behavior. It can be used with children experiencing school learning difficulties as well as with children and adults attempting to recover from effects of traumatic brain injury. The first component of the model is training cognitive skills with cognitive training exercises on a computer as a method to increase attention, decrease processing speed variability, decrease impulsivity, and increase accuracy of responding. The use of computer-based cognitive exercises was reviewed by the National Academy of Neuropsychology (NAN) (2002), which led to the statement: "NAN supports such empirically and rationally based cognitive rehabilitation techniques that have been designed to improve the quality of life and functional outcomes for individuals with acquired brain injuries." However, there remains a need for more evidence-based work to further define and tailor cost-effective cognitive rehabilitation interventions (Ricker, 1998) and for expanded academic curricula to offer training courses in rehabilitation to treat individuals with brain injuries (Uzzell, 2000). An extensive review suggested that treatment aimed at helping people learn or relearn skills after an acquired brain injury will probably be effective, particularly if the skill being learned has a substantial attentional component. The most rewarding programs will likely be those that focus on training skills that also are of great functional importance to the individual participants (Park & Ingles, 2001). A meta-analysis showed that attention deficits after acquired brain injury can be effectively treated (i.e., improved) using attention-demanding tasks (Park & Ingles, 2001). Another extensive review of research on Cognitive Rehabilitation by Cicerone et al. (2000) concluded that computer-based interventions are effective if they include active therapist involvement to foster insight into cognitive strengths and weaknesses, to develop compensation strategies, and to facilitate transfer of skills into real-life situations. They did not recommend sole reliance on repeated exposure and practice on computer-based tasks without extensive involvement and intervention by a therapist. Several studies have found that the benefits of attention training are greater on more complex tasks that require selective or divided attention than on basic tasks of reaction time and vigilance (Gray, Robertson, Peatland, & Anderson, 1992; Sturm & Wilmes, 1991; Sturm, Wilmes, & Orgass, 1997).

The second component is the use of neurofeedback to increase physiological arousal so that the client can note EEG changes in real time (feedback) as they complete cognitive tasks. The client can note the changes, and the trainer can observe the changes and comment on them based upon the type of task, electrode location, and brainwave that is monitored. These psychophysiological data provide quick identification of very subtle changes in attention and teach the client how his or her brain is working during tasks. The reader is referred to a bibliography of outcome studies on neurofeedback (Hammond, 2001) for a comprehensive list of published studies. For example, there are outcome data for children with attention deficit hyperactivity disorder (ADHD) (Linden, Habib, & Redojevic, 1996) and a large study showing changes in attention after neurofeedback (Kaiser & Othmer, 2000).

The third component is teaching clients how to "think" with metacognition techniques, defined as one's knowledge concerning one's own cognitive processes or anything related to them (Flavell, 1976, 1979). As children get older, they demonstrate more awareness of their thinking processes (Duell, 1986), and metacognition is important for the continuing development of critical thinking and self-reliant learning (Larkin, 2000). Metacognition may explain why children of different ages deal with learning tasks in different ways (Flavell, 1976).

These processes can include the regulation of one's own thinking processes in order to cope with changing situational demands, monitoring of the available information during the course of thinking and using this information to regulate subsequent memory processes (Kluwe, 1982; Schneider, 1985; Schoenfeld, 1987), or the use of problem solving or plans that learners make before tackling a task, the adjustments they make as they work, and the revisions they make afterward (Paris & Winograd, 1990). Clients with a mild traumatic brain injury (mTBI) or ADHD and various learning disorders often do not utilize such strategies and shortcuts to solve problems. The specific metacognitive skills taught can include encouraging the client to think about a task before starting it so that they can learn to solve the task accurately and quickly, developing a strategy during the completion of the task, and learning to modify a strategy as the task progresses. The trainer is vital to teaching these skills to the client through constant feedback about cognitive and emotional changes while completing cognitive exercises, and about the physiological data from the EEG equipment. Early research combined cognitive rehabilitation with personalized treatment procedures including therapist feedback and "confidence building" by monitoring the subject's emotional reaction to deficits (Wilson & Robertson, 1992). Others allocated time in training sessions to give the client feedback on their performance, and actively teaching learning strategies to improve their functioning during cognitive rehabilitation (Niemann, Ruff, & Baser, 1990). Most recently, Thompson and Thompson (1998) taught metacognitive strategies related to academic tasks when the feedback indicated that the person was focused, and suggested the combination of metacognitive strategies and neurofeedback was a useful intervention. Although computer-based exercises are effective, the exercises alone do not facilitate cognitive functioning (Cicerone, 2000), and there is a similar conclusion about neurofeedback in that a computer software, and auditory or visual feedback concerning EEG changes do not, by themselves, change symptoms or facilitate performance on tasks. For optimal results, there must be a human interaction during cognitive retraining and neurofeedback that uses encouragement and metacognitive strategies to assist the client to make a connection between the auditory and visual feedback from the two computers and his or her own internal processes.

The fourth component is the use of a variety of tasks and distractions while the client is completing cognitive training exercises. This could involve focusing on two tasks simultaneously (sometimes referred to as dual processing or multitasking). This can be accomplished by talking to the client during the training, and usually is implemented after several training sessions. Another method to teach increased attention during cognitive exercises is for the trainer to talk to a parent or other person in the background while the client is completing cognitive tasks. They are required to complete the cognitive tasks while blocking out or ignoring the background noise in the room. This is a real-world component in which the client must complete tasks with background noise in a classroom.

IMPLEMENTATION OF TREATMENT METHOD

The specific treatment method developed by the author will be described in the following text. This is a typical setup and there is plenty of room for variation depending upon office space and personal preference.

Computer Setup

Two separate computers are placed side-by-side in an office with one computer dedicated solely to the feedback of EEG, and the second to the cognitive retraining exercises, that is, Captain's Log. In the early DOS version of Captain's Log (Sandford, Browne, & Turner, 1993), the computer speaker was connected to a Soundblaster card so there was some control of the volume of auditory feedback. The recently released version of Captain's Log, called Captain's Log for Windows (Sandford, 2005), is much more flexible, contains more exercises, uses the audio sound card more efficiently, and the programs are also administered in hierarchically structured automated protocols.

Neurofeedback Program

The Lexicor Biolex program is used for training, but any of the newer neurofeedback programs can be used. One advantage of the Lexicor program is that the auto threshold is used so the trainer does not have to monitor the level of feedback throughout the session. There is a significant level of auditory and visual stimuli from the two computers during treatment. Therefore, as a general rule of thumb, the treatment's auditory feedback should use just one tone (e.g., indicating increase SMR or decrease theta). Multiple tone combinations or band change tones should be avoided. A feedback percentage equal to or greater than 85 percent will help the client become aware of his or her performance. The exact electrode placement may be secondary as the focus on cognitive exercises results in a high demand for cognitive processes and changing of them. As a rule of thumb, if the client's Integrated Visual and Auditory Continuous Performance Test (IVA) shows poor visual attention, an electrode can be placed on the right hemisphere (C4 or F4) (Sandford & Turner, 1995). A majority of visual cognitive training exercises involve visual spatial perception, facial recognition, shape discrimination, and directionality as are processed primarily in the right hemisphere (Parker, 1990). If the IVA showed low scores on auditory attention, an electrode can be placed on the left hemisphere (C3 or F3). A majority of auditory cognitive training exercises are related to verbal processing and analysis of auditory input as processed largely at locations such as left temporal gyri (Parker, 1990).

Progression of Sessions

During session 1 through session 7, the main focus is on cognitive exercises, and the client needs to be reminded often to listen for the EEG feedback tone. Amplitude threshold levels of targeted EEG frequencies can be adjusted during training to insure that the client does not receive too much or too little feedback. This can be done manually by the trainer, but also can be done through the EEG equipment by use of "automatic threshold," which will lower thresholds if too little feedback is being attained and raise them when too much feedback is being received. Metacognition techniques are very important here to educate the client about changes in physiology and cognitive processing. For example, with a simple "decrease theta" neurofeedback training protocol, the microvolts of theta generally will increase in the early sessions, but by as early as three sessions, there can be a significant decrease in levels. The client should be educated on the importance of starting to decrease theta. Cognitive training should focus on accurate, attentive responding on tasks of visual attention, with occasional addition of frontal lobe tasks that emphasize the effect of attention skills on problem solving. It is not recommended to start auditory training at this point, as it is likely to be too confusing for the client.

During the middle of training (session 8 through session 14), the main emphasis is on the inclusion of auditory training with the Sound-Smart Program (Sandford, 2002) in the cognitive training. Mixing the visual and auditory stimuli gives a large variety of tasks to take advantage of changing responses and modality quickly. It is important to start talking to a client about paying attention to any changes they may be experiencing in their environment. The subtle changes are important as you point out that these are changes one should look for in the real world.

During the final training (session 16 through session 20), the emphasis is on quickly changing tasks, talking to the clients about their performances and keeping them continuously performing on tasks for 40 to 45 minutes. The trainer should help them recall that they could not complete this kind of performance during the early eight sessions, and remind them of their earlier performances on visual scanning and color discrimination. In the last two to three sessions, let the client (especially children) pick the cognitive training exercises or use reading, math problems, or video games. Additional tasks such as Tetris, reading, and homework also can be used anytime after 12 to 15 sessions. And, with younger children, these can be used as reinforcement tasks for earlier sessions. It is important to start introducing schoolwork at this point in the training so that a transition is made from training attention and information processing to more traditional educational information.

Important Training Decisions

Throughout the 20 sessions of treatment, the trainer must make every effort to help the client become aware of the feedback from the computer that is providing the neurofeedback while completing cognitive exercises on the other computer, and of metacognitive techniques after exercises. One technique is to remind clients to remember the sound of the neurofeedback during the session, and when in a demanding condition such as school, they can re-create and imagine that sound in their minds. Remind them that the sound is telling them that they are doing the right process or they are in the correct mind state, and that their performance is increasing on the task. Another technique is to have the clients remember the office surroundings and, in their minds, re-create those surroundings when they are completing complicated tasks such as reading or homework. This will take into account the contextual cues, which they can use to re-create the environment where they had performed during training when they are in new environments. The trainer also must continue to promote multisensory processing, ignoring external environmental stimuli, and monitoring internal thoughts and self-talk. As noted earlier, there are various ways to add environmental stimuli such as bringing a family into the room or talking to the client during the exercises.

Specific Cognitive Exercises

Previous research has shown that attention retraining typically requires participants to complete a series of exercises in which they respond to visual or auditory stimuli, often classifying items on the basis of a rule (Park & Ingles, 2001). These exercises rely upon repetition, drill, and practice to facilitate processing speed, focused attention, and divided attention (Cicerone et al., 2000). Similarly, the author's treatment method uses a large variety of cognitive exercises to facilitate attention and other cognitive processes through repetition, drills, and teaching quick classification of information within a two-minute time period. The cognitive exercises in the Captain's Log for Windows (Sandford, 2005) provide a wide variety of exercises for all ages from six years to older adults. Each task has various requirements (levels of difficulty) that can be changed depending upon the age and cognitive problems of the client.

In the cognitive training used by the author, there are three areas to be trained and monitored throughout the training. First and most importantly, the client must maintain near perfect accuracy (100 percent performance) in order to decrease impulsivity and make accurate decision responses, with less emphasis on reaction time. This principle is based upon the conclusion that a person can naturally overcome slow processing with consistent accurate responses to stimuli; or, in other words, it is better to be accurate, and less variable in reaction time at the cost of initially slower overall response speed. The difficulty of the exercises can be changed and distractibility stimuli added as needed within the two-minute exercises. While completing two minutes on a task, the client can develop self-awareness or metacognition about performance while interacting with the trainer. If necessary, the trainer can extend the length of the task when trying to develop greater awareness of a state of processing and/or of the feedback from the neurofeedback computer, or when training specifically to extend sustained attention over a period of three minutes or greater. The time between the two-minute tasks allows the trainer to talk about the client's performance and make adjustments in neurofeedback protocols. The clients can learn about their processing of information by making mistakes, observing their mistakes, and talking with the trainer about it. But, most importantly, they are given other trials to learn how to *not* make mistakes and see success instantly.

The order of selection of exercises by the trainer is probably less important to improvement in attention because the most important part of the treatment method may be the client's focus on their performance and awareness of cognitive, emotional, and physiological changes before, during, and after the cognitive exercise. The cognitive exercises from the Captain's Log for Windows are listed in Table 6.1, along with a brief description of each task. These exercises provide a very large source of tasks. The following guidelines list the tasks found particularly helpful.

During the early sessions of treatment, two specific exercises (Cat's Pay or Visual Scanning and Match Point or Color Discrimination) are used primarily to decrease inattention and impulsivity. Within these programs, the client learns to make accurate responses by making choices in a discriminatory manner. The stimuli presentation length is changed across sessions so the client is shaped over time from a long duration of three seconds (i.e., must respond in less than three seconds) to a shorter duration of one second (must respond in less than one second). The client learns to master accuracy and make a correct response to quickly changing stimuli over two-minute periods. If the client is inattentive for even three stimuli during any two-minute training, they are made aware of the inattention and how they can use

TABLE 6.1. Captain's Log program descriptions with a brief description of each task.

DOS name	Captain's Log for Windows	Description
Attention skills: Developmental		
Auditory discrimination/rhythm	Drum Signals	Determine whether rhythm patterns are the same or different
Auditory discrimination/tones	Musical Pairs	Determine whether tone patterns are the same or different
Color discrimination/inhibition	Match Point	Distinguish between the color/size/shape of sets
Scanning reaction time	Cat's Play	Match pictured objects to featured picture
Scanning reaction/inhibition	Mouse Hunt	Match color of object to color of the border
Stimulus reaction time	Target Practice	Find target objects
Stimulus reaction/fields	Watchdog	Help cat locate yard
Stimulus reaction/inhibition	Red Light, Green Light	Match color of shapes to the border
Conceptual/memory skills		
Conceptual discrimination	The Ugly Duckling	Find different images in boxes
Numeric skills	Total Recall	Count the number of the shapes
Pattern display match	Domino Dynamite	Find differences between picture set
Size discrimination	Tower Power	Find images based on size
Symbolic display match	Max's Match	Organize pictures into boxes
Logical sequences (Trail A & B)	Happy Trails	Put letters in order of appearance
Visual pattern recognition	What's Next?	Figure out patterns with changing rules
Numeric concepts/memory skills		
Numeric classifications	Bits and Pieces	Find number of shapes based on changing rules
Numeric combinations	Matchmaker	Match by number patterns

TABLE 6.1 *(continued)*

DOS name	Captain's Log for Windows	Description
Numeric discrimination	City Lights	Pick out boxes by quantity of images
Numeric distinctions	Counting Critters	Determine number of spaces between objects
Numeric recall	Happy Hunter	Remember the numbers on the screen
Visual/motor skills		
Maze learning	Great Escape	Go through maze to find destination
Visuospatial memory	Concentration	Match objects two at a time
Visual categorization	PickQuick	Locate target object from behind pictures
Visual response time	Pop-N-Zap	Doors slide open and click on car that appears
Visual timing	Darts	Send dart to catch objects
Visual tracking/discrimination	On the Road	Drive and pick up target objects
Visual tracking/response	Hide and Seek	Find objects while avoiding harmful stimulus
Attention skills: The next generation		
Auditory patterns/rhythms (scanning)	Mystery Messages	Match the tone of bars to rhythm patterns
Scanning location (symbol search?)	The Great Hunt	Find target letters
Image scanning/inhibition	Smart Detective	Find target shapes
Logic skills		
None	Conceptor	Which image does not belong
None	Eagle Eye	Click when letters of numbers are the same
None	Pick and Pop	Pick the missing image
None	Figure It Out	Pick the missing image
None	What's missing?	Identify the missing number

the neurofeedback to become aware of the inattention and teach themselves to refocus on the stimuli. The tasks can increase accuracy by decreasing impulsivity and increasing quick decision making within one to three seconds. This requires rapid decisions while attending to determine which stimuli are relevant or important for a response and which are not. Exercises such as Symbolic Display Match (Max's Match) and Conceptual Discrimination (Ugly Duckling) especially challenge frontal lobe function to increase problem solving, decision making, rapid determination of rules, and concept formation. In the Captain's Log for Windows, the initial reaction times are averaged and the response latency time is adjusted so that a correct response requires a faster reaction time. Also, the response time latency is adjusted to slow when incorrect responses are made.

In latter training sessions, the focus should be on increasing the speed of responding. This should only be completed after accuracy (over time) has been sustained, and the client is able to understand that speed should not sacrifice accuracy. After impulsivity and inattention are decreased and becomes less of a problem, tasks of processing speed can be introduced. These tasks can include numeric skills (Total Recall), image scanning/inhibition (Smart Detective) and visual-spatial memory (Concentration).

Measuring Treatment Change

The IVA (Sandford & Turner, 1995a), Wisconsin Card Sorting Test (Heaton et al., 1993), Neuropsychological Impairment Scale (O'Donnell et al., 1984), and a Quantitative EEG are completed prior to treatment. The IVA can be readministered after 10 sessions to assess improvement and provide the client with feedback. The post testing includes the same tests, plus meeting with the client, spouse, or family to review results. The author has found that in persons with ADHD, 20 sessions usually are enough to achieve the goals, while for persons with mTBI, another 10 sessions are often necessary.

OUTCOME DATA

Outcome data from this treatment model in adults diagnosed with ADHD and mTBI was published by Tinius and Tinius (2000). The specific treatment protocol for each client was listed in that publication. Overall, results showed that after treatment, both groups with ADHD and mTBI performed very similarly to a nonimpaired control group on a measure of sustained attention (IVA), but the mTBI group continued to report more significant symptoms after treatment compared to the control and ADHD groups. No EEG data were analyzed; however, Stathapoulou and Lubar (2004) found significant QEEG changes in a small group of college students who completed only cognitive exercises with Captain's Log. This suggests that QEEG may assist in measuring effects of use of this treatment model. This model has been used with children and adolescents, but there has not been enough outcome data to show effectiveness compared to a control group. Further data is required to assess the effectiveness of this treatment with specific population groups.

SUMMARY AND CONCLUSIONS

This chapter discussed how cognitive training exercises can be combined with neurofeedback treatment. Published outcome data (Tinius & Tinius, 2000) has shown the effectiveness of such treatment. As with most treatments, a client with average to higher interest, motivation, and willingness to commit time can be expected to show the greatest benefit. This treatment does not necessarily eliminate symptoms, but teaches the management of symptoms and commonly results in a decrease of symptoms. The author's clients generally belong in one of three groups during treatment. The first group consists of persons with a mild head injury after a high school or post high school education. These individuals lost their skills from the neurological trauma, and treatment can assist them to recover the skills. The retraining serves to help develop compensation skills and greater success on rapidly changing tasks. The second group consists of clients with a TBI and less than a 12th-grade education. They may have never acquired skills because of a learning disability or ADHD prior to a mild TBI. These groups may need many repetitions on cognitive exercises to learn even some basic skills. Finally, the third group consists of clients with ADHD who never had some of these skills, need to learn the skills, and probably have developed ineffective compensation strategies prior to training.

Data analysis from clients in our office found that, for adults with ADHD, the Full Scale Attention Quotient of the IVA was significantly correlated with Scale 2 (Depression) of the Minnesota Multiphasic Personality Inventory—2 (MMPI-2; Hathaway & McKinley, 1989), but was not correlated in adults with mTBI. This suggests that depression needs to be taken into account during training of adults with ADHD. Neurofeedback for symptoms of depression, chronic pain, or anxiety could be used during early training sessions for symptom reduction when using this cognitive training model.

There is a lack of QEEG or other data showing physiological changes from this treatment procedure. Stathapoulou and Lubar (2004) showed some EEG changes in a very small group who completed only cognitive retraining exercises with the Captain's Log System. After reviewing the literature, Thornton (2000) concluded that neurofeedback interventions have proved to be a useful approach to remediation of cognitive difficulties in patients with TBI, whether the approach was directed toward coherence or magnitude measures. The limitations of these studies, however, included a lack of specificity of relationships between the cognitive difficulties and QEEG variables, failure to obtain or indicate that the cognitive improvements were concomitant with changes in the QEEG measures, lack of high EEG frequency analysis, and lack of long-term follow-up (Thornton, 2000).

The treatment model described in this chapter is consistent with the recommendations of the National Institutes of Health (NIH) Consensus Statement (1998), which concluded there should be more focus on research-based treatment, less focus on medical outcome, and focus on approaches that are more integrative and based upon an empirical and rational theory. Riccio and French (2004) reviewed over 80 published studies on the treatment of attention, and concluded that, there is a need for more research on the efficacy of treatment programs. The quality of therapeutic intervention beyond the specific training tasks may be an important variable to consider in the effectiveness of treatment (Cicerone et al., 2000). The treatment procedure described in this chapter is a therapeutic intervention using computerized training tasks, EEG biofeedback, and metacognition as tools to facilitate changes in brain functioning. It can increase attention on a variety of cognitive tasks, and has a theoretical basis gleaned from the best available research models.

REFERENCES

American Psychiatric Association. (1994). *Diagnostic and statistical manual of mental disorders*, (4th ed.). Washington, DC: Author.

Cicerone, K. D., Dahlberg, C., Kalmar, L., Langenbahn, D., Malec, J. F., Berquist, T. F., Felicetti, T., Giacino, J. T., Harley, J. P., Harrington, D. E., Herzog, J., Kneipp, S., Laatsch, L., & Morse, P. (2000). Evidence-based cognitive rehabilitation: Recommendations for clinical practice. *Archives of Physical Medicine and Rehabilitation, 81,* 1596-1615.

Duell, O. K. (1986). Metacognitive skills. In G. Phye & T. Andre (Eds.), *Cognitive classroom learning*. Orlando, FL: Academic Press.

Flavell, J. H. (1976). Metacognitive aspects of problem solving. In L. B. Resnick (Ed.), *The nature of intelligence*. Hillsdale, NJ: Erlbaum.

Flavell, J. H. (1979). Metacognition and cognitive monitoring: A new area of cognitive-developmental inquiry. *American Psychologist, 34,* 906-911.

Gray, J. M., Robertson, I., Peatland, B., & Anderson, S. (1992). Microcomputer-based attentional retraining after brain damage: A randomized trial. *Neuropsychological Rehabilitation, 2,* 97-115.

Hammond, D. C. (2001). Comprehensive neurofeedback bibliography. *Journal of Neurotherapy, 5,* 113-128.

Hathaway, S. R. & McKinley, J. C. (1989). *MMPI-2 manual for administration and scoring*. Minneapolis: University of Minnesota Press.

Heaton, R. K., Chelune, G. J., Talley, J. L., Kay, G. G., & Curtiss, G. (1993). *Wisconsin card sorting test: Revised and expanded*. Odessa, FL: Psychological Assessment Resources Inc. (Manual).

Kaiser, D. A. & Othmer, S. (2000). Effect of neurofeedback on variables of attention in a large multicenter trial. *Journal of Neurotherapy, 4*(1), 5-15.

Kluwe, R. H. (1982). Cognitive knowledge and executive control: Metacognition. In D. R. Griffin (Ed.), *Animal mind—Human mind*. New York: Springer-Verlag.

Larkin, S. (2000). *How can we discern metacognition in year one children from interactions between students and teacher?* Paper presented at ESRC Teaching and Learning Research Program Conference.

Linden, M., Habib, T., & Radojevic, V. (1996). A controlled study of the effects of EEG biofeedback on cognition and behavior of children with attention deficit disorder and learning disabilities. *Biofeedback and Self-Regulation, 21*(1), 35-49.

National Academy of Neuropsychology. (2002). *Cognitive Rehabilitation: Official Statement of the National Academy of Neuropsychology,* www.nanonline.org.

National Institutes of Health (NIH) Consensus Statement. (1998). *Rehabilitation of Persons with Traumatic Brain Injury, 16*(1), 1-49.

Neath, I. & Surprenant, A. M. (2003). *Human Memory* (2nd ed.), Wadsworth/ Thomson Learning: Belmont California.

Niemann, H., Ruff, R. M., & Baser, C. A. (1990). Computer-assisted attention retraining in head injured individuals: A controlled study of an outpatient program. *Journal of Consulting and Clinical Psychology, 58,* 811-817.

O'Donnell, W. E., DeSoto, C. B., DeSoto, J. L., & Reynolds, D. McQ. (1984). *Neuropsychological impairment scales (NIS) manual.* Annapolis, MD: Annapolis Neuropsychological Services.

Paris, S. G. & Winograd, P. (1990). How metacognition can promote academic learning and instruction. In B. F. Jones & L. Idol (Eds.), *Dimensions of thinking and cognitive instruction* (pp. 15-51). Hillsdale, NJ: Erlbaum.

Park, N. W. & Ingles, J. L. (2001). Effectiveness of attention rehabilitation after an acquired brain injury: A meta-analysis, *Neuropsychology, 15*(2), 199-210.

Parker, R. S. (1990). *Traumatic brain injury and neuropsychological impairment.* New York: Springer-Verlag.

Riccio, C. A. & French, C. L. (2004). The status of empirical supports for treatments of attention deficits. *The Clinical Neuropsychologist, 18,* 528-588.

Ricker, J. H. (1998). Traumatic brain injury rehabilitation: Is it worth the cost? *Applied Neuropsychology, 5,* 184-193.

Sandford, J. A. (2005). *Captain's log for windows* (Computer Program). Richmond VA: Braintrain Inc.

Sandford, J. A., Browne, R. J., & Turner, A. (1993). *Captain's log cognitive training system* (Computer Program). Richmond VA: Braintrain Inc.

Sandford, J.A. & Turner, A. (1995a). *Intermediate visual and auditory continuous performance test* (Computer Program). Richmond VA: Braintrain Inc.

Sandford, J.A. & Turner, A. (1995b). *Manual for the integrated visual and auditory continuous performance test.* Richmond, VA: Braintrain Inc.

Sandford, J. A. & Turner, A. (1996). *Alphabet bingo* (Computer Program). Richmond VA: Braintrain Inc.

Schneider, W. (1985). Developmental trends in the metamemory-memory behavior relationship: An integrative review. In D. L. Forrest-Pressley, G. E. MacKinnon, & T. G. Waller (Eds.), *Metacognition, cognition, and human performance*, Vol. 1. New York: Academic Press.

Schoenfeld, A. H. (1987). What's all the fuss about metacognition? In A. H. Schoenfeld (Ed.), *Cognitive science and mathematics education.* Hillsdale, NJ: Erlbaum.

Stathopoulou, S. & Lubar, J. F. (2004). EEG changes in traumatic brain injured patients after cognitive rehabilitation. *Journal of Neurotherapy, 8*(2), 21-51.

Sturm, W. & Wilmes, K. (1991). Efficacy of reaction training on various attentional and cognitive functions in stroke patients. *Neuropsychological Rehabilitation, 1,* 259-280.

Sturm, W., Wilmes, K., & Orgass, B. (1997). Do specific attention deficits need specific training? *Neuropsychological Rehabilitation, 7,* 81-103.

Thompson, L. & Thompson, M. (1998). Neurofeedback combined with training in metacognitive strategies: Effectiveness in students with ADD. *Applied Psychophysiology and Biofeedback, 23*(4), 243-263.

Thornton, K. (2000). Rehabilitation of memory functioning in brain injured subjects with EEG bio-feedback. *Journal of Head Trauma Rehabilitation, 15*(6), 1285-1296.

Tinius, T. P. & Tinius, K. A. (2000). Changes after EEG biofeedback and cognitive retraining in adults with mild traumatic brain injury and attention deficit hyperactivity disorder. *Journal of Neurotherapy, 4*(2), 27-44.

Uzzell, B. P. (2000). Neuropsychological rehabilitation. In A. L. Christensen and B. P. Uzzell (Eds.), *International handbook of neuropsychological rehabilitation*. The Netherlands: Kluwer Academic/Plenum Publishers.

Wilson, B. & Robertson, I. H. (1992). A home-based intervention for attentional slips during reading following head injury: A single case study. *Neuropsychological Rehabilitation, 2*, 193-205.

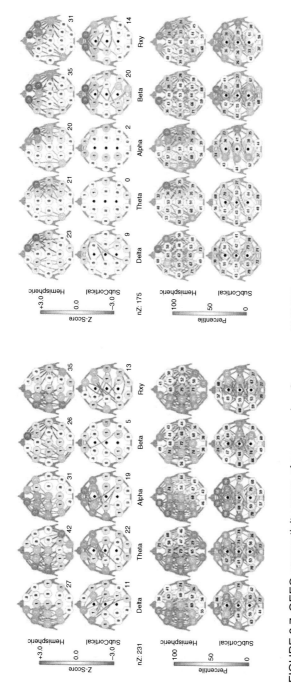

FIGURE 8.7. QEEG connectivity maps of case number 6, eyes closed (EC) shows, in the upper panel, the Z-score (nZ = 231) as average of duplicate recordings. *Source: ROSHI Journal, 3(1): 1-7, January 2006.*

FIGURE 8.8. QEEG connectivity maps of case number 6, eyes open (EO) shows the Z-score (nZ = 175) as average of duplicate recordings. *Source: ROSHI Journal, 3(1): 1-7, January 2006.*

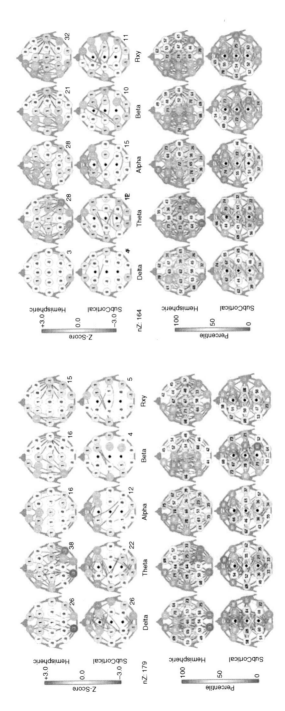

FIGURE 8.9. QEEG connectivity maps of case number 6, eyes closed (EC) during ROSHI light training shows the Z-scores. The nZ = 179 is significantly lower than during the EC baseline (nZ = 231) (see Figure 8.7). *Source: ROSHI Journal, 3(1): 1-7, January 2006.*

FIGURE 8.10. QEEG connectivity maps of case number 6, eyes closed (EC) after ROSHI training, shows the Z-scores. The nZ = 164 is still significantly lower than the EC baseline (nZ = 231). *Source: ROSHI Journal, 3(1): 1-7, January 2006.*

Patient ID: CCHNEC_0
Z-Values of EEG Features Referenced to Norms

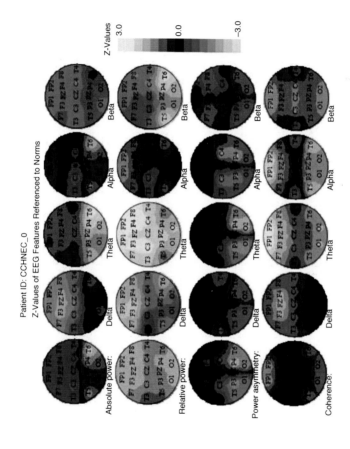

FIGURE 11.2. QEEG hyperactive/impulsive type ADHD protocol (Hypo-aroused).

Patient ID: TLFNEC_0

Z-Values of EEG Features Referenced to Norms

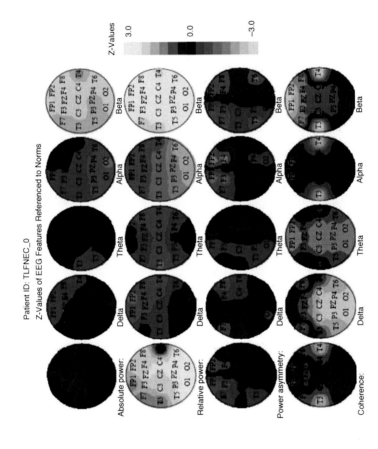

FIGURE 11.3. QEEG hyperactive/impulsive type ADHD protocol hyper-aroused inattentive protocol targeting hypo-arousal: increase beta-1/decrease theta.

Patient ID: HGSNEC_0

Z-Values of EEG Features Referenced to Norms

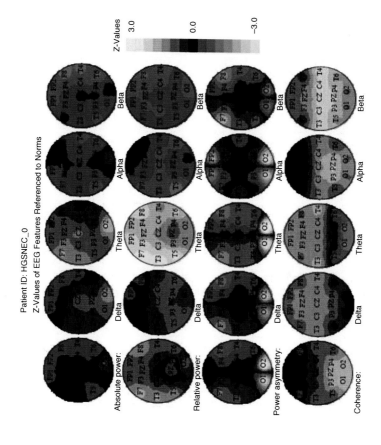

FIGURE 11.4. QEEG inattentive ADHD protocol hypo-aroused protocols modified from the three basic "Tried and True Trio."

Patient ID: CCHNEC_0

Z-Values of EEG Features Referenced to Norms

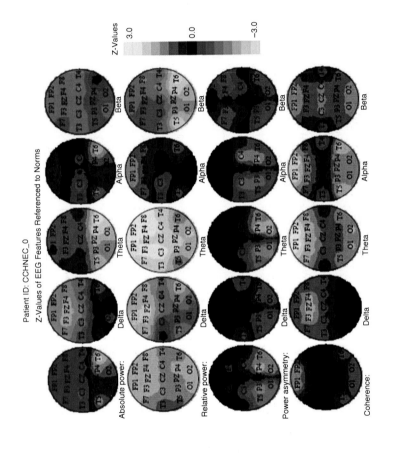

FIGURE 11.5. QEEG cortical hypo-arousal.

Patient ID: CHPEECA_0

Z-Values of EEG Features Referenced to Norms

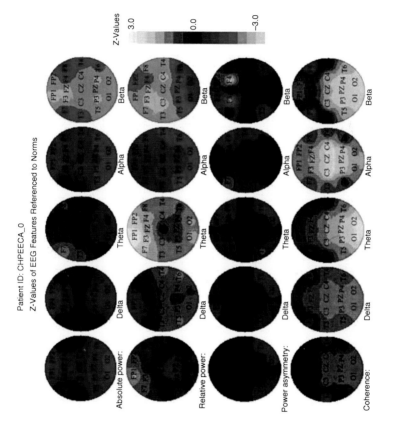

FIGURE 11.6. QEEG Maturational Lag.

Patient ID: TLPNEC_0
Z-Values of EEG Features Referenced to Norms

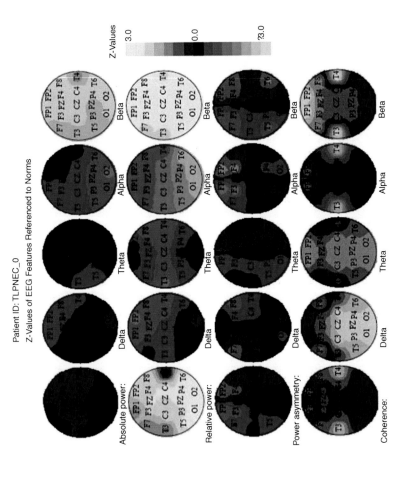

Z-Values

3.0

0.0

3.0

FIGURE 11.7. QEEG hyper-arousal, "short-fuse" subtype.

Chapter 7

Audio-Visual Entrainment: History, Physiology, and Clinical Studies

David Siever

HISTORY

Clinical reports of flicker stimulation appear as far back as the dawn of modern medicine. It was at the turn of the twentieth century when Pierre Janet, at the Salpêtrière Hospital in France, reported that when he had his patients gaze into the flickering light produced from a spinning spoked wheel in front of a kerosene lantern, the effect lowered their depression, tension, and hysteria (Pieron, 1982). With the development of the EEG, Adrian and Matthews published their results showing that the alpha rhythm could be "driven" above and below the natural frequency with photic stimulation (Adrian & Matthews, 1934). This discovery propagated a flurry of small physiological outcome studies on the "flicker following response," the brain's electrical response to visual and/or auditory stimulation (Bartley, 1934, 1937; Durup & Fessard, 1935; Jasper, 1936; Goldman, Segal, & Segalis, 1938; Jung, 1939; Toman, 1941).

In 1956, W. Gray Walter published the first results on thousands of test subjects comparing flicker stimulation with the *subjective* emotional feelings produced. Test subjects reported all types of visual illusions and in particular the "whirling spiral," which was significant with alpha production. In the late 1950s, as a result of Kroger's

Handbook of Neurofeedback
© 2007 by The Haworth Press, Inc. All rights reserved.
doi:10.1300/5889_07

research on why US military radar operators often drifted into trance (Kroger & Schneider, 1959), Kroger teamed with Sidney Schneider of the Schneider Instrument Company in Ohio, and, utilizing his electronic know-how, created the world's first electronic clinical photic stimulator—the "Brainwave Synchronizer." It consisted of a neon strobe light, which was later upgraded to a xenon strobe light. It included a dial that could be set to flash at any frequency coincident with the standard four brain wave rhythms. It had powerful hypnotic qualities and soon studies on hypnotic induction (Kroger & Schneider, 1959; Lewerenz, 1963; Sadove, 1963; Margolis, 1966) as well as altered perception and consciousness (Freedman & Marks, 1965; Glicksohn, 1986; Richardson & McAndrew, 1990) were published.

As EEG equipment improved, there was a renewed interest in the brain's evoked electrical response to photic stimulation, and a flurry of studies were completed (Barlow, 1960; Van der Tweel, 1965; Kinney, McKay, Mensch, & Luria, 1973; Townsend, 1973; Donker et al., 1978; Frederick et al., 1999). Studies into evoked potentials from auditory stimulation also generated interest, although not to the same degree as studies involving photic stimulation (Chatrian, Petersen, & Lazarte, 1959).

Additional studies explored the use of photic stimulation to induce hypnotic trance (Kroger & Schneider, 1959; Lewerenz, 1963), to augment anesthesia during surgery (Sadove, 1963) and to reduce pain, control gagging, and accelerate healing in dentistry (Margolos, 1966). More recently, the induction of dissociation was explored (Leonard, Telch, & Harrington, 1999, 2000). This provided an improved understanding to the process of helping persons with dissociative pathology to desensitize and to the development of better techniques for rapidly relaxing people suffering from trauma and posttraumatic stress disorder (Siever, 2003).

In 1984, Comptronic Devices Limited of Edmonton, Alberta, Canada (presently named "Mind Alive, Inc.") released the "Digital Audio-Visual Integration Device" (DAVID1), which was initially used for hypnotic induction, and to reduce anxiety and stage fright in performing arts students at the University of Alberta. The "light and sound" (L&S) market, as it was known at that time, was in its infancy then, and resided primarily within the unscientific "new age" sector. However, since the discovery of entrainment by Adrian and Matthews, a considerable number of clinical L&S studies have been published. Nonetheless, entrainment has yet to receive significant acceptance in medical arena, despite much off-label prescriptions by medical doctors. This prompted the author to write a book *The Rediscovery of Audio-Visual Entrainment Technology* (Siever, 2000). As reflected in the title, I have since renamed this phenomenon "audio-visual entrainment" or AVE, which occurs when any given frequency of stimulation is reflected in coincident brain wave activity, as observable in a QEEG record, and also often observable on a traditional EEG.

CLINICAL OUTCOMES

AVE studies are far more prolific than some might imagine. Many clinical studies on AVE exist today, encompassing pain (Twittey & Siever, 1998) and fibromyalgia (Berg et al., 1999), Seasonal Affective Disorder (Siever, 2004), and attentional disorders (Carter & Russell, 1993; Budzynski & Tang, 1998; Joyce, 2001). One study of 99 children showed that treatment with AVE was more effective for inattention than psychostimulant medications such as Ritalin and Adderall (Micheletti, 1998). Another study (n = 30) provided group treatment for ten children at a time who had attention deficits (Joyce & Siever, 2000). Pre and post treatment results based on overall Test of Variables of Attention (TOVA) scores are shown in Figure 7.1. The results exceeded those of six leading neurofeedback studies (Siever, 2003) and at 10 percent of the cost of neurofeedback, as ten children were being treated simultaneously (Figure 7.2).

Jaw tension and degradation of the joint and its cartilage, more formally known as temporo-mandibular dysfunction (TMD), is often a direct physiological outcome in response to stress (Yemm, 1969). Figure 7.3 shows nighttime teeth grinding, or bruxism, of an individual in relation to daily stress. Audio entrainment plus EMG biofeedback has been shown to directly reduce the symptoms of TMD (Manns, Miralles, & Adrian, 1981). Many of those with TMD show dysponesis or bracing (tensing up) when asked to relax (Thomas & Siever, 1989). This can be seen in Figure 7.4, which shows finger cooling and increased masseter muscle tension during the "relaxation request" portion of the study. Note that AVE applied at 10 Hz produced rapid muscle relaxation and finger temperature warming.

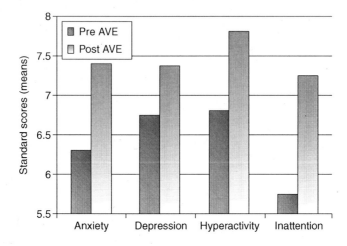

FIGURE 7.1. Results of the "Joyce" study.

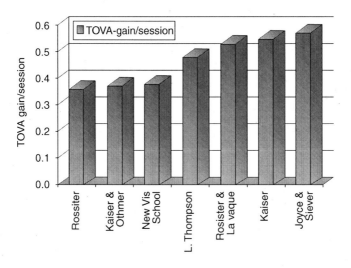

FIGURE 7.2. Comparison of NF & AVE studies.

AVE has also been shown to reduce jaw tension (Siever, 2003) during wide-mouth opening. AVE has been used to reduce jaw pain, patient anxiety, and heart rate during dental procedures (Morse & Chow, 1993). Results for heart are shown in Figure 7.5. With alpha AVE

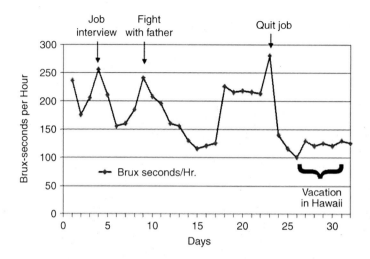

FIGURE 7.3. Daily stress and nocturnal bruxism.

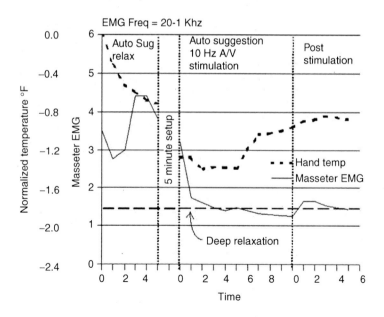

FIGURE 7.4. Masseter muscle tension.

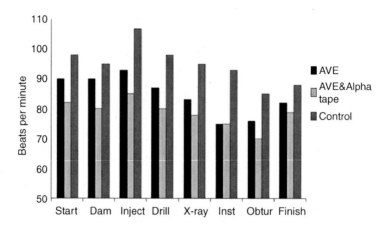

FIGURE 7.5. Heart rate during a root-canal procedure.

alone, heart rate was reduced significantly. With increased dissociation by listening to a relaxation tape, heart rate was further reduced.

AVE lends itself very well to stabilizing panic and anxiety. When using white light as the stimulus, all measures of finger temperature, EMG, EDR, and heart-rate variability (HRV) are dramatically improved within ten minutes. HRV has been shown to be a powerful indicator of autonomic arousal (McCraty, Atkinson, & Tiller, 1995; Moss, 2004). HRV training was based on paced breathing in ten-second (0.1 Hz) breath cycles. Combining AVE at alpha frequencies with breathing paced from a timed heartbeat sound, heard through headphones, has provided reason to believe that this combination produces much better outcomes in heart-rate variability (HRV) than HRV training alone and is therefore a powerful treatment modality in the treatment of anxiety.

The following graphs from the Freeze Framer system are divided into four quadrants. The upper left window shows raw data of actual heart rate fluctuations. In the lower left window is a graphical "score" of one's HRV. The lower right window depicts the heart rate in beats per minute plus an "entrainment ratio," which is based on smoothness of the heart rate variance, the steadiness of that variance and the amount of consistence of variance with breathing (10 to 15 bpm swing). The upper right window shows a spectral analysis. Power at various frequencies indicates breathing power and autonomic arousal.

Shown in Figure 7.6 are the pre-AVE findings of a woman suffering from both high anxiety and posttraumatic stress disorder (PTSD). Her life was disrupted when police charged her husband with molesting two girls (of ages six and eight years) and possessing explicit child pornography on their computer. She moved away and filed for divorce. Her "ex" is aggressive and blames her for his "problem," contending he had done nothing wrong and that, in actuality, the girls seemed interested. The court has awarded him alternate weekends with her eight-year old son and six-year old daughter. Figure 7.7 shows her rapid relaxation response to AVE at an alpha/theta frequency.

Figures 7.8 and 7.9 show a 31-year old woman with a history of shyness and a trauma in grade 3 induced by a cruel teacher, who singled out and berated her on a constant basis. As the girl "fell to pieces," she became the target of other children, and was eventually unable to ride the school bus. As an adult, she continues to see herself as a failure in all aspects of her life. Upon her first arrival for therapy, she was crying and mildly hysterical, lashing out at any hint that she might be a worthwhile human being. She was given two 5-minute, 10-second

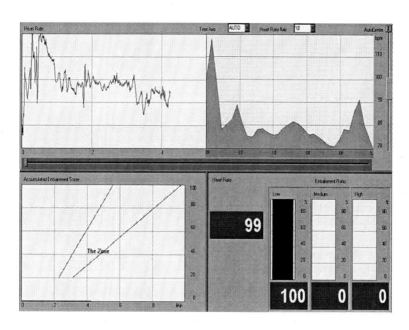

FIGURE 7.6. HRV pre AVE.

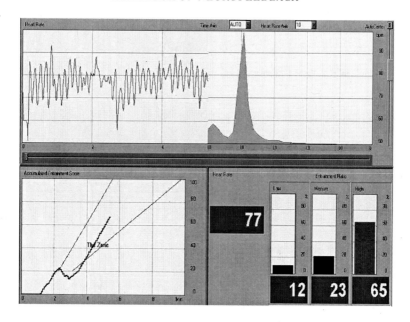

FIGURE 7.7. HRV during alpha AVE.

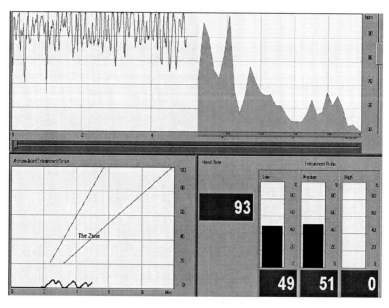

FIGURE 7.8. Trial #2-HRV profile with paced breathing during alpha AVE.

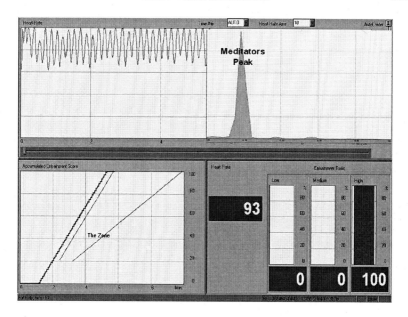

FIGURE 7.9. HRV profile following one week of paced breathing during alpha AVE.

breathing cycle AVE sessions in succession. Her performance was considerably poorer on the second trial, as her fear of failure increased (as shown in Figure 7.8). However, following one week of practice at home, during an alpha/theta AVE session with paced breathing, she showed an ability to relax and had mastered her breathing and HRV (Figure 7.9).

Cognitive decline in older adults is an ever-growing problem, because not only the numbers of older adults are expanding, but also longer life increases the likelihood of loss of memory and decline in cognitive performance. Cerebral blood flow has been shown to drop with age (Hagstadius & Risberg, 1989; Gur et al., 1987), as shown in Figure 7.10. It has also been shown that an increase in overall theta activity is the best and earliest indicator of cognitive decline (Prichep, et al., 1994). Budzynski and Budzynski (2001) have shown that randomized AVE or more appropriately audio-visual stimulation (AVS) produces pronounced cognitive improvements in seniors with age-related cognitive decline (Figure 7.11).

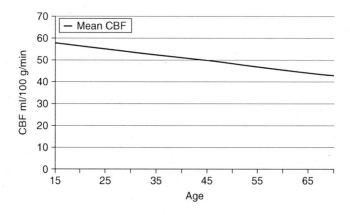

FIGURE 7.10. CBF with age.

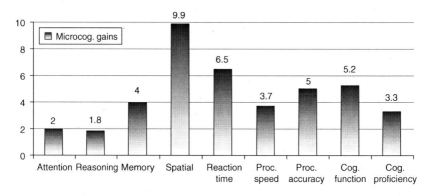

FIGURE 7.11. Microcog results following AVE.

Falls are the leading cause of injuries and injury-related deaths among persons aged 65 years and older (Fife & Barancik, 1985; Hoyert, Kochanek, & Murphy, 1999). They are the cause of 95 percent of hip fractures in senior women (Stevens & Olsen, 1999). Hip fractures, in turn, are associated with decreased mobility, onset of depression (Scaf-Klomp et al., 2003), diminished quality of life, and premature death (Zuckerman, 1996). A study by Berg and Siever (2004), with results shown in Figures 7.12 and 7.13, utilized a stimulus at 18 Hz in the right visual fields and right headphone (left brain stimulation) and a stimulus at 10 Hz in the left visual fields and left headphone (right

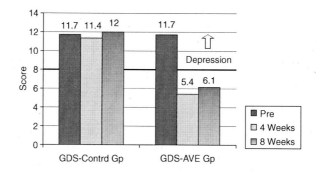

FIGURE 7.12. Geriatric depression scale.

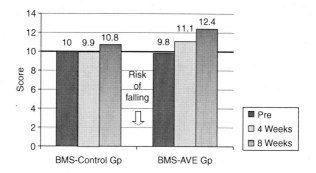

FIGURE 7.13. Balance mean scores.

brain stimulation) during a 30-minute preprogrammed session. This approach normalized the asymmetry in brain "alpha" activity that is typical of depression (Rosenfeld, 1997). This was seen 20 minutes later in QEEG records; and subjective case reports suggest the effects may last up to three or four days. Depression as recorded on the Geriatric Depression Scale (GDS) was reduced significantly (Figure 7.12). Balance and gait were measured using the Tinetti Assessment Tool (Tinetti, 1986). Figure 7.13 shows the improvement in balance as seen on the Balance Mean Scores (BMS). As depression lifted, balance and gait improved.

A study of change during fifty migraine headaches of seven migraine sufferers (all with premigraine auras and periodic vomiting) showed that thirty-minute AVE sessions reduced migraine duration from a pretreatment average of 6 to 35 minutes (Anderson, 1989). Forty-nine of the migraines were decreased in severity and 36 were stopped. The participants generally preferred alpha frequencies and brighter intensity of the lights. Since then, some clinicians have successfully treated hundreds of migraine sufferers with alpha or alpha/theta AVE.

To date, a great number of AVE related clinical studies have been completed and more studies are in progress. Studies, with clinical implications, including sample sizes and participant ages, are listed in Table 7.1.

APPLYING AVE WITH NEUROFEEDBACK

Neurofeedback (NF) and AVE complement each other. Many practitioners use photic entraining eyesets with view holes during NF sessions. By manually adjusting the AVE frequency to be the same as the NF augment (reward) frequency, a patient can get a sense of what it "feels" like to produce that particular frequency, which in turn speeds

TABLE 7.1. AVE related clinical implications including sample sizes and participant ages.

Participant category	Sample size
Attention deficit disorder	4 (n = 359, school children)
Academic performance in college students	2 (n = 22, college students)
Improved cognitive performance in seniors	1 (n = 40, from two seniors' homes)
Reduced falling in seniors	1 (n = 80, seniors)
Dental—during dental procedures	2 (n = 36)
Temporo-mandibular dysfunction	2 (n = 43, middle-aged)
Seasonal affective disorder	1 (n =74, middle-aged)
Pain and fibromyalgia	3 (n = 66, middle-aged)
Insomnia	1 (n = 0, middle-aged)
PTSD	~600 cases (public, police, and military)
Migraine headache	1 (n = 7)
Hypertension	1 (n = 28)

up the NF process considerably. Other clinicians have their patients use AVE on a take-home basis. Regardless of the approach, clinicians who combine AVE with NF report that the typical forty-session NF process often may be reduced to ten NF sessions. This, of course, saves the client money and allows the practitioner a much greater percentage of the population that can now afford neurotherapy. Many people are also too tense to relax and/or too unstable to practice NF. The use of AVE in the first couple of weeks of training can sharply decrease their tension and reduce the frustration that many patients experience during the early sessions of NF. The new generation of AVE equipment now allows the clinician to install only those sessions desired and the number of times the session may be replayed, at which time the session stops running, and the patient must return for a "recharge."

PSYCHOPHYSIOLOGY OF AUDIO-VISUAL ENTRAINMENT

AVE is believed to achieve its effects through several mechanisms simultaneously. These include the following:

1. altered EEG activity
2. dissociation/hypnotic induction
3. limbic stabilization
4. increases in neurotransmitters
5. (possible) increased dendritic growth
6. altered cerebral blood flow

Mechanisms of Audio-Visual Entrainment

All sensory information, except that of smell, must pass through the thalamus in order to gain access into other brain regions. Audio, visual, and tactile stimulation all excite electrical potentials within the thalamus and this is loosely known as brain wave entrainment. AVE of course, does not include tactile stimulation. In order for entrainment to occur, one must present constant, repetitive stimuli of proper frequency and sufficient strength to "excite" the thalamus. These stimuli do not transfer energy directly into the cortex as TV and radio waves do into a tuned circuit, nor in the same manner as placing a tuning fork near another tuning fork that is vibrating at the same frequency thus making the silent fork "hum" as well. The direct transmission of energy from AVE only goes so far as to excite retinal cells in the eyes and pressure sensitive cilia within the cochlea of the ears. The nerve pathways from the eyes and ears carry the elicited electrical potentials into the thalamus. From there, the entrained electrical activity within the thalamus is "amplified" and distributed throughout other limbic areas and the cerebral cortex via the *cortical thalamic loop*. In essence, AVE involves the continuous electrical response of the brain in relation to the stimulus frequency, plus the mathematical representation (harmonics) of the stimulus wave shape. Figure 7.14 shows the visual pathways for visual entrainment. Figure 7.15 shows an occipital record of square wave visual entrainment at 2, 4, 8, 12, and 20 Hz.

Effects of Audio-Visual Entrainment

Altered EEG Activity

AVE effects on the EEG are primarily found frontally, over the sensorimotor strip, and in parietal (somatosensory) regions, and slightly less within the prefrontal cortex. It is within these areas where executive function, motor activation, and somatosensory (body) awareness

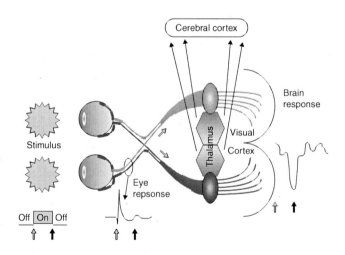

FIGURE 7.14. Visual pathways.

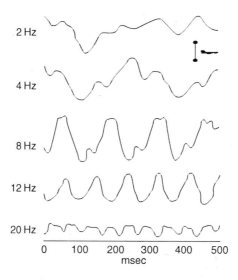

FIGURE 7.15. Visual entrainment.

are primarily mediated. It is believed this is why AVE lends itself well for the treatment of such a wide variety of disorders including PTSD, panic, anxiety, depression, cognitive decline, and attentional disorders. Eyes-closed AVE at 18.5 Hz has been shown to increase EEG brain wave activity by 49 percent at the vertex (CZ) (the only site examined in this study). Auditory entrainment at the vertex (with the eyes closed) produced an increase in EEG brain wave activity by 21 percent (Frederick et al., 1999).

Figure 7.16 shows the thalamic distribution of EEG signal during AVE (visual and auditory stimulation) at 8 Hz. Notice that the highest activity is in frontal, central, and parietal areas as indicated on the legend. Because square/sine wave photic stimulation was used (Figure 7.17), a smaller magnitude, second harmonic appears at 16 Hz.

Dissociation

Dissociation occurs in varying degrees: when we meditate, exercise, enter a hypnotic trance, read a good book, become involved in a movie, or enjoy a sporting event. We get drawn into the present moment and let go of thoughts relating to our daily hassles, hectic schedules, paying rent, urban noise, worries, threats, or anxieties and

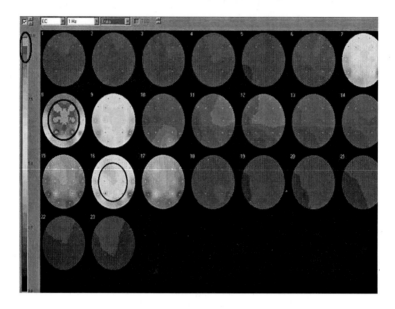

FIGURE 7.16. Brain map in 1Hz bins during 8 Hz AVE (SKIL database-eyes closed).

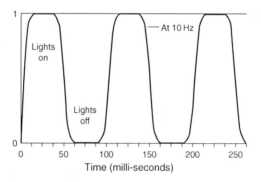

FIGURE 7.17. Semi-sine waveform.

the accompanying, often unhealthy, mental chatter. Dissociation involves a "disconnection" of self from thoughts and somatic awareness, for example, as is experienced during deep meditation. As dissociation begins (after approximately four to eight minutes) from properly applied AVE, a *restabilization* effect occurs—where muscles relax, electrodermal activity decreases, peripheral blood flow stabilizes (hand temperature normalizes to 32 to 33°C), breathing becomes diaphragmatic and slow, and heart rate becomes uniform and smooth. Visual entrainment alone, in the lower alpha frequency range (7 to 10 Hz), has been shown to easily induce hypnosis (Lewerenz, 1963); and it has been shown that nearly 80 percent of subjects entered into either a light or deep hypnotic trance within six minutes during alpha AVE (Kroger & Schneider, 1959), as shown in Figure 7.18. Additional studies have shown that AVE provides an excellent medium for achieving an altered state of consciousness (Glicksohn, 1987).

Psychologists often look for ways to induce dissociation in their clients as a part of fear and phobia treatment. Inducing dissociation using AVE delivered by the DAVID1 was found to be more effective than dot staring or stimulus deprivation for both high and low dissociators (Leonard, Telch, & Harrington, 1999) in raising dissociative scores on the Acute Dissociation Index (as shown in Figure 7.19).

Furthermore, Leonard completed a second study with people who experience dissociative anxiety (Leonard, Telch, & Harrington, 2000) as measured on the Dissociative Sensitivity Index (DSI). People with dissociative anxiety feel a need to have a sense of control in their lives and become anxious or panicky when they dissociate, be it driving home, at the office, or in a clinical setting. Leonard and her colleagues clinically dissociated people who become anxious when dissociating,

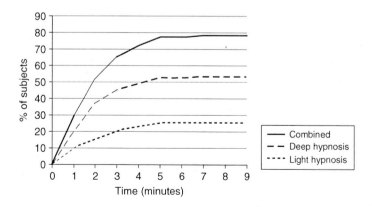

FIGURE 7.18. Photic stimulation induction of hypnotic trance (Kroger & Schneider, 1959).

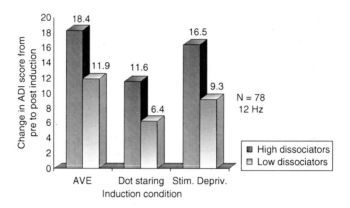

FIGURE 7.19. AVE induced dissociation (Leonard et al., 1999).

by using a DAVID *Paradise* Hemistep alpha session. As expected, the participants' perceived anxiety (ADI-Anx) had almost doubled by the end of the AVE session. The surprise, however, was that the participants' heart rate actually decreased, contrary to normal anxiety reactions (Figure 7.20). Thus, AVE may prove useful as a means of decreasing the somatic components of anxiety even during perceived anxiety.

Limbic Stabilization

Because AVE produces hand-temperature normalization, muscle relaxation, reduced electrodermal activity, reduced heart rate, and reduced hypertension, it is speculated that AVE may produce a calming effect on limbic structures, particularly the amygdala and hypothalamus.

The amygdala is responsible for the activation of the fight-or-flight response, and the hypothalamus controls all autonomic functioning including muscle tension, electrodermal response, heart rate, arterial tone, body temperature, eating, and satiety, all of which are dramatically affected during fear, anxiety, and stress (McClintic, 1978). Figure 7.21 shows increased finger temperature. Figure 7.22 shows reduced forearm tension, and Figure 7.23 shows decreased electrodermal response using white-light AVE (DAVID system) at alpha frequencies. Notice how the normalization effect begins to take place after roughly six minutes of AVE.

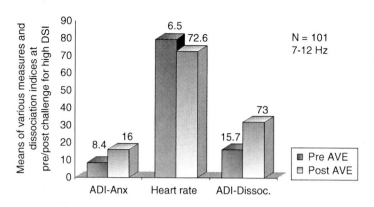

FIGURE 7.20. Dissociative anxiety and somatic arousal (Leonard et al., 2000).

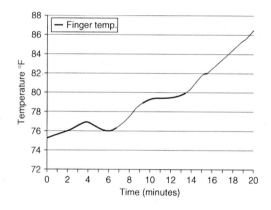

FIGURE 7.21. Finger temperature levels.

NEUROTRANSMITTER CHANGES

People under the influence of long-term anxiety eventually develop hypoadrenalis or *adrenal fatigue* as they slip into depression and lethargy. This depressed, lethargic condition is highly correlated with a loss of both serotonin and norepinephrine. In one AVE study, blood serum levels of serotonin, endorphine, and melatonin all rose considerably (Shealy et al., 1989), following 10 Hz, white-light photic stimulation (as shown in Figure 7.24). Several clinical studies showed

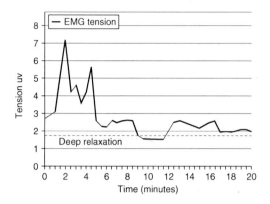

FIGURE 7.22. Forearm EMG levels.

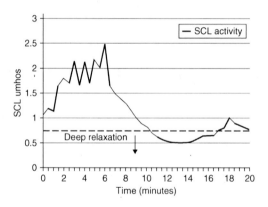

FIGURE 7.23. Reduced electrodermal activity during alpha AVE.

declines in depression, anxiety, and/or suicidal ideation following a treatment program using AVE (e.g., Gagnon & Boersma, 1992; Berg & Siever, 2004).

Dendritic Growth

There is evidence that stimulating neurons with mild electrical stimulation promotes growth of dendrites and dendritic shaft synapses in the cells being stimulated (Beardsley, 1999; Lee, Schottler,

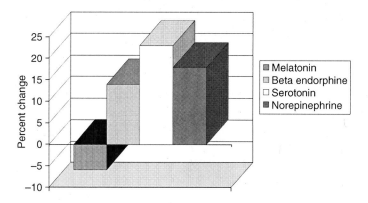

FIGURE 7.24. Changes in neurotransmitter activity following 10 Hz photic stimulation for 30 minutes.

Oliver, & Lynch, 1980). Studies do not yet exist on the influence of AVE on dendritic growth, although it is suspected because many people with autism, palsy, stroke, and aneurysm have regained significant motor and cognitive function following a treatment program of AVE (Russell, 1996).

Changes in Cerebral Blood Flow and Metabolism

SPECT and FMRI imaging show that hypoperfusion of cerebral blood flow (CBF) is associated with many forms of mental disorders (Rubin, Sacheim, Nobler, & Moeller, 1994), including anxiety, depression (Wu et al., 1992; Cohen et al., 1992), attentional problems (Teicher et al., 2000), behavior disorders, and impaired cognitive function (Mortel et al., 1994; Hirsch et al., 1997). AVE has been shown to increase brain glucose metabolism overall by 5 percent, and to increase CBF in the striate cortex, peaking with a 28 percent increase at 7.8 Hz (Fox & Raichle, 1985) as shown in Figure 7.25. This, coincidentally, is the *Schumann Resonance,* the frequency that electromagnetic radiation propagates around the earth (Schumann, 1952; Bliokh, Nikolaenko, & Filippov, 1980; Sentman, 1987). In addition, AVE has been shown to increase CBF throughout various other brain regions, including frontal areas (Mentis et al., 1997; Sappey-Marinier et al., 1992).

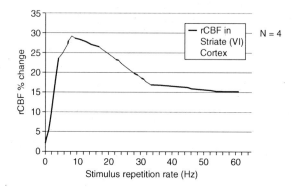

FIGURE 7.25. Changes in CBF following photic stimulation at various frequencies.

SIDE EFFECTS OF AVE

Side effects from exposure to AVE are relatively few. The most common may be a mild headache during the first few times of use, which may easily be eliminated by drinking a large glass of water 15 minutes prior to an AVE session. Another side effect may be orthostatic hypotension or low blood pressure from being extremely relaxed. This too, is easily eliminated by allowing the user a few minutes to "wake up" at the end of a session before standing. People with dissociative anxiety have a tendency to get anxious during an AVE session. These people need to be eased into the AVE experience by first learning to relax and breathe, and perhaps experience dual-induction hypnosis or alpha/theta training. A more serious reaction to AVE is that of improved organ functioning. On occasion, people with Type 2 diabetes or hypothyroidism, as is sometimes seen in those with fibromyalgia, have experienced a return of organ function and had an abreaction to their medications.

The fact that AVE is able to easily and dramatically affect brain wave activity also allows it to generate an epileptic seizures or photoconvulsive response (PCR) in those who are prone. Photic-induced seizures in adults are roughly 1 in 10,000 (Jeavons, Bishop, & Harding, 1986), and about 1 in 4,000 of those aged from 5 to 24 years (Newmark & Penry, 1979). Care must, therefore, be taken when delivering photic stimulation. Physiological photic stimulators generally used to induce seizures employ a Xenon strobe light that reaches maximum brightness within 50 microseconds at intensities of 10,000-300,000 lux. Harding and Jeavons (1994) found that peak photo-convulsive response (PCR) sensitivity occurs from 15 to 20 flashes per second. Red flicker in particular provokes an increased PCR relative to other wavelengths (Carterette & Symmes, 1952; Bickford, Daly, & Keith, 1953; Marshall, Walker, & Livingston, 1953; Pantelakis, Bower, & Jones, 1962; Brausch & Ferguson, 1965; Harley, Baird, & Freedman, 1967; Takahashi & Tsukahara, 1972a, 1973, 1976). Ruuskanen-Uoti (1994) reported on a person who developed seizure while using a "light and sound" machine utilizing square wave stimulation delivered by red light emitting diodes (LEDs). Takahashi and Tsukahara (1976) also observed that red light stimulation was superior in producing PCRs than stroboscopic (white) light. They also found that emerging spike and wave activity associated with the onset of a seizure could be inhibited by low levels of blue light. In addition to increased risk of seizure, square wave photic stimulation produces harmonic activity in the brain, whereas sine wave stimulation produces a sine wave-like response (insignificant harmonic activity). Van der Tweel and Lunel (1965), Townsend (1973), Donker et al. (1978) and Regan (1965) all agree that sine-wave modulated light eliminates the problem of anxiety-producing harmonics generated within the neocortex. Of these sine wave stimulation studies, the concern of inducing seizures is completely omitted from the studies. In the raw EEGs shown in the studies, there are no signs of epileptiform activity or any discussion about it. To address the concerns of eliciting a photic-induced seizure, the eyesets used in the DAVID systems have a slowed turn-on and turn-off time of about 15 msec. Recently, a sine wave stimulation option has been added to the programming of a session.

SUMMARY AND CONCLUSIONS

In conclusion, a large and growing body of research and clinical experience demonstrates that AVE quickly and effectively modifies conditions of high autonomic (sympathetic and parasympathetic) activation and under- and over-aroused states of mind, bringing about a return to homeostasis. AVE may be used alone or with hypnotic suggestions on tape or CD, with live suggestions via a microphone, in conjunction with neurofeedback or along with breathing exercises. AVE is believed to exert a powerful influence on brain/mind stabilization and normalization by means of increased cerebral blood flow, increased levels of certain neurotransmitters, and by normalizing EEG activity. AVE is proving to be a safe and cost-effective treatment, especially for the large number of disorders associated with dysfunctions of the central and autonomic nervous systems.

REFERENCES

Adrian, E. & Matthews, B. (1934). The Berger rhythm: Potential changes from the occipital lobes in man. *Brain, 57,* 355-384.

Anderson, D. (1989). The treatment of migraine with variable frequency photic stimulation. *Headache, 29,* 154-155.

Barlow, J. (1960). Rhythmic activity induced by photic stimulation in relation to intrinsic alpha activity of the brain in man. *Electroencephalography and Clinical Neurophysiology, 12,* 317-326.

Bartley, S. (1934). Relation of intensity and duration of brief retinal stimulation by light to the electrical response of the optic cortex of the rabbit. *American Journal of Physiology, 108,* 397-408.

Bartley, S. (1937). Some observations on the organization of the retinal response. *American Journal of Physiology, 120,* 184-189.

Beardsley, T. (1999). Getting wired. *Scientific American, 280,* 6, 24-25.

Berg, K., Mueller, H., Seibel, D., & Siever, D. (1999). Outcome of medical methods, audio-visual entrainment, and nutritional supplementation in the treatment of fibromyalgia syndrome. In-house manuscript. Mind Alive Inc., Edmonton, Alberta, Canada.

Berg, K. & Siever, D. (2004). The effect of audio-visual entrainment in depressed community-dwelling senior citizens who fall. *In-house manuscript.* Mind Alive Inc., Edmonton, Alberta, Canada.

Bickford, R., Daly, D., & Keith, H. M. (1953). Convulsive effects of light stimulation in children. *American Journal of Diseases of Children, 86,*170-183.

Bliokh, P., Nikolaenko, A., & Filippov, Y. (1980). *Schumann resonances in the earth-ionosphere cavity.* London: Peter Perigrinus.

Brausch, C. & Ferguson, J. (1965). Color as a factor in light-sensitive epilepsy. *Neurology, 15,* 154-164.

Budzynski, T. H. & Tang, J. (1998). Biolight effects on the EEG. *SynchroMed Report.* Seattle, WA.

Budzynski, T. & Budzynski, H. (2001). Brain brightening—preliminary report, December 2001. In-house manuscript. Mind Alive Inc. Edmonton, Alberta, Canada.

Carter, J. & Russell, H. (1993). A pilot investigation of auditory and visual entrainment of brain wave activity in learning disabled boys. *Texas Researcher, 4,* 65-72.

Carterette, E. C. & Symmes, D. (1952). Symposium: Photo-metrazol activation of electroencephalogram; Color as experimental variable in photic stimulation. *Electroencephalography and Clinical Neurophysiology, 4,* 289-296.

Chatrian, G., Petersen, M., & Lazarte, J. (1959). Response to clicks from the human brain: Some depth electrographic observations. *Electroencephalography and Clinical Neurophysiology, 12,* 479-489.

Cohen, R. Gross, M., & Nordahl, T. (1992). Preliminary data on the metabolic brain pattern of patients with winter seasonal affective disorder. *Archives of General Psychiatry, 49,* 545-552.

Donker, D., Njio, L., Storm Van Leewan, W., & Wieneke, G. (1978). Interhemispheric relationships of responses to sine wave modulated light in normal subjects and patients. *Encephalography and Clinical Neurophysiology, 44,* 479-489.

Durup, G. & Fessard, A. (1935). L'electroencephalogramme de l'homme (The human electroencephalogram). *Annale Psychologie, 36,* 1-32.

Fife, D. & Barancik, J. I. (1985). Northeastern Ohio trauma study, 3: Incidence of fractures. *Annals of Emergency Medicine, 14,* 244-248.

Fox, P. & Raichle, M. (1985). Stimulus rate determines regional blood flow in striate cortex. *Annals of Neurology, 17*(3), 303-305.

Frederick, J., Lubar, J., Rasey, H., Brim, S., & Blackburn, J. (1999). Effects of 18.5 Hz audio-visual stimulation on EEG amplitude at the vertex. *Journal of Neurotherapy, 3*(3), 23-27.

Freedman, S. & Marks, P. (1965). Visual imagery produced by rhythmic photic stimulation: Personality correlates and phenomenology. *British Journal of Psychology, 56*(1), 95-112.

Gagnon, C. & Boersma, F. (1992). The use of repetitive audio-visual entrainment in the management of chronic pain. *Medical Hypnoanalysis Journal, 7,* 462-468.

Glicksohn, J. (1986-1987). Photic driving and altered states of consciousness: An exploratory study. *Imagination, Cognition, and Personality, 6*(2), 167-182.

Goldman, G., Segal, J., & Segalis, M. (1938). L'action d'une excitation inermittente sur le rythme de Berger. (The effects of intermittent excitation on the Berger rhythms (EEG rhythms). *C.R. Societe de Biologie Paris, 127,* 1217-1220.

Gur, R. C., Gur, R. E., Obrist, W., Skolnick, B., & Reivich, M. (1987). Age and regional blood flow at rest and during cognitive activity. *Archives of General Psychiatry, 44,* 617-621.

Hagstadius, S. & Risberg, J. (1989). Regional cerebral blood flow characteristics and variations with age in resting normal subjects. *Brain and Cognition, 10,* 28-43.

Harding, F. A. & Jeavons, P. M. (1994). *Photosensitive epilepsy, New Edition.* Suffolk: Lavenham Press Ltd.

Harley, R., Baird, H., & Freedman, R. (1967). Self-induced photogenic epilepsy. Report of four cases. *Archives of Opthalmology, 78,* 730-737.

Hirsch, C., Bartenstein, P., Minoshima, S., Willoch, F., Buch, K., Schad, D., Schwaiger, M., & Kurk, A. (1997). Reduction of regional cerebral blood flow and cognitive impairment in patients with Alzheimer's disease: Evaluation of an observer independent analytic approach. *Dementia and Geriatric Cognitive Disorders, 8,* 98-104.

Hoyert, D. L., Kochanek, K. D., & Murphy, S. L. (1999). Deaths: Final data for 1997. *National Vital Statistics Report 1999, 47,* 1-104.

Jasper, H. H. (1936). Cortical excitatory state and synchronism in the control of bioelectric autonomous rhythms. *Cold Spring Harbor Symposia in Quantitative Biology, 4,* 32-338.

Jeavons, P. M., Bishop, A. & Harding, G. F. A. (1986). The prognosis of photo-sensitivity. *Epliepsia, 27*(5), 569-575.

Joyce, M. (2001). New Vision School: Report to the Minnesota Department of Education, unpublished.

Joyce, M. & Siever, D. (2000). Audio-visual entrainment program as a treatment for behavior disorders in a school setting. *Journal of Neurotherapy, 4*(2) 9-15.

Jung, R. (1939). *Das Elektroencephalogram und seine klinische Anwendung.* (The electroencephalogram and its clinical application). *Nervenarzt, 12,* 569-591.

Kinney, J. A., McKay, C., Mensch, A., & Luria, S. (1973). Visual evoked responses elicited by rapid stimulation. *Encephalography and Clinical Neurophysiology, 34,* 7-13.

Kroger, W. S. & Schneider, S. A. (1959). An electronic aid for hypnotic induction: A preliminary report. *International Journal of Clinical and Experimental Hypnosis, 7,* 93-98.

Lee, K., Schottler, F., Oliver, M., & Lynch, G. (1980). Brief bursts of high-frequency stimulation produce two types of structural change in rat hippocampus. *Journal of Neurophysiology, 44*(2), 247-258.

Leonard, K., Telch, M., & Harrington, P. (1999). Dissociation in the laboratory: A comparison of strategies. *Behaviour Research and Therapy, 37,* 49-61.

Leonard, K., Telch, M., & Harrington, P. (2000). Fear response to dissociation challenge. *Anxiety, Stress, and Coping, 13,* 355-369.

Lewerenz, C. (1963). A factual report on the brain wave synchronizer. *Hypnosis Quarterly, 6*(4), 23.

Manns, A., Miralles, R., & Adrian, H. (1981). The application of audiostimulation and electromyographic biofeedback to bruxism and myofascial pain-dysfunction syndrome. *Oral Surgery, 52*(3), 247-252.

Margolis, B. (1966, June). A technique for rapidly inducing hypnosis. *CAL (Certified Akers Laboratories),* 21-24.

Marshall, C., Walker, A. E., & Livingston, S. (1953). Photgenic epilepsy: Parameters of activation. *Archives of Neurology (Chicago), 69,* 760-765.

McClintic, J. (1978). *Physiology of the human body* (p. 127). New York: John Wiley & Sons.

McCraty, R., Atkinson, M., & Tiller, W. (1995). The effects of emotion on short term heart rate variability using power spectrum analysis. *American Journal of Cardiology, 76*(14), 1089-1093.

Mentis, M., Alexander, G., Grady, C., Krasuski, J., Pietrini, P., Strassburger, T., Hampel, H., Schapiro, M., & Rapoport, S. (1997). Frequency variation of a pattern-flash visual stimulus during PET differentially activates brain from striate through frontal cortex. *Neuroimage, 5,* 116-128.

Micheletti, L. (1998). PhD dissertation, unpublished. Available through Mind Alive Inc. Edmonton, Alberta, Canada.

Morse, D. & Chow, E. (1993). The effect of the Relaxodont™ brain wave synchronizer on endodontic anxiety: Evaluation by galvanic skin resistance, pulse rate, physical reactions, and questionnaire responses. *International Journal of Psychosomatics, 40*(1-4), 68-76.

Mortel, K., Pavol, A., Wood, S., Meyer, J., Terayama, Y., Rexer, J., & Herod, B. (1994). Perspective studies of cerebral perfusion and cognitive testing among elderly normal volunteers and patients with ischemic vascular dementia and Alzheimer's disease. *Journal of Vascular Diseases, 45,* 171-180.

Moss, D. (2004). Heart rate variability (HRV) biofeedback. *Psychophysiology today. 1/2004,* 4-11.

Newmark, M. & Penry, J. (1979). *Photosensitivity and epilepsy: A review.* New York: Raven Press.

Pantelakis, S. N., Bower, B. D., & Jones, H. D. (1962). Convulsions and television viewing. *British Medical Journal, 2,* 633-638.

Pieron, H. (1982). Melanges dedicated to Monsieur Pierre Janet. *Acta Psychiatrica Belgica, 1,* 7-112.

Prichep, L., John, E., Ferris, S., Reisberg, B., Almas, M., Alper, K., & Cancro, R. (1994). Quantitative EEG correlates of cognitive deterioration in the elderly. *Neurobiology Of Aging, 15*(1), 85-90.

Regan, D. (1965). Some characteristics of average steady-state and transient responses evoked by modulated light. *Electroencephalography and Clinical Neurophysiology, 20,* 238-248.

Richardson, A. & McAndrew, F. (1990). The effects of photic stimulation and private self-consciousness on the complexity of visual imagination imagery. *British Journal of Psychology, 81,* 381-394.

Rosenfeld, P. (1997). EEG biofeedback of frontal alpha asymmetry in affective disorders. *Biofeedback, 25*(1), 8-12.

Rubin, E., Sackeim, H., Nobler, M., & Moeller, J. (1994). Brain imaging studies of antidepressant treatments. *Psychiatric Annals, 24*(12), 653-658.

Russell, H. (1996). Entrainment combined with multimodal rehabilitation of a 43-year-old severely impaired postaneurysm patient. *Biofeedback and Self Regulation, 21,* 4.

Ruuskanen-Uoti, H. & Salmi, T. (1994). Epileptic seizure induced by a product marketer as a "Brainwave Synchronizer." *Neurology, 44,* 180.

Sadove, M. S. (1963). Hypnosis in anaesthesiology. *Illinois Medical Journal,* 39-42.

Sappey-Marinier, D., Calabrese, G., Fein, G., Hugg, J., Biggins, C., & Weiner, M. (1992). Effect of photic stimulation on human visual cortex lactate and phosphates using 1H and 31P magnetic resonance spectroscopy. *Journal of Cerebral Blood Flow and Metabolism, 12*(4), 584-592.

Scaf-Klomp, W., Sanderman, R., Ormel, J., & Kempen, G. (2003). Depression in older person after fall-related injuries: a prospective study. *Age and Aging, 32,* 88-94.

Schumann, W. O. (1952). Uber die strahlungslosen eigenschwingungen einer leitenden kugel, die von einer luftshicht und einer ionospharenhulle umgeben ist. *Zeitschrift fur Naturforsch, 7a,* 149.

Sentman, D. (1987). Magnetic polarization of Schumann Resonances. *Radio Science, 22,* 595-606.

Shealy, N., Cady, R., Cox, R., Liss, S., Clossen, W., & Veehoff, D. (1989). A comparison of depths of relaxation produced by various techniques and neurotransmitters produced by brainwave entrainment. *Shealy and Forest Institute of Professional Psychology.* A study done for Comprehensive Health Care, Unpublished.

Siever, D. (1992). Jaw tension in masseter muscle during wide mandibular opening. In house manuscript. Mind Alive Inc. Edmonton, Alberta, Canada.

Siever, D. (2000). The Rediscovery of Audio-Visual Entrainment Technology. Unpublished manuscript. Available from Mind Alive Inc., Edmonton, Alberta, Canada.

Siever, D. (2003). Applying audio-visual entrainment technology for attention and learning-part III. *Biofeedback, 31,* 4, 24-29.

Siever, D. (2003). Audio visual entrainment: II. Dental studies. *Biofeedback, 31*(3), 29-32.

Siever, D. (2003) Techtalk: Matters of the heart. Spring, 2003 newsletter. Available from: http://www.mindalive.com/1_0/spring03.htm.

Siever, D. (2004). The application of audio-visual entrainment for the treatment of seasonal affective disorder, *Biofeedback, 32*(3), 32-35.

Stevens, J. & Olsen, S. (1999). Reducing falls and resulting hip fractures among older women. *Home Care Provider, 5,* 134-141.

Takahashi, T. & Tsukahara, Y. (1972a). EEG Activation by red color (in Japanese). *Igaku No Ayumi, 83,* 25-26.

Takahashi, T. & Tsukahara, Y. (1972b). Inhibitory effect of blue color on seizure discharges (in Japanese). *Igaku No Ayumi, 83,* 81-82.

Takahashi, T. & Tsukahara, Y. (1973). Study of visual epilepsy—red flicker activation and clinical EEG findings (in Japanese). *Clinical Neurology, 13,* 697-704.

Takahashi, T. & Tsukahara, Y. (1976). Influence of color on the photoconvulsive response. *Electroencephalography and Clinical Neurophysiology, 41,* 124-136.

Teicher, M., Anderson, C., Polcari, A., Glod, C., Maas, L., & Renshaw, P. (2000). Functional deficits in basal ganglia of children with attention-deficit/hyperactivity disorder shown with functional magnetic resonance imaging relaxometry. *Nature Medicine, 6*(4), 470-473.

Thomas, N. & Siever, D. (1989). The effect of repetitive audio/visual stimulation on skeletomotor and vasomotor activity. In D. Waxman, D. Pederson, I. Wilkie, & P. Meller (Eds.). *Hypnosis: 4th European congress at Oxford* (pp. 238-245). London: Whurr Publishers.

Tinetti, M. F. (1986). Performance-oriented assessment of mobility problems in elderly patients. *Journal of American Geriatric Society, 34,* 119-126.

Toman, J. (1941). Flicker potentials and the alpha rhythm in man. *Journal of Neurophysiology, 4,* 51-61.

Townsend, R. (1973). A device for generation and presentation of modulated light stimuli. *Electroencephalography and Clinical Neurophysiology, 34,* 97-99.

Twittey, M. & Siever, D. (1998). Audio/visual stimulation as a treatment for chronic pain. In-house manuscript. Mind Alive Inc. Edmonton, Alberta, Canada.

Van Der Tweel, L., & Lunel, H. (1965). Human visual responses to sinusoidally modulated light. *Encephalography and Clinical Neurophysiology, 18,* 587-598.

Walter, W. G. (1956). Color illusions and aberrations during stimulation by flickering light. *Nature, 177,* 710.

Wu, J., Gillin, J., Buchsbaum, M., Hershey, T., Johnson, J., & Bunney, W. (1992). Effect of sleep deprivation on brain metabolism of depressed patients. *American Journal of Psychiatry, 149,* 538-543.

Yemm, R. (1969). Variations in the electrical activity of the human masseter muscle occurring in association with emotional stress. *Archives of Oral Biology, 14,* 873-878.

Zuckerman, J. D. (1996). Hip fracture. *New England Journal of Medicine, 334,* 1519-1525.

Chapter 8

The ROSHI in Neurofeedback

Victoria L. Ibric
Charles J. Davis

INTRODUCTION

There are several neurofeedback-related approaches that make use of auditory and/or visual stimulation (AVS) to entrain or disentrain brain electrical activity. Some of these are used independently (see Siever, this volume), while others are used in conjunction with neurofeedback. Some of the latter employ separate equipment that simply presents light flashes from light emitting diodes (LED) embedded in goggles (or coordinated light and auditory tone stimuli) of a frequency at which it is considered important to entrain the client's brain waves for the purpose of speeding up, or assisting, neurofeedback training. For example, it might be considered important to entrain a higher concentration of the alpha frequency to expedite relaxation, or to disentrain excessive theta when excessive theta power seems to be contributing to problems with sustained attention. In other approaches, equipment detects the client's EEG activity and then adjusts light and/or sound stimuli in a manner designed to decrease abnormalities such as excessive amplitude at certain frequencies. One of the better known and unique of these is the ROSHI, which involves not only EEG-guided light stimulation to adjust both amplitude and phase, but also makes use of electromagnetic stimulation (EM) to modify abnormal brain electrical activity. The purpose of this chapter is to introduce the reader to this enhanced type of neurofeedback. Some of the rationale behind the ROSHI approach and a brief history of the evolution of

Handbook of Neurofeedback
© 2007 by The Haworth Press, Inc. All rights reserved.
doi:10.1300/5889_08

ROSHI instruments will be presented, followed by discussion of some basic details of the process, and presentation of a few case histories, which illustrate the effectiveness of this approach with a variety of client types.

THEORETICAL VIEWPOINT

An essential aspect of the theory behind the ROSHI approach is that all of one's EEG activity is a reflection of his or her life experiences. Abnormal EEG activity reflects abnormal, undesirable experiences, and can take the form of excessive amplitude and chaotic phase relationships. Such EEG abnormalities frequently are associated with fatigue, anger, anxiety, depression, sleep disorders, problems with sustained attention, and/or memory loss. By using equipment that provides feedback concerning when abnormal EEG activity is decreasing, and uses light or EM stimulation to, for example, "squash" excessive power and build greater phase synchrony, one can experience positive life changes, including removal of disease symptoms and greater voluntary control of future behaviors. In other words, the ROSHI task is to normalize and stabilize one's brain electrical activity for improved, clearer thinking and more stable performance. By doing ROSHI training, a person, is, in fact, on the way to peak performance.

HISTORICAL DEVELOPMENTS

Mr. Davis, the co-author of this chapter, began writing the computer code for ROSHI in 1988. Originally, he named his invention TALOS4 MindWorks, but changed it to ROSHI after a visit to Japan where he met a Zen master referred to as ROSHI. If one remembers, TALOS4 in *Star Trek* was the land of Illusion. When he learned about the master's ability to keep his student's in the "now" or present, he decided to create a computer program that would imitate the master. Similar to being coached by a Zen master, the computer program was designed to train one's brain and "toughen you up." Most of the feedback modes embedded in this and subsequent programs are based on ideas and previous research of the following persons: Ochs (1992), Patton (1993, 1995), Peniston and Kulkowsky (1991), Lubar (1991), Green, Green, and Walters (1970), Pfurtscheller and Aranibar

(1977), Cade and Coxhead (1989), Fried (1989), Tansey (1984), Tachiki, Ochs, and Weiler (1994), Gevins et al. (1979, 1995), Monroe (1971), Fehmi (1978), and Sterman (1972, 1973). The authors apologize if others have been inadvertently omitted from this list.

There have been three generations of ROSHI instruments and procedures.

First Generation

In 1992, a company known as Advanced Neurotechnologies, Inc. was involved with training of Olympic and professional athletes using its BrainLink neurofeedback system, which incorporated the so-called Patton Protocol (Patton, 1993). This process, with its associated hardware and software, was licensed to RoshiCorp of Los Angeles for the manufacture and distribution of a fully integrated unit that would automatically implement the Patton Protocol. The resulting ROSHI system (ROSHI I) utilized an Amiga desktop computer and carried the BrainLink logo. It was featured in hundreds of publications, radio shows, and television programs worldwide. ROSHI/BrainLink training protocols for developing peak performance were used with athletes from many sports including karate, golf, baseball, ice-skating, and kayaking, and several controlled research studies were completed. In addition to the Patton Protocol, there were some 20 other preprogrammed protocols that could be explored, including enhance or inhibit protocols for beta, theta, alpha/theta, and synchrony training.

In particular, as the ROSHI/Amiga software was some of the earliest interhemispheric neurofeedback training software, which included the fastest response times available, Dick Patton felt that this software would be a perfect platform in which to embed his BrainLink peak performance training protocol. This protocol entailed the use of three proprietary frequencies that had to give feedback within 16 msec of crossing a given training threshold, putting this training beyond human volition, that is, beyond human ability to consciously thwart its effects.

In 1995, ROSHI/BrainLink began to investigate EEG in relationship to chaos theory and complex chaos "audio-visual stimulation." This came to involve EEG coupled with photostimulation (light) or electromagnetic stimulation (EM). We now refer to this as "neurofeedback enhanced by light or electromagnetic closed-loop EEG" (Ibric, 2001, 2002a,b). As initially used in the ROSHI I, this involved what we term the "discrete adaptive modality" of stimulation. The latter term was first used by Len Ochs (1992). It refers to modification of brain electrical activity by use of a program, which detects, follows, and discourages the dominant EEG frequency by use of photostimulation. The coauthor created and used a modified version of this in the ROSHI I. In that version, training was accomplished by following the dominant frequency and switching light frequency up and down a few Hertz from the dominant one every fifteen seconds. In this manner, the dominant frequency was inhibited. Since the glasses (goggles) used in presentation of the light stimuli had LEDs on each side, it was possible to also program phase relationships between the right- and left-side lights such that appropriate entrainment of phase relationships (synchrony) within a client's EEG could occur. Although this type of training has been reported to be effective (e.g., Hammond, 2000), the author has found that it produces adverse reactions in some clients with posttraumatic brain injury symptoms.

Instead of the discrete adaptive, the complex adaptive modality came to be preferred. This complex adaptive modality was the coauthor's brainchild. It involves extracting the error aspects of one's EEG, for example, features such as transients, from the wideband EEG, and feeding back to the client nonerror features of his or her brain electrical activity in the form of light flashes very much in real time. This is referred to here as "NF (neurofeedback) closed loop EEG" because the EEG activity of the client is delivered back in a closed loop mode to his or her eyes and brain as light flashes and electromagnetic waves respectively. The computer can be set to enhance or inhibit, as appropriate, any particular frequency or frequency band, thus encouraging or discouraging some particular feature of the EEG. A similar process is true for phase conjugation protocols. Phase synchrony is closely associated with "coherence," or point-to-point information transfer and agreement within the brain's neurology. This type of procedure proved to be very powerful and is usually readily accepted by clients.

Second Generation

The Standalone/ROSHI II and II+ had a new configuration, which allowed the equipment to be used with or without the ROSHI computer-driven software. In 2000, under the coauthor's supervision, the chief engineer at Photosonix was contracted to move what we refer to as complex (adaptive) routines to the then new EEG-driven ROSHI II unit. ROSHI II+ differs from the ROSHI II in that the system contains one complex (adaptive) and one discrete modality, instead of two complex (adaptive) modalities. The discrete was set to stimulate only the 40 Hz frequency.

Third Generation

The newest in the ROSHI line is the pROSHI/BB (personal ROSHI/ Brain Brightener). It was created by the second author as an entraining/ disentraining instrument, following the idea that a "good" brain should be a flexible brain. Its algorithms are based on a concept of chaos theory. Light or EM waves are presented to the client in a standardized complex (adaptive) mode as mentioned earlier for purposes of entrainment/disentrainment. This is designed to encourage the brain to imitate the sequence of frequencies presented by the pROSHI in a flexible, yet not abnormally variable manner. Therefore, the pROSHI uses the very advanced concept that the brain itself can become its own neurofeedback device, correcting its own internal errors, given the proper external (proprietary) neurostimulus.

ROSHI is the first neurofeedback instrument that used EM as closed loop-EEG-EM. Among the "Roshinis," the author is believed to have been the first to use EM for prolonged times. Specifics of several applications and protocols have been presented at conferences (Ibric, 1998, 1999, 2000, 2001, 2002a, 2004). Applications have included drug resistant sleep disorders, addictions, head injuries, and tremor.

We now use EEG-EM at low energy levels. Initially, we tried following the work of Reuven Sandyk who used picoTesla levels of pulsating transcranial stimulation, and reported good results in cases of Parkinson's disease (Sandyk, 1997a, b, c), multiple sclerosis (Sandyk, 1997d), and central pain (Sandyk, 1995). However, we noted while monitoring clients' brain electrical activity during training on the ROSHI I that the higher EM fields disturbed the activity. By lowering the EM field and keeping it between 2 and 10 mGauss, such disturbance was not noted, yet positive effects were found. For example, the tremor of one patient was observed to subside. Furthermore, use of EM at these levels was noted to coincide with stabilization of coherence measures.

Since 2001, the author has had an opportunity to apply closed loop-EEG-EM in several cases of Parkinson's disease and sleep disorders. Such electromagnetic-enhanced neurofeedback seems to produce desired outcomes especially in those cases where reaching deeper structures of the brain such as the basal ganglia, inferior olive, or pineal gland is called for, and where light stimulation proved insufficient to produce significant change. [See Ibric (1999, 2000, 2001, 2002a) for more details.]

MISCELLANEOUS INFORMATION ON ROSHI

Certain questions and concerns are among the most frequently voiced in regard to ROSHI. These will be addressed in this section from the authors' perspectives.

We often are asked about specific training protocols and electrode positions. These are chosen by taking into consideration the subjective complaints of individual patients, along with more objective data collected by cognitive testing (e.g., Test of Variables of Attention (TOVA) or Integrated Visual and Auditory Continuous Performance Test (IVA), QEEG results, and/or inspection of the EEG power presentations over the sensorimotor integration area of the cortex. Further pretraining diagnostic information is obtained by observing the Neural Efficiency Index (NEI) shown in the neural efficiency window of ROSHI equipment (sometimes referred to as the "third eye" by ROSHI users). There are many possibilities for training to enhance or inhibit EEG features that can be applied [see ROSHI manual and ROSHI on Bioexplorer (Ibric & Martin, 2002)]. More details regarding specific training modalities (protocols) will follow in the case presentations of later sections of this chapter.

How many sessions of ROSHI training are required for positive results is a frequently asked question and that is quite complicated to answer. However, the author has found that when the neurofeedback training experience is enhanced by ROSHI equipment, the number of sessions needed is lower than with traditional types of neurofeedback. In general, our approach is to train for 20 sessions, which enables establishment of a learning curve [as demonstrated by Marzano (2000)]. We then reevaluate to determine degree of progress. In more complex cases, where more than one brain area or EEG feature is in need of training the number of sessions can be as high as 100 or more. Protocols are adjusted during training to be in concordance with patient symptoms and/or QEEG information.

Another question pertains to how long positive results of ROSHI training last. From our experience, we can say that changes accomplished through such enhanced neurofeedback can be sustained for at least eight years after training is discontinued (Ibric, 2004, 2005).

Many practitioners considering using ROSHI are concerned about adverse side effects. The authors have found any such effects to be temporary and readily corrected by modifying the training protocol. Most common examples are (1) irritability during or following beta enhancement or alpha inhibition; (2) heightened sensitivity to light or sound in brain injury cases; (3) nightmares and/or flashbacks in clients suffering from post traumatic stress disorder; (4) insomnia or decreased need for sleep where protocols include beta enhancement or alpha inhibition; and (5) temporary sadness, especially following sensorimotor rhythm (SMR) (12-15 Hz) or alpha enhancement. There are some reactions occasionally seen especially with use of the pROSHI BB. There are some very sensitive individuals who cannot train for long periods of time with this equipment. They often are individuals who have sustained mechanical or chemical head injuries or who have eye disorders such as cataracts or glaucoma. In such cases, shorter training sessions should be recommended, and the light stimulation used with caution or replaced with EM.

Some pROSHI BB users report anxiety or sleep disturbances at the beginning of daily use of this equipment. In such cases, it is recommended that they train in the morning and for shorter lengths of time. Also, it is very important to consider the color of the lenses or glasses used with light stimulation in order to optimize positive effects and prevent negative effects. The authors have found that red is indicated in cases of chronic fatigue or depression, while blue-green is more useful for anxiety and certain sleep disorders.

Finally, there is the question of how ROSHI training affects the EEG and specific patient symptoms. To try to answer this, we studied effects under the following conditions:

1. ROSHI I training while EEG recorded using Neurocybernetics equipment.

2. ROSHI I training with evaluation and reevaluation using Neuro-cybernetics equipment, before and after the ROSHI I training.
3. Continuing training on Neurocybernetics equipment, but with addition of ROSHI II+ standalone.
4. Continuing Neurocybernetics training, but with addition of pROSHI.
5. QEEG recordings before, during, and after ROSHI I training.
6. QEEG recordings before, during, and after pROSHI training.

Results from each of these conditions will be discussed later in the form of case studies.

Training on Neurocybernetics Equipment Followed by Subsequent Roshi Training While Recorded on Neurocybernetics Equipment

Two case examples using this condition are presented here. The first case was of a twenty-nine year old drama student who presented with stage fright, bruxism, temporo-mandibular joint (TMJ) problems, anxiety, and panic attacks. She was taking no medications at the time of the initial evaluation. She completed 133 neurofeedback sessions, 88 using Neurocybernetics equipment and 45 with ROSHI I. Protocols used with Neurocybernetics were enhancing SMR (12-15 Hz) at sites CZ or C4, or enhancing the alpha/theta frequency at site O1. During ROSHI training, electrode positions were: (1) bilateral at F3/F4, and enhancing SMR 14 or beta 16; or (2) bilateral at C3/C4 with SMR or SMR14 enhanced; or (3) bilateral at P3/P4 with alpha (only) enhanced. The ROSHI I training was accompanied by changes in brain electrical activity (see Figure 8.1), and there were positive changes in this woman's emotional makeup. After the ROSHI experience, the patient recognized that she also suffered from posttraumatic stress disorder, and worked with a psychotherapist in regard to that. At the physical level, the bruxism and the TMJ pain were substantially lowered. She improved cognitively as well, as evidenced by the fact that she was able to finish acting school and start a brilliant drama/comedy career.

The second case or this type was an eleven-year old boy. He had a history of repeated head traumas from birth, having been born as a "blue baby," and having fallen 16 feet from a window at the age of

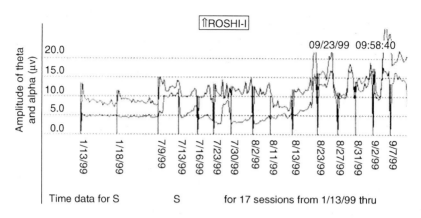

FIGURE 8.1. Case 1 on neurocybernetics (NC), alpha/theta training and ROSHI I added and NC recording continued. (In this spectral display, the theta wave is above, at about 10 μV and the alpha below, at about 5 μV).

18 months. He became a "risk-taker," and experienced numerous other accidents. His symptoms included severe dyslexia, other learning disabilities, asthma, excessive anger, depression, aggressive behaviors, and night terrors. He had been taking Ritalin, but this was stopped at the time of the initial evaluation for neurofeedback. With the eight sessions on Neurocybernetics equipment, electrodes were at C3 or F3 positions and 15-18 Hz beta was enhanced, or were placed at CZ or C4 and SMR was enhanced. The twenty-two ROSHI I sessions involved electrodes positioned bilaterally at C3/C4 with SMR or SMR14 enhanced, or at F3/F4 either inhibiting theta or enhancing beta 16. As shown in Figure 8.2, there were definite and almost immediate decreases in theta power when the ROSHI I training was initiated. An enhanced academic performance (from 1.8 to 3.4 GPA) as well as sports (golf) improvement and elimination of his asthma attacks were only some of the consequences of his NF training. This case was the subject of an article in the *ROSHI Journal, 1*(5): 1-2, June 2004.

ROSHI I Training with Evaluation and Reevaluation on Neurocybernetics, before and after the ROSHI I sessions

Case 3 involved a 78-year old man with a complex medical history. He had past surgeries for prostate/bladder cancers and heart valve re-

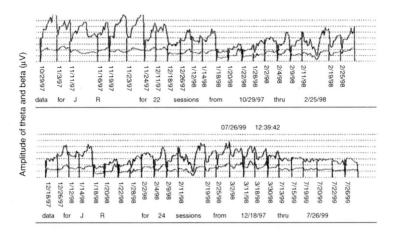

FIGURE 8.2. Case 2 on neurocybernetics (NC) beta/theta training and ROSHI I added and NC recording continued (In this spectral display theta in above and beta below). *Source: ROSHI Journal*, 1(5): 1-2, June 2004.

placement, and had suffered from Parkinson's disease for 13 years. He was on dopamine replacement therapy, and other medications: Miramex, Cinemet, Atenolol, Furosemide, potassium, and aspirin. At intake, he had the following symptoms: neck and postural distortion, shuffling gait, and resting tremor of both hands, more marked on the left. Although he reported mild stress, no cognitive or emotional dysfunctions were mentioned or noted. The neurofeedback training was done for 40 sessions, two on Neurocybernetics equipment and 38 on ROSHI I. Protocols were as follows: On Neurocybernetics, SMR was enhanced at site CZ. On ROSHI I, using electromagnetic and light closed loop EEG, SMR was enhanced at C1/C2 or C3/C4, and alpha only was enhanced at C3/C4, while high beta only was inhibited at F3/F4 or F7/F8 or Sync enhanced.

After the 38 ROSHI I sessions, this man's brain electrical activity changed significantly as can be seen in the comparison between Figures 8.3 and 8.4. These figures represent "snapshots" taken with use of Neurocybernetics equipment during the early Neurocybernetics training and after 38 ROSHI I sessions, respectively. The patient's spasticity, gait, and tremor improved. The tremor was checked session-by-session by having the patient draw the Archimedes spirals before

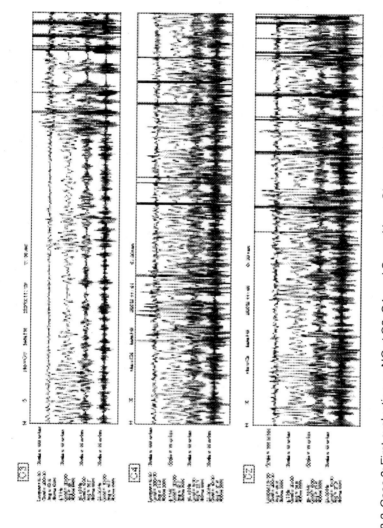

FIGURE 8.3. Case 3: First evaluation on NC at C3, C4, and Cz positions. Observe the variability over the left hemisphere, and high amplitudes of theta, beta, and high beta, mostly over the right hemisphere and at vertex. *Note:* Snapshot was recoded on Neurocybernetics.

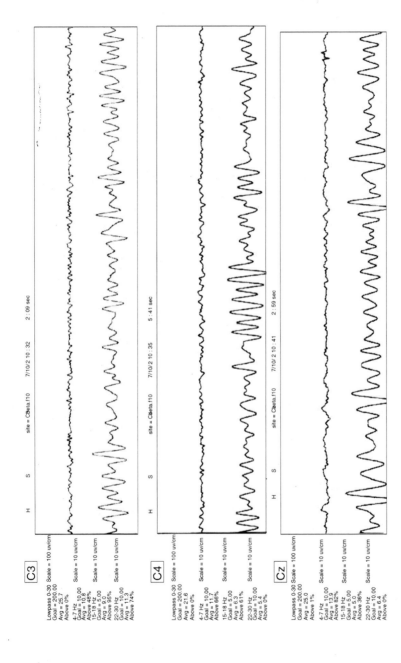

FIGURE 8.4. Case 3: Re-Evaluation on NC post 38 sessions of ROSHI-I. Observe the overall normalization of this patient's EEG. *Note:* Snapshots was recorded on Neurocybernetics.

and after each session with both right and left hands. Details of this case were presented at the tenth annual conference of the Society for Neuronal Regulation (Ibric, 2002b).

Training on Neurocybernetics Equipment, but with Addition of ROSHI II+ (Standalone)

Case 4 concerned a 24-year old female entrepreneur with a history of Grave's disease, and who also had been diagnosed with temporal lobe epilepsy post-thyroid radioablation in 1996. She had tried a variety of other therapies without resolution of her symptoms, including chiropractic, acupuncture, acupressure, and various medical procedures. She had been prescribed Carbatrol and Phenobarbital. At intake, she reported the following symptoms: daily seizures, sleep disorders, forgetfulness, and sweaty palms. Results of various subjective tests indicated a very low level of stress. Results of the Integrated Visual and Auditory Continuous Performance Test (IVA) indicated that the cognitive abilities it measures were not adversely affected by her condition or medications. Protocols used with Neurocybernetics equipment included the following: electrode placement at site T3, CZ, or C3, and SMR enhanced while theta and high beta were inhibited. While on ROSHI I or II training, (1) electrodes were at CZ/C3, F3/T3, or FP1/T3, and theta (only) inhibited; or (2) electrodes were placed at F3/F4 or C3/C4 and theta (only) inhibited; or (3) electrodes were at C3/C4 with theta (only) or high beta (22 Hz and above) inhibited. Training was conducted with her eyes open, and with "true-white" glasses plugged into the ROSHI II+ standalone. As shown in Figure 8.5, there was a dramatic decrease in theta amplitude when ROSHI II+ training began, that is, after 14:21 min into the session. The frequencies of her seizures reduced (from one per day to one every other month or less). The intensity of her seizures decreased mostly while on ROSHI I, but not on ROSHI II+ standalone. Although the EEG changes were dramatic, the standalone modality was discontinued because we suspected that ROSHI II+ standalone, in feeding-back her brain waves without blocking the unhealthy frequencies, (as set by the computer) was capable of producing kindling, and thus causing seizures.

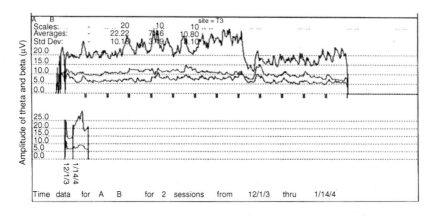

FIGURE 8.5. Case 4: Training on NC and ROSHI II+ standalone, eyes open with true white glasses was added after 14:21 min into the session.

Training on Neurocybernetics Equipment with Addition of pROSHI

Case 5 is included only to illustrate the similar effects of use of ROSHI I and pROSHI. Figure 8.6 shows effects of addition of pROSHI training 16 minutes into a training session. Comparison of Figure 8.5 with Figure 8.6 permits observation of the similar effects of the two ROSHI procedures on theta suppression and separation between beta and high beta amplitudes.

ROSHI II and pROSHI Training, with QEEG Recording Before, During, and After Training

The data on the following cases were collected in the office of the first author, and processed by Dr. William Hudspeth using his method of connectivities analysis (Hudspeth & Ibric, 2004). Three-minute samples of QEEG data were collected using Lexicor Neurosearch-24 equipment during eyes closed and/or eyes open conditions. During the ROSHI I neurofeedback, active electrodes of the ROSHI instrument were positioned at FP1/F7 and FP2/F8 (or F5/F6). Neurofeedback was enhanced by light closed loop-EEG or electromagnetic closed loop-EEG. Electrode placements were the same during pROSHI stimulation. Specific ROSHI training protocols varied, as dictated by the EEG

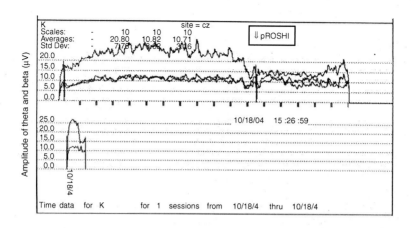

FIGURE 8.6. Case 5: Training on NC and pROSHI added after 16 min into the session, eyes open with true white glasses.

presentations on the ROSHI screen, for example, SYNC up, alpha (only) inhibit, and theta (only) inhibit. The data involving pROSHI were presented at a past conference (Hudspeth et al., 2005).

A single case study, case number 6, will be presented here to illustrate use of QEEG in planning treatment protocols, as well as QEEG changes, which can result from ROSHI training.

A 42-year old carpenter with a history of asthma, mild traumatic brain injury, left inguinal hernia, mild chronic ulcerative colitis, chronic urogenital inflammation, and chronic cocaine and marijuana use was seen for chronic pain and severe depression. Prior to neurofeedback training, he had followed medical, surgical, and acupuncture therapies. After neurofeedback training was started, medications were stopped including ibuprofen, morphine, and epinephrine for asthma. Various training protocols were used. There were nine sessions on a Neurocybernetics instrument involving SMR, beta, and alpha training and sites C4, C3, and P3. This was followed by 81 sessions with ROSHI-enhanced neurofeedback using light and electromagnetic closed loop EEG. Electrode placement/frequency combinations used were as follows: (1) electrodes at F3/F4 while inhibiting alpha only, theta only, or theta 4; (2) electrodes at P3/P4 and enhancing alpha only; (3) electrodes at C3/C4 while SMR was enhanced; (4) electrodes at

F3/F7 (or FP1/T3) and synchrony inhibited. Specific protocols were guided by initial QEEG results.

The QEEG connectivity mapping based on the eyes closed (EC) and eyes open (EO) conditions respectively are shown in Figures 8.7 and 8.8. Both indicated that the patient had a previous head injury of the coup contre-coup type. This conclusion was drawn from the presentation of hyperconnectivity over the FP1 and F7 sites and hypoconnectivity over T6 and O2, along with the location of his reported head injury, that is, impact (coup) in the right parietal/occipital area, and contre-coup in the left frontal area. Analysis done with the EC data shows that this hyper- and hypoconnectivity were present at the cortical level for all bands except beta. Subcortically, there was an extension of the hyperconnectivity to the right frontal region in the delta,

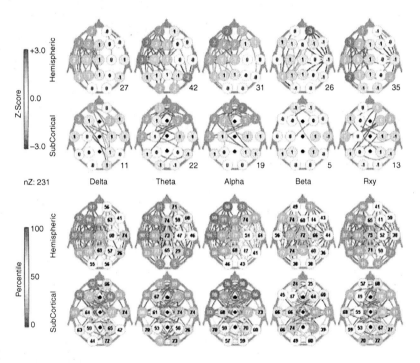

FIGURE 8.7. QEEG connectivity maps of case number 6, eyes closed (EC) shows, in the upper panel, the Z-score (nZ = 231) as average of duplicate recordings. (See also color gallery.) *Source: ROSHI Journal, 3*(1): 1-7, January 2006.

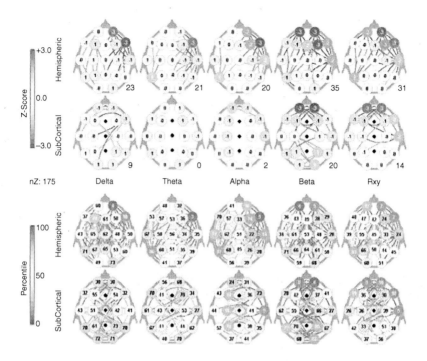

FIGURE 8.8. QEEG connectivity maps of case number 6, eyes open (EO) shows the Z-score (nZ = 175) as average of duplicate recordings. (See also color gallery.) *Source: ROSHI Journal, 3*(1): 1-7, January 2006.

theta, and alpha frequencies. The Z scores changed from EO to EC condition.

Comparisons were made between eyes closed QEEG results obtained during and after ROSHI neurofeedback training. It is obvious from comparing data shown in Figure 8.9 (during training) to that in Figure 8.10 (after ROSHI training) that Z scores were lower after training.

Comparison of coefficients of variability (CV) found before training (see Figure 8.11a and b) to those found during and after training (see Figure 8.12a and b) indicates a trend in reduction of variability. CV reduced from 105.4 pretreatment to 83.1 and 84.2 during and after treatment respectively.

The ROSHI training with this man was followed by reports of significant reduction of pain and increased ability to control pain without

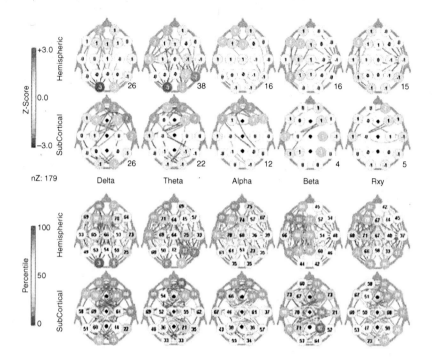

FIGURE 8.9. QEEG connectivity maps of case number 6, eyes closed (EC) during ROSHI light training shows the Z-scores. The nZ = 179 is significantly lower than during the EC baseline (nZ = 231) (see Figure 8.7). (See also color gallery.) *Source: ROSHI Journal, 3*(1): 1-7, January 2006.

medication. His depression was resolved, and he was able to finish a computer school training program and compose a number of songs.

LONGITUDINAL STUDIES

In this section, two more case histories of ROSHI-treated persons will be discussed, which have been followed-up for several years.

The seventh case involved a 27-year old male student translator at UCLA who experienced a severe motor vehicle accident, which left him in coma for four months. When he regained consciousness, he was paralyzed over the left side, was aphasic, and developed a seizure disorder. He also experienced deep depression, memory impairment, and a sleep disorder. Two years after the accident, he started neuro-

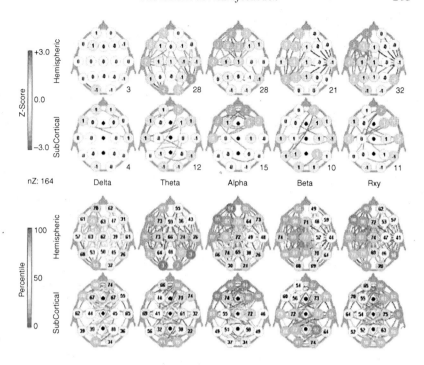

FIGURE 8.10. QEEG connectivity maps of case number 6, eyes closed (EC) after ROSHI training, shows the Z-scores. The nZ = 164 is still significantly lower than EC baseline (nZ = 231). (See also color gallery.) *Source: ROSHI Journal, 3*(1): 1-7, January 2006.

feedback training under the supervision of the first author. Over an approximately six-year interval between the middle of 1998 and 2004, he completed 360 neurofeedback sessions. ROSHI training began near the end of 1999. As can be seen in Figure 8.13, the numbers of sessions needed to sustain the learning process through neurofeedback were reduced yearly from 70 in 1998 to less than 20 in 2004. This case was presented in more detail at various conferences and was published in *ROSHI Journal, 1*(11): 1-10, December 2004.

At intake, this patient was on Tegretol, 200 mg b.i.d., Dilantin, 300 mg per night, Celexa, Serozone, and Zoloft. For the last four years of treatment, he was under the supervision of a neurologist associate who reduced medications to only Dilantin and folic acid. Training started with Neurocybernetics equipment following a Sterman protocol

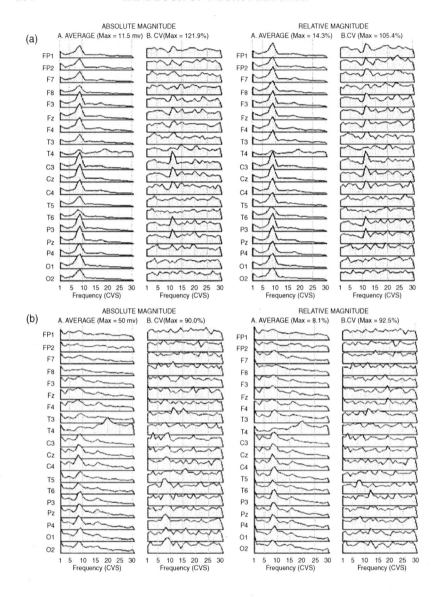

FIGURE 8.11. Power Spectrum Display and the Coefficient of Variation (CV) in eyes closed (a) and eyes open (b) conditions. CV in EC condition is 105.4% versus 92.5% in EO condition. *Source: ROSHI Journal, 3*(1): 1-7, January 2006.

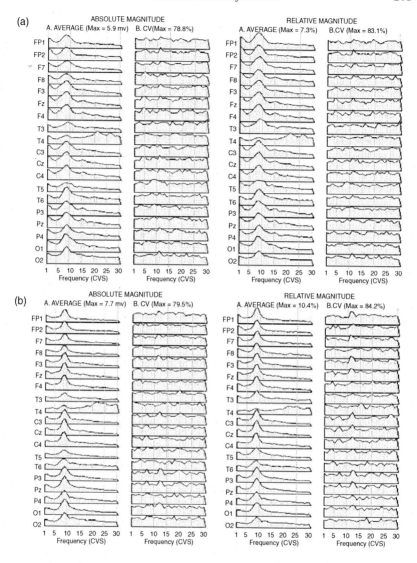

FIGURE 8.12. Power Spectrum Display and the Coefficient of Variation (CV) in eyes closed (EC) condition during ROSHI (a) and post ROSHI (b). During the ROSHI training the CV was 83.1% and post ROSHI, 84.2%, both significantly lower than the EC baseline condition, CV of 105.4 (see Figure 8.11a). *Source: ROSHI Journal, 3*(1): 1-7, January 2006.

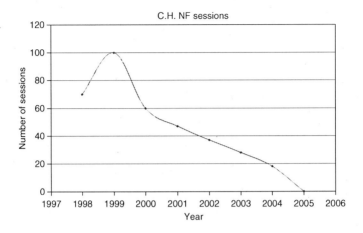

FIGURE 8.13. The number of NF sessions per each year that case 7 needed in order to obtain and maintain the maximum benefit from the neuromodulation effect of the NF. Special notes: his training was only for half a year in 1998 and his ROSHI training started at the end of 1999. Since year 2000 patient became and remained seizure free. *Source: ROSHI Journal, 1*(11): 1-10, December 2004.

(Sterman & Friar, 1972), with electrodes at Cz or C4 while enhancing SMR and suppressing theta and high beta. This was done to address his physical impairments and seizure disorder. ROSHI training was done at various electrode locations to inhibit or enhance certain frequencies, including theta only (inhibit) and SMR (enhance), or to modify coherence abnormalities found in prior QEEG evaluations. Protocols were (1) with electrodes at C1/C2 (or, more often, over the Cz position), inhibiting theta only or enhancing SMR; (2) with electrodes at Cz/C4, inhibiting theta only or enhancing synchrony (sync) between Cz and C4; (3) with electrodes at C3/C4, enhancing SMR and 14 Hz, or sync between C3 and C4; (4) with electrodes at F3/F4, or F4/T4 inhibiting theta only, or enhancing sync between F4 and T4.

Progress was monitored by repeated subjective tests such as the Beck Inventory, the SCL-90R, and other tests of stress, and objective tests such as the Test of Variables of Attention (TOVA) and Integrated Visual and Auditory Continuous Performance Test (IVA). Scores on these tests normalized as has been reported previously (Ibric, 2002a, 2003, 2004, 2005). After the ROSHI training started, seizure activity reduced and then completely subsided. He has been seizure-free for the past five years. He returned to school and is earning high grades, and was able to regain his driver's license. He enjoys a normal, productive life.

The eighth case is that of a 42-year old housewife who came for neurofeedback training due to depression and problems with weight control. She was first diagnosed with depression and prescribed antidepressants at age of 12 years after her father died. She was medicated and self-medicated with psychoactive drugs for almost 30 years, except for the two times she was pregnant. At the time of the initial evaluation, her depression and anxiety were enhanced by the fact that her mother had developed Alzheimer's disease. When neurofeedback training began, she was taking tranquilizer medication and lithium, which may have contributed to her weight gain, problems with mobility, and increased intake of food and alcohol. The latter likely helped perpetuate her preexisting depression. There also was a family history of depression and suicide. Testing revealed several marked psychological and cognitive disabilities along with severe impairments on all measures of interpersonal, intrapsychic, and attentional function. She was unable to carry out many activities of daily living. During training, multiple food allergies were detected and subsequently addressed.

Over a seven-year interval, this woman completed 191 neurofeedback sessions—68 on Neurocybernetics equipment and 123 with ROSHI. The distribution of these sessions over the years is shown in Figure 8.14. As can be seen, except for 2001 when her mother died, the number of sessions declined year by year. Despite declining numbers of sessions, there were no relapses and during later years, training was done only on an as-needed basis—much like "booster" sessions.

Neurofeedback protocols varied in terms of both electrode locations and frequencies, inhibited or enhanced. Training with NeuroCybernetics equipment mainly was at C3 and enhancing 15-18 Hz or at C4 with enhancement of 12-15 Hz. During these early months of training, she seemed unable to stay awake, even though she persisted in trying to do so. ROSHI training was introduced with electrodes at F3/F4 and discouraging theta (or alpha), or enhancing 16 or 17 Hz beta. Combining this with red glasses and the complex adaptive modality had a positive impact, and she progressed much faster. After one and one half months of training, this patient stopped smoking cigarettes; and during the first year of training, she was able to completely stop using

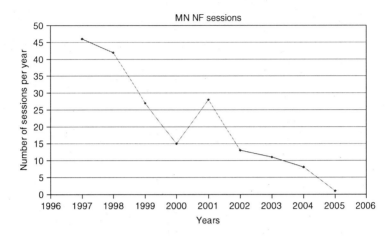

FIGURE 8.14. The NF training sessions per year that case 8 needed to obtain and maintain maximum benefit from the neuromodulation effect of the NF. Special notes: First year, 1997 was only for the last half a year, and in 2001, the number of sessions increased due to the patient's need to control her stress, when her mother, with advanced Alzheimer passed away. *Source: ROSHI Journal, 1(1): 1-2, February 2004.*

all her medications. There were distinctive changes in her ability to stay awake, and she showed increased zest for life. Both subjective and objective test scores normalized, and have remained normal for the past three years. By the time the neurofeedback treatment, nutritional adjustments (specific amino acids regimen), and detoxification programs were completed, this client had regained her zest for life. More details concerning this case have been presented at professional conferences (Ibric, Kaur, & Davis, 1998; Ibric & McCourt, 2002a,b), and it was published in *ROSHI Journal, 1*(1): 1-2, February 2004 and in the BSC Newsletter, 20(1): 6-7, Spring 2004.

SUMMARY AND CONCLUSIONS

Over the years, neurofeedback enhanced by the light and/or electromagnetic closed loop-EEG of ROSHI instruments has proven to be very beneficial with a variety of conditions. Our use of ROSHI has been associated with corrections of cognitive, emotional, and physical dysfunctions. Examples include improvements in organizational and memory skills in persons diagnosed with ADHD, decreases in anxiety, stabilization of mood, improvement in sleep patterns, pain control, decreased tinnitus, decreasing addictive behaviors, and assisting with neuromuscular reeducation. It has been our experience that symptom alleviation using ROSHI has proven to be much faster, and effects were longer lasting than obtained through traditional neurofeedback. Although there continues to be a need for controlled scientific research, enhanced neurofeedback training using ROSHI instruments appears to be an efficacious, safe, and, in the long run, cost-effective approach, which allows patients with a wide variety of symptoms to live normal, self-sufficient lives, often independently of pharmacological intervention.

REFERENCES

Cade, C.M. & Coxhead, N. (1989). *The awakened mind: Biofeedback and the development of higher states of awareness.* New York: Dell.

Fehmi, L.G. (1978). EEG biofeedback, multichannel synchrony training, and attention. In A. A. Sugarman & R. E. Tarter (Eds.), *Expanding dimensions of consciousness.* New York: Springer.

Fried, R. (1989). *EEG in clinical psychophysiology: Application in migraine.* [Abstract]. Proceedings of the 20th Annual Meeting of the Association for Applied Psychophysiology and Biofeedback, 70-73.

Gevins, A., Leong, H., Smith, M.E., Le, J., et al. (1995). Mapping cognitive brain function with modern high-resolution electroencephalography. *Trends in Neurosciences, 18*(10), 429-436.

Gevins, A.S., Zeitlin, G.M., Yingling, C.D., Doyle, J.C., Dedon, M.F., Schaffer, R.E, Rousmasset, J.T., & Yeager, C.L. (1979). EEG patterns during "cognitive" tasks: I-Methodology and analysis of complex behaviors. *Electroencephalography and Clinical Neurophysiology, 47,* 693-703.

Green, E.E., Green, A.M., & Walters, E.D. (1970). Self-regulation of internal states. In J. Rose (Ed.), *Progress of Cybernetics,* Proceedings of the International Congress of Cybernetics (pp. 1299-1327). London: Gordon & Breach.

Hammond, C. (2000). Neurofeedback treatment of depression with the ROSHI, *Journal of Neurotherapy, 4*(2), 45-55.

Hudspeth, W.J. & Ibric, V.L. (2004). QEEG and Behavioral Indices for Neurofeedback Effectiveness, [Abstract] Proceedings, *Journal of ECNS Conference, 5*(4), 213-214.

Hudspeth, W.J., Ibric, V.L., Coben, R., & Gunkelman, (2005). *Journal of Symposium: Advances in the assessment of brain functioning,* [Abstract] Proceedings of AAPB 36th Annual Meeting, Austin, TX.

Ibric, V.L. (1999). *AVS/EEG training on ROSHI/BrainLink® instrument and proto-cols (I),* [Abstract] Proceedings for the workshop presented at the 7th annual meeting of SNR.

Ibric, V.L. (2001). *AVS/EEG training on ROSHI/BrainLink® instrument and proto-cols (III),* [Abstract] Proceedings for the workshop presented at the 9th Annual Meeting of SNR, Monterey, CA.

Ibric, V.L. (2002a). *AVS/EEG training on ROSHI/BrainLink® instrument and proto-cols (IV),* [Abstract] Proceedings for the workshop presented at the 10th Annual Meeting of SNR, Scottsdale, AZ.

Ibric, V.L. (2002b). *Neurofeedback enhanced by light and electromagnetic closed loop EEG in Parkinson's disease,* [Abstract] Proceedings for Lecture presented at the 10th Annual Meeting of SNR, Scottsdale, AZ.

Ibric, V.L. (2003). *ROSHI and applications—Longitudinal studies,* [Abstract] Pro-ceedings for workshop presented at Winter Brain Conference, Palm Springs, CA.

Ibric, V.L. (Spring 2004). Bipolar depression and addictions—Seven-year success. *California Biofeedback Newsletter, 20*(1), 6-7.

Ibric, V.L. (2005). *Enhanced types of neurofeedback,* [Abstract] Proceedings for Lecture presented at Winter Brain Conference, Palm Springs, CA.

Ibric, V.L. & Davis, C.J. (2000). *AVS/EEG training on ROSHI/BrainLink® in-strument and protocols (II),* [Abstract] Proceedings for the workshop presented with Chuck Davis at the 8th Annual Meeting of SNR, St-Paul, MN.

Ibric, V.L., Kaur, S., & Davis, C. (1998). *Various diagnostic cases treated using ROSHI/Neurocybernetics—Preliminary results,* [Abstract] Proceedings for the 6th Annual Meeting of SSNR, Austin TX.

Ibric, V.L. & Martin, G. (2002). *ROSHI manual and ROSHI on bioexplorer,* (Eds) at Therapy and Prevention Center, in house press.

Ibric, V.L. & McCourt, J.L. (2002a). *ROSHI as a diagnostic tool,* [Abstract] Pro-ceedings for workshop presented at the 10th Annual Conference of SNR, Scottsdale, AZ.

Ibric, V.L. & McCourt, J.L. (2002b). Neurofeedback training: Intergration with diet and detoxification programs, *Journal of Neurotherapy, 6*(4) 25-38.

Kolbinger, H., Hoflich, G., Hufnagel, A., Moller, H., & Kasper, S. (1995). Trans-cranial Magnetic Stimulation (TMS) in the treatment of major depression— A pilot study. *Human Psychopharmacology, 10,* 305-310.

Lubar, J.F. (1991). Discourse on the development of EEG diagnostics and biofeed-back for attention-deficit/hyperactivity disorders. *Biofeedback & Self-Regulation, 16*(3), 201-225.

Marzano, R.J. (2000). *Transforming classroom grading.* Alexandria, VA, USA: Copyright 2000 by McREL Institute ASCD publications.

Monroe, R.A. (1971). *Journeys out of the body.* New York: Random House.

Ochs, L. (1992). EEG Treatment of addictions. *Biofeedback & Self Regulation, 20*(1), 8-16.

Patton, R. (1993). *Peak performance.* [Abstract] Proceedings at the First Meet-ing of the Society for the Study of Neuronal Regulation Annual Conference, Catalina, CA.

Patton R. (1995). *Neuroregulation to optimize sports performance.* Paper presented at the American Volleyball Coaches Association National Convention, Springfield, MA.

Peniston-Kulkowsky, Peniston, E. G., & Kulkosky, P. J. (1991). Alpha-theta brainwave neuro-feedback therapy for Vietnam veterans with combat-related posttraumatic stress disorder. *Medical Psychotherapy, 4,* 47-60.

Pfurtscheller, G. & Aranibar, A. (1977). Event related cortical desynchronization detected by power measurements of scalp EEG. *Electroencephalography and Clinical Neurophysiology, 42,* 817-826.

Sandyk, R. (1995). Transcranial magnetic coil stimulation in patients with central pain. *International Journal of Neuroscience, 36,*1037-1040.

Sandyk, R. (1997a). Treatment with weak electromagnetic fields restores dream recall in a parkinsonian patient. *International Journal of Neuroscience, 90,* 75-86.

Sandyk, R. (1997b). Reversal of cognitive impairment in an elderly parkinsonian patient by transcranial application of picotesla electromagnetic fields. *International Journal of Neuroscience, 91,* 57-68.

Sandyk, R. (1997c). Treatment with AC pulsed electromagnetic fields improves the response to levodopa in Parkinson's disease. *International Journal of Neuroscience, 91,* 189-197.

Sandyk, R. (1997d). Treatment with electromagnetic fields improves dual-task performance (talking while walking) in multiple sclerosis. *International Journal of Neuroscience, 92*(1-2): 95-102.

Sterman, M.B. (1973). Neurophysiological and clinical studies of sensory-motor EEG biofeedback training: Some effects on epilepsy. *Seminars in Psychiatry, 5*(4), 507-525.

Sterman, M.B. & Friar, L. (1972). Suppression of seizures in epileptics following sensorimotor EEG feedback training. *Electroencephalography & Clinical Neurophysiology, 33,* 89-95.

Tachiki, K.H., Ochs, L., & Weiler, E. (1994). *Brain Entrainment as a tool in brainwave retraining,* [Abstract] Proceedings for paper presented at the 2nd Annual Conference of the Society for the Study of Neuronal Regulation, Las Vegas, NV.

Tansey, M.A. (1984). EEG sensorimotor rhythm biofeedback training: Some effects on the neurological precursors of learning disabilities. *International Journal of Psychophysiology, 3.*

Chapter 9

Coherence and the Quirks of Coherence/Phase Training: A Clinical Perspective

Joseph J. Horvat

INTRODUCTION

When the author first became interested in EEG coherence training several years ago, it was a time when virtually no neurotherapists were talking about such training. At that time, I was doing quite a bit of work with mild traumatic brain injury (MTBI), and most of my treatment procedures were commonly used ones in the field of neurotherapy. Basically, these involved decreasing or increasing relative EEG power using protocols recommended by pioneers in the field such as Ayers, the Lubars, or the Othmers. As these protocols are quite similar, the ones used at any particular point in time generally depended on whose introductory workshop most recently had been attended.

Although having considerable success with these protocols, the concept of coherence kept coming up. Primarily this was because when working with MTBI patients, I regularly completed a quantitative EEG (QEEG) evaluation, and processed the scores through the Thatcher database (Thatcher, 1987) and associated MTBI discriminant analysis. At that time, the clinician had to calculate the probability of MTBI from a list of variables with highest loadings in the discriminant analysis, and coherence measures constituted several of these variables. Thus, with each patient's QEEG evaluation, I was reminded of

Handbook of Neurofeedback
© 2007 by The Haworth Press, Inc. All rights reserved.
doi:10.1300/5889_09

the importance of coherence. Furthermore, I was fully aware that Thatcher and other researchers have for years considered coherence abnormalities to be closely associated with brain injury.

My first actual use of a coherence training protocol came in the later stages of work with a six-year old child who had fallen from a second floor balcony. The child's mother had been happy with the treatment as he had only some very mild symptoms remaining. On his final QEEG "mapping," however, there were a number of coherence deviations. Reasoning that the remaining symptoms might respond to coherence training, and knowing that my neurofeedback equipment had coherence training capability, a decision was made to give it a try. Perhaps I have so successfully blocked what followed from my mind, that I do not remember exactly which coherence abnormalities were being trained. But, at any rate, the mother bitterly complained that many of the child's previous symptoms were returning. Treatment was stopped immediately, and another QEEG evaluation was completed. There had been a major change from excessive coherence to abnormally decreased coherence at the same sites and frequency after just three treatment sessions. Although I did not try coherence training again for several years, I continued to notice the prominence of coherence abnormalities in the QEEG evaluations of my MTBI patients, and to wonder at the speed with which coherence scores had responded to treatment the one and only time I had tried it. Eventually I came back to trying to understand the "quirks" of coherence training.

DEFINITIONS OF COHERENCE

Among the many definitions of coherence and the related concept of phase reviewed by the author, the clearest and most helpful were taken from an unpublished manuscript by Hammond (2003). Definitions and related information from the same source are presented in the next paragraphs.

Coherence refers to the connectivity between different parts of the brain. It is a cross correlation between two electrode sites in a given frequency band, indicating the extent to which two waveforms are similar in shape (synchrony). It represents the degree of joint variation between the electrode pairs. Electrode sites closer together have more coherence. Significant decreases in coherence are often correlated with increased phase delays. A statistically significant reduction in coherence is more serious clinically than excessive coherence. Hyper-coherence suggests inadequate differentiation of function. The areas are too similar, and the activity in the spans is excessively synchro-nized or coupled. The sites are doing too much of the same thing at the same time. Hypocoherence indicates that the two sites are out of syn-chrony with each other, and are not doing enough of the same thing at the same time. Thus, if these are homologous sites, it indicates that the activity in the bands is poorly synchronized between the hemispheres. This lack of relationship may indicate a functional uncoupling of the shared source generator within or between the hemispheres. They are not doing the same thing and there is less integration. With either too much or too little coherence, there is no optimally efficient cortical function and different brain areas are not working with each other at an optimal level.

Phase refers to relationships between a point on an EEG wave and the identical point on the same wave recorded simultaneously at an-other electrode site. Phase represents covariation in time or conduc-tion time. Does it arrive at the same point in time or is it too soon or too late? A high phase lag means there is a time delay and conduction time, and communication efficiency are delayed. Low phase lag means the speed of conduction is rapid and there is good efficiency and com-munication. Reduced coherence and/or increased phase delay often is related to reduced connectivity between two brain regions, and of-ten is clinically correlated with white matter or axonal injury as well as gray matter dysfunction. Significant decreases in coherence are often correlated with increased phase delays. Because of the short, medium, and long-distance fibers that interconnect regions of the cor-tex, normal cortical integration is characterized by a stable set of rela-tionships (coherence) and conduction times (phase) among the EEG waveforms from each electrode site.

COHERENCE TRAINING

Within the field of coherence training, there is an unresearched area that remains one of the greatest potential problems with such training. The specific software formulae for calculating coherence dif-fer among the various equipment manufacturers and QEEG databases.

Coherence is not defined in the same way mathematically by, for example, the NX Link database (1999) and the Thatcher database (Thatcher, 1987). Usually the differences center on whether or not phase and phase shifts are included in the formulae for calculating coherence. This problem is further complicated by the fact that the mathematical definitions of coherence built into neurofeedback instruments used to train coherence usually are different from those involved in the databases. Again, how phase is handled or excluded in the calculations is usually the issue. For example, in the author's early work with coherence, the definition of coherence in the Thatcher database used to determine need for coherence training differed from the definition used with the Lexicor Medical Technology equipment employed for neurofeedback training. The Lexicor equipment used a correlation that included average amplitude in calculating coherence, whereas the Thatcher database did not. To the author's knowledge, only the Lexicor and Brain Master neurofeedback equipment are designed to permit coherence training at this time. The Brain Master equipment allows one to choose between two different definitions of coherence. However, the author is aware of no published research showing that one or the other is more or less effective when combined with any specific QEEG equipment or database.

Although the definitions of abnormal coherence in databases used and those in the neurofeedback equipment software being used by the author to train coherence differ, clients' symptoms usually are reduced. It is not known at this time which definition may be better for identifying abnormalities related to client's specific symptoms or enable more efficient neurofeedback training. As long as equipment manufacturers develop something new, better, and different without getting together to agree on similar definitions of coherence, this situation will continue. From the author's perspective, it seems rather simple: just promote research to determine which definition is most related to symptomatology and treatment efficacy, agree upon a single definition, and use it. (However, I have often been accused of oversimplifying complex matters!)

It should be mentioned here that neurofeedback treatment issues around coherence and phase are inextricably related. Both are measures of connectivity and conductivity, and, as noted earlier, there is a moderately strong inverse relationship between them. Due to this commonly observed inverse relationship between coherence and phase, when one changes, the other also often changes. Thus, in many cases, a neurotherapist may treat only coherence abnormalities, yet also help bring about effective changes in phase. Few clinicians treat phase directly. Perhaps this is because, as has been the author's experience, phase changes are unstable.

It should be obvious by now that the author feels coherence/phase neurofeedback treatment should not be attempted without a QEEG evaluation, with obtained measures referenced to a normative database to determine areas of abnormality. Nevertheless, there are times, when, after looking at a particularly complicated QEEG-based brain map, I wish I could totally accept the concept of symptom-driven treatment. In fact, with frequency training, I do sometimes use commonly used symptom-based ("canned") treatment protocols, especially for sleep disorders, depression (increase left hemisphere beta), and attention deficit disorder (decrease theta/beta or theta/SMR ratios). However, without QEEG evaluations and associated mapping/remapping, one would not know whether or not to treat coherence, which frequency bandwidth(s) to treat, and if and when coherence had been normalized (or made more abnormal) through neurofeedback treatment.

COMMON PATTERNS OF COHERENCE DEVIATION

The most common coherence abnormality observed by the author involves excessive coherence and decreased phase delay or lag (insufficient delay). This particular situation occurred in a case where an inexperienced neurofeedback provider had given a client a number of theta/beta ratio reduction type training sessions, but was not making progress. This was a 16-year old boy with a diagnosis of attention deficit disorder who also had problems with depression, headaches, sleep, anger control, and academic achievement and was repeating the ninth grade. Relative power deviations had all been normalized, yet coherence deviations and symptoms remained. The previous treatment provider used "canned" treatment protocols rather than QEEG-guided treatment. Thus, it was not known whether the observed coherence deviations preceded or were causally related to the previous treatment.

In any event, coherence treatment by the author was associated with resolution of his symptomatology.

Treatment for this type coherence deviation always involves training to reduce coherence. However, due to the commonly seen inverse relationship between coherence and phase, as excessive coherence decreases phase deviations usually also change, that is, there is an increase in phase delay (or lag) toward more normal degrees. As was true for this example, coherence deviations may not exist in only one frequency bandwidth, and may not be associated with abnormalities of phase. The author considers a preferred situation to be one in which an observed coherence deviation in a specific frequency band is accompanied by an inverse-type phase abnormality in the same band. This is because there are then two measures rather than only one indicating connectivity abnormality, thus providing some degree of verification of the validity of the deviations. In the author's opinion, these will be the type abnormalities with the most associated symptoms.

A few years ago, Thatcher (2003) stated that we are making an assumption (although a good assumption) that the highest levels of deviation from normality of various EEG measures probably have the highest levels of symptoms associated with them. However, he also pointed out that there is not much difference between say a Z score deviation of 1.94 and 1.97. While the latter is considered significant and the former is not, nonsignificant scores also can be associated with symptomatology. As an aside, he noted it was only necessary to reduce any Z score deviation by approximately 10 percent in order to produce a positive change, that is, remove or decrease symptomatology. Whether the latter statement was based on research or on a theoretical position he held is unknown to the author. However, it seems commensurate with a statement Margaret Ayers made some time ago, that the brain "has a natural desire to get well," and what neurofeedback does is "show it the way" (perhaps with only a 10 percent change) (Ayers, 1993). At any rate, it is possible to have an excessive coherence/decreased phase lag situation where the coherence abnormality is statistically significant, while the phase deviation is not sufficiently great to reach statistical significance.

The second most common (and second easiest to treat) coherence deviation, in the author's opinion, involves decreased (insufficient) or normal coherence and increased phase delay or lag. Here, one is more likely to see increased phase delay without significant coherence deviation than abnormal coherence with normal phase, indicating that the inverse coherence/phase relationship is not as consistent in this type deviation. An example of this, from our clinic, was a 15-year old boy with significant attention deficit/hyperactivity disorder, problems with anger control, learning problems, and obsessive-compulsive tendencies. Again using the inverse relationship between coherence and phase and not directly treating phase alone, the neurofeedback protocol for this type deviation would always involve training to increase coherence. This would be true whether or not there is statistically significant decreased coherence or increased phase delay. In this particular case, however, there was an exception to designing a neurofeedback training protocol based strictly on QEEG findings regarding coherence abnormalities. Here, there was significantly decreased coherence in the delta frequency range between some right hemisphere sites. In the author's opinion, one should never increase delta frequency coherence regardless of degree or location of decreased delta observed. In fact, the author never trains to increase delta whether it is coherence, phase, amplitude asymmetry, or relative power. Even if there were no deviations observed anywhere, except in the delta range, the author would refrain from training increases in that frequency, and would use symptom-driven protocols. It is widely accepted that delta in the awake state commonly is associated with pathological symptoms. Therefore, training delta increases could be dangerous for the client.

Sometimes, unusual and often complex coherence/phase relationships are found. In the author's experience, these are more often noted, and are more complex, when midline scalp sites are involved in coherence measures. More recent database score presentations, for example, NeuroGuide Deluxe (2003) include coherence between midline sites as well as between midline sites and both left and right side sites. As difficult as it may be to design protocols for these complex situations, the same general rules mentioned earlier regarding the inverse relationship between coherence and phase still apply.

The author have not yet decided whether it is better to treat only intrahemispheric coherence abnormalities and just ignore those involving central sites. In the past, client's symptoms usually improved without ever addressing central location abnormalities. And, there is no published research known to the author, which compares intrahemispheric coherence treatment efficacy with interhemispheric treatment or that which involves midline sites. Nevertheless, some leaders in the field of neurofeedback now routinely do cross-hemisphere training of power (e.g., Othmer, 1994) and of coherence (Walker, 1994), and report favorable results. This seems to be a viable treatment approach in some cases despite the fact that only 25-30 percent of neural connections are interhemispheric (Lubar & Lubar, 1994). The author has not yet tried working with some coherence training protocols that involve midline sites. But, unless more significant differences in symptoms are seen with interhemispheric protocols than with intrahemispheric protocols, the relative simplicity of the latter will remain a strong argument in favor of staying with them.

VARIOUS RANDOM TREATMENT PRINCIPLES

The principles discussed in this section are not necessarily based on research (although some are), and are not necessarily "industry-accepted" (although some are), but, rather, are based primarily on what the author has tried and found effective in his clinical work.

Neurofeedback Treatment and Unexpected QEEG Mapping Changes

During the early days of the author's neurofeedback career, it was his policy to complete further QEEGs and "mappings" during treatment to determine what changes in brain function might be occurring. This sometimes produced distressing results. Often, there would be very significant abnormalities noted which were not present at the initial evaluation. And, this often occurred even when the client's symptoms were diminishing. It was difficult trying to explain to clients why their symptoms were less, but some QEEG findings were more deviant.

To investigate this phenomenon further, the author retrieved and studied all the cases where he had trained coherence in the delta, theta, or beta frequency ranges. When delta training was involved, it was to decrease abnormally high coherence in the delta frequency band. As noted, the author never trains increases in the delta band. None of these involved the alpha band or coherence training designed to modify phase. Most of the clients were MTBI cases, two suffered from chronic fatigue syndrome, three from attention problems, and one from a learning disability. Number of treatment sessions was variable. There were 31 cases. In all cases, Lexicor equipment had been used to gather QEEG data and train coherence. Average coherence deviations of pre- and posttreatment measures were calculated regardless of sign (i.e., disregarding whether a Z score was negative or positive), and t tests of significance of differences between measures were run (see Table 9.1).

As can be seen, treatment, overall, was effective in normalizing initial coherence deviations. Following this analysis, changes in another QEEG measure, power (amplitude) asymmetry, was investigated. Very significant increases in power asymmetry between several sites were found within the delta frequency band regardless of the frequency bands that were involved in the coherence training protocols. Many such asymmetry changes were in the delta band, although there were some significant changes in the theta frequency band as well. Despite these asymmetry changes, clients were showing decreases in presenting symptoms and no other new symptoms. Thus, it seems that the changes were asymptomatic.

After observing the asymmetry changes noted earlier, the author questioned whether training EEG power might work in the opposite direction, that is, produces changes in coherence. To investigate this, 50 cases were studied where there had been significant deviations in

TABLE 9.1. Pre-post coherence and asymmetry means.

	Delta	Theta	Alpha	Beta
Coherence				
Pre-treat	21.380	14.480	7.680	17.440
Post-treat	−.140	.760	3.630	2.130
SIG.	.001	.002	.063	.004
Asymmetry				
Pre-treat	13.490	1.730	12.230	3.280
Post-treat	27.390	7.140	13.970	4.720
SIG.	.008	.030	.3950	.375

coherence and phase, but neurofeedback treatment had involved only protocols designed to change theta/beta or theta/SMR power ratios. Roughly, two-thirds of the cases showed increases in number of coherence abnormalities, most often within the delta frequency band. The remaining third had either no change or a decrease in coherence deviations. However, the changes in coherence Z scores did not reach statistical significance. The reason why the power asymmetry changes following coherence training seemed more pronounced and less random than the changes in coherence observed following power training is unknown. In any event, what is known is that coherence training or power training often is associated with various EEG changes. These changes may be at nontreated sites and/or at frequencies not involved in the training protocol, and appear to be asymptomatic. Perhaps, they simply should be considered treatment "artifacts," or due to lack of test-retest reliability in the QEEG measures. Such changes could, however, become an important issue if they persisted and were seen as significant abnormalities at a later QEEG evaluation. A different neurotherapist might then inappropriately orient treatment around normalizing them. Clearly, this is an area worthy of further research.

Over-Training

It is very important to consider that in any kind of coherence/phase treatment, it is possible to go "too far." As noted earlier, this obviously is what happened with the author the very first time he tried such training. In the following paragraph, another case will be discussed where over-training led to trouble.

A second-grade child was brought to the clinic because of attention problems and an expressive language disorder. The first QEEG map appeared initially to show very few abnormalities. However, closer inspection revealed many deviant coherence Z scores, which only approached statistical significance. A decision was made to train coherence, and the child's parents soon noticed positive changes. However, these began to decrease and disappear. A second QEEG evaluation was completed after 20 treatment sessions. Results showed more abnormalities than initially seen. By hindsight, it is apparent that a second QEEG evaluation should have been completed after no more than 10 sessions. Had that been done, it is likely that the coherence abnormalities of borderline significance would have been found to be normalized and coherence training would have been discontinued. The main point here is that with coherence/phase training, it can be easy to get "too much of a good thing." In the author's opinion, there is a positive (but certainly not perfect) relationship between number of neurotherapy sessions and speed with which coherence changes occur. And, this appears to be true regardless of whether coherence is being directly trained or whether training of power is involved.

Treatment Order and Priorities

In workshops conducted by the author, the questions of order of treatment and treatment priority often come up. In this section, the procedure followed by the author is discussed, although readers should bear in mind that there are frequent exceptions depending on the nature of particular cases.

With certain conditions that affect brain wave patterns, the author considers it important to treat the disorder before completing a QEEG evaluation and preparing treatment protocols based on database abnormalities. In such conditions, some QEEG abnormalities are likely to be due to the disorder rather than a cause of it, and using QEEG-driven protocols could be useless. The author considers sleep disorders and posttraumatic stress disorder (PTSD) to be examples of these. Use of "canned" training protocols in the treatment of sleep disorders generally has proven successful, for example, reducing theta power and increasing SMR power at site CZ in cases of initial insomnia, and reducing theta while increasing beta power at the same site in cases of middle insomnia. In cases of PTSD, it has been the author's experience that eye movement desensitization and reprocessing (EMDR) not only is an effective treatment, but also leads to changes in brain wave patterns. The author routinely observes this when comparing pre- and post-EDMR QEEG results. Treating sleep disorders and PTSD in these ways may lead to cessation of symptoms and make QEEG-based coherence training or other neurofeedback training unnecessary. However, in many cases (e.g., MTBI), there will be other symptoms that will relate to QEEG findings and will require further neurofeedback treatment.

Sometimes during the pretreatment QEEG evaluation, visual inspection of the raw EEG waveforms will reveal significant sharp wave activity. In such cases, it is the author's practice to try to eliminate this, prior to any further training. This is done by identifying the locations and frequency bands where sharp wave activity is predominant and reducing power at these sites and frequencies. Very often, this involves training to decrease theta power and increase power in the SMR frequency band at the appropriate site(s). When symptoms persist even after the aforementioned treatment of any sleep disorder, PTSD, or sharp wave activity, and with most of all other clients, I proceed with neurofeedback treatment.

With most of the neurotherapy clients, the author begins with coherence training and tries to get coherence and phase scores at least moderately improved before going on to power training. (Incidentally, some others do not. Walker [1994], for instance, does exactly the opposite, working with power before coherence.) The author notes that improvement in presenting symptoms often begins during the early coherence training and occasionally all symptoms vanish. Unless all symptoms cease, or the symptoms are of a nature indicating need for further coherence training sessions, power training is initiated. After about 10 sessions, a second QEEG and "mapping" are completed if treatment has been at exactly the same location and within the same frequency band during all sessions. If not, the second evaluation is completed after about 15 sessions.

While the specific order of neurofeedback sessions varies depending on individuals' QEEG findings, the following is a commonly used order (1) reduce delta coherence; (2) reduce theta coherence; (3) reduce beta coherence; (4) increase beta coherence; (5) decrease or increase relative power at specific locations guided by QEEG results, or by symptomatology and use of standard "canned" protocols such as decrease theta/raise beta (or SMR). Of course, this exact order would not be strictly followed unless relevant abnormalities were present. Furthermore, treating one frequency band or electrode location often produces changes in others, making it unnecessary to strictly follow the sequence. Ordinarily, however, the author prefers to treat in this order when indicated because he believes it is the order that usually causes most symptoms. In other words, delta produces more symptoms than theta, and theta more than beta, etc. This is based only on the author's clinical experience, and has no knowledge of published research to support it.

QEEG Score Improvement with No Change in Symptoms

Occasionally after coherence (or power) training, there is no improvement noted in presenting symptoms, despite progress toward normalization of the statistically significant deviations observed at an initial QEEG evaluation. In such cases, it may be that the deviations treated were not related to the symptomatology. When this occurs, it is recommended that the QEEG findings be inspected for abnormalities of "borderline" significance, that is, deviations that may be significant at 0.05 to 0.10 levels rather than below 0.05 (or whatever level of significance had been used earlier). Despite the usual assumption that the greatest deviations from database norms are most likely to be the ones related to symptoms, this may not always be the case. The less significant abnormalities may be the ones causally related to presenting symptoms, and the ones that should be treated.

Plasticity of the Brain During Neurofeedback Treatment

During neurofeedback treatment, it may be that there is increased brain plasticity. This is based only on the author's clinical experience, and he has no knowledge of published research to support it. An example of this involved a 58-year old male whose symptoms included dyslexia, difficulty with memory and concentration, irritability and low energy, and who had a history of traumatic brain injury at age 19. Following treatment sequence principles as enumerated earlier, the author began treatment with reducing theta coherence, alternating between left and right hemisphere sites. After 12 sessions, abnormalities in the theta, alpha, and beta frequencies noted at the initial QEEG evaluation were normalizing. Unfortunately, however, at about this point in time, he suffered another serious head injury. A subsequent QEEG evaluation revealed a return of the theta frequency coherence deviations, as well as development of very significant coherence abnormalities in the alpha frequency band. A new treatment program was started in which alpha coherence was reduced during one-half of each training session and theta coherence during the second half.

After only three such sessions (two involving left hemisphere and one involving right hemisphere sites), there were major reductions in coherence deviations. The author has observed similar developments with several other cases as well. It seems that, because of enhanced neural plasticity during coherence training, effects of brain injury experienced during such treatment can be more rapidly reversed than effects of pretreatment injuries. This is another area in need of serious research.

SUMMARY AND CONCLUSIONS

Coherence/phase training certainly is not a panacea for all disorders referred to neurotherapists. In the author's opinion, it should never completely take the place of other forms of therapy, which have been clinically proven to be useful, and/or have research-based evidence to support their efficacy. However, particularly in cases of epilepsy and MTBI, and those cases of learning disability and attention deficit disorder where there is a history of head injury or poor response to other forms of therapy, the author has found that evaluating and treating coherence/phase abnormalities makes good sense. With appropriate coherence/phase training, such cases often respond very rapidly.

One potential drawback to coherence/phase training in the past has been the need for several QEEG evaluations during the course of treatment. This is more of an issue with this type training as opposed to other neurotherapy training because of the speed with which changes can occur and lead to "over-training." The financial costs of multiple QEEG evaluations can present a hardship for many clients. Now, however, Brain Master Technology's "mini-mapper" or "mini-Q" software allows users of their equipment to not only train coherence, but also gather small time samples of EEG and process them through a database to determine coherence scores. This makes it feasible to quickly and frequently monitor treatment progress during a training session without having to change electrode sites. Although a full QEEG evaluation can provide much additional and potentially useful information, use of the "mini-Q" should make coherence training more efficient, less costly, and more appealing to both clients and practitioners.

REFERENCES

Ayers, M.E. (1993). Controlled study of EEG neurofeedback training and clinical psychotherapy for right hemispheric closed head injury. AAPB Conference Seminar on neurofeedback treatment modalities.

Hammond, D.C. (2003). "Compendium of common terms in EEG and neurofeedback." Unpublished manuscript.

John, E.R. (1999). *Neurometric analysis system.* Richmond, WA: NxLink, Ltd.

Lubar, J.F., & Lubar, J.O. (1994). *Seminar presentation: New treatments for ADD/ADHD.*

Othmer, S. (1994). "A discussion of alpha/theta training and SMR/beta training and their respective roles." Unpublished manuscript.

Thatcher, R.W. (1988). *A life span EEG normative database.* Copyright TXu 347.139. Washington, DC: US Copyright Office.

Thatcher, R.W. (2003). *Neuroguide deluxe.* St. Petersburg, FL: Applied Neuroscience, Inc.

Walker, J.M. (1994). Personal communication.

SECTION IV:
SPECIFIC CLINICAL
APPLICATIONS

Chapter 10

Brain Brightening:
Restoring the Aging Mind

Thomas Budzynski
Helen K. Budzynski
Hsin-Yi Tang

OVERVIEW: AN ORIENTATION TO AGING

The fundamental issue about aging in this day and age is have we gained enough knowledge about the mechanisms of aging so that we have a coherent view of how aging progresses? Furthermore, has our information countered our stereotypes about aging so that we will apply appropriate treatments to extend the lives of the elderly in a fulfilling way?

If only it were so. As it is, the advances in the knowledge base have developed so rapidly and in such a piecemeal form that there is a kind of incoherence about which treatments are valid and how they should be offered. Only reluctantly have we given up beliefs depicting the aging processes as simply a downward linear trajectory. For example, do we yet believe that cognitive impairment is the precursor to eventual dementia or possibly Alzheimer's disease? And that, once the functional neural processes are lost, they are gone forever? Present understanding about neurologic functioning and neurogenesis would suggest that we should believe otherwise.

Do we believe that cell death in skin, organs, and brains is inevitable and irreversible? The emerging field of glycoscience suggests that cell functioning may be restored by metabolic means, even as the

Handbook of Neurofeedback
doi:10.1300/5889_10

structure of cells age. Glyconutrients missing from our modern diet can be used to restore the natural immune responses of the body, re-placing/augmenting the myriad of drugs now used for pneumonia and possibly other serious generalized infections that plague vulnerable elderly (Maeder, 2002; Elkins, 2002; Rudd et al., 2001).

Advances in basic beliefs about our bioelectrical and bioenergy systems suggest new possibilities for elder care. Appropriate forms of externally presented bioelectrical energy can restore cell structure and alter metabolic functioning. A more noninvasive care, incorporating what is now known about resonant frequency responses of the body, can be applied to unhealthy cell activity with new instrumentation. Eastern and Western medicine are beginning to meld, knowing now that the bioelectric and magnetic energy structure of our tissues as recognized by ancient oriental medicine offers alternative types of noninvasive, nonpharmaceutical relief from chronic symptoms (Oschman, 2000; Kirsch, 2001).

Clues to the link between psychological stress and cellular aging are becoming far more specific through the work of Epel and others (2004). Cellular senescence is evidenced by the shortening of telemeres and the reduction of telemerase activity, thus leading to potential chronic disease among those who live a long enduring stressful life. The cellular environment plays an important role in regulating telemere length and telemerase activity. Sapolsky (2004) offers illustrations from the scientific literature showing psychological and physiologic challenges to metabolism to be the basis for the acceleration of aging. The work of Epel and others (2004) now documents just how brain senescence occurs at the cellular level under psychologically stressful conditions.

Of great concern among elderly is the potential for irreversible deterioration of brain functioning in the course of an increasingly longer life span. But it has been seen that neurostimulation and neurofeedback have made inroads in changing the circulatory, metabolic, and functional activity of brain and the nervous system. A most exciting possibility is in the findings emerging since the late 1990s that improving the neural environment (such as with stimulation) can activate stem cell activity and produce neurogenesis in the hippocampus, thus improving memory functions (Diamond, 1988; Gage, 2002; Nottebohm,

2002; Reh, 2002; Peterson, 2002; Parent, 2003; Kokaia & Lindvall, 2003; Kemperman et al., 2004).

This chapter addresses a number of advances in knowledge about brain functioning in older ages so that elder care regarding cognitive impairment can be addressed in a substantial way. The potential for preventing and/or halting further cognitive decline and dementia is within our grasp, and not only by pharmaceuticals. Knowledge about cell oxidation and structural brain changes, for example, demonstrate the role that both play in degrading brain cells as well as restoring functioning. Certainly, the research demonstrating that new neural tissue can be generated is the most startling finding of all. The recognition that the brain performs self-repair through neurogenesis helps to forge a new goal of achieving understanding about conditions under which these self-repair actions can occur. Among aging elders are thousands of instances where people are debilitated and losing cognitive function—probably due to lack of healthy cellular conditions for restoration of cells and neural tissue. Although, it need not be.

This chapter traces the process of cognitive aging, including mild forgetfulness as well as the various forms of dementia. The diagnosis of dementia may or may not, upon autopsy, involve structural change of tangles and plaque formation. Furthermore, when tangles and plaques do characterize the Alzheimer's diagnosis at autopsy, they cannot always explain the level of functional disability of the brain. In his longitudinal study of nuns, Snowden (2001) reported on the pathology findings of 102 sisters who had died by 1995. Of the 102 sisters, 45 had been classified as demented based on mental exams. Within the demented group, only 57 percent had the classic tangles and plaque formation in gray matter of the brain, indicative of Alzheimer's. The others (with the exception of one) did not feature the extensive pathology of Alzheimer's, but showed white matter lesions indicative of stroke.

These findings indicate that areas of white matter destroyed by lack of cerebral flow due to strokes, contributed to the disruption of communication between parts of the brain. This lack of high correlation between Alzheimer's structural pathology in gray matter and disabled mental functions, suggests that circulatory and metabolic damage to the elderly brain white matter may also be at fault in cognitive impairment. It also suggests that treatment focused upon increasing blood flow and glycogen could produce some restoration of cognitive functioning, even in the face of structural brain changes. The property of the brain's ability to change functionally is referred to as plasticity. The hope for restoration of functioning may be in capitalizing on the conditions that promote plasticity.

Prevalence of Age-Related Cognitive Decline (ARCD)

Cognitive decline in elders is marked by some researchers as generalized lower functioning in the domains of short-term memory, resulting in delayed recall, loss of sustained attention, perceptual-motor skills, executive function, problem solving, and speed of performance (Petersen et al., 1992; Craik et al., 1990; Rapp & Heindel, 1994). But not all impaired cognitive processes are necessarily associated with short-term memory, such as temporal orientation and verbal reasoning (Howieson et al., 1993). How much does lower cognitive functioning impact a population? The Canadian Study of Health and Aging (Ebly, Hogan, & Parhad, 1995), using direct testing, documented the prevalence of cognitive impairment in a community sample of persons older than 65 years. Of 10,263 persons, 2,914 (28.3 percent) were identified with cognitive impairment. Upon further breakdown of the cognitively impaired, a mildly impaired subgroup constituted 30 percent of the cognitively impaired group. Thus, about two-thirds of those complaining of cognitive impairment are a serious public health problem. They represent a particularly vulnerable group of persons who are at risk for physical decline (given the association of cognitive impairment with mortality), high use of health services, and major disabilities.

Many active, healthy, persons over the age of 65 years complain of some memory loss, but generally have adequate cognitive functioning. As noted in the Canadian Study documenting the presence of a large proportion of slightly cognitively compromised persons in an aging group, an ever-increasing proportion of elderly persons are living longer and reported to be generally feeling better (Howieson et al., 1993; Jagger, Clarke, & Clarke, 1991). Such a status is believed to be largely due to awareness of the importance of a healthy lifestyle, as well as due to control of infectious diseases and management of structural pathology such as cancer and heart disease. Nevertheless, functional dysregulations such as hypertension, arthritis, chronic fatigue, tremors, chronic pain, irritable bowel syndrome, asthma, insomnia, and diabetes, all directly related to brain function, continue to plague the elderly (Ornstein & Sobel, 1987). The relationship between chronic disability/mortality and cognitive impairment is not surprising (Branch & Jette, 1982; Boaz, 1994; Hanninen et al., 1995; Kelman et al., 1994; Swan, Carmelli, & LaRue, 1995). Thus, our attention to mild cognitive impairment goes hand in hand with an increase in helping patients find relief from nagging physical chronic symptoms. Chronic stress responses have been identified etiologically with cognitive impairment and physical decline (Sapolsky, 1992, 1994; Sapolsky, Krey, & MacEwen, 1986; Orrell & O'Dwyer, 1995; Gilad & Gilad, 1995). This finding, therefore, may be a key to treatment.

Because cognitive impairment seemed to be causally linked to both physical and psychological disorders (Elby, Hogan, & Parhad, 1995; Perls et al., 1993) and because milder impairment may be easier to prevent, decrease, or reverse, the treatment of mild cognitive problems is the focal point of this chapter. No rigorous studies have traced these causal relationships, nor has it been documented that these mild or slight impairments translate into dementia over time. In fact, a recent longitudinal study found that slight cognitive impairments are not presymptomatic of dementia. The quest becomes to limit these mild age-related cognitive deficits so that they are only temporarily dysfunctional and are reversible (Youngjohn & Crook, 1993).

MEMORY AND COGNITIVE PROCESSES IN AGING

The major domains of cognitive functioning usually fall under the general headings of attention, memory, language processing, visuospatial processing, abstraction, and conceptual flexibility. Within these domains are such attributes as information processing speed (response time), accuracy, and quantity of information (Wisocki, 1991). Most cognitive training efforts focus upon memory and manipulation of the processes called "fluid intelligence." Fluid intelligence refers to performance involving sustained attention, perceptual-motor skills, strategic planning and organization, problem solving, and speed of performance (Horn, 1982). This fluid intelligence is noted to be influenced by stress conditions and aging (Willis, 1982). Fluid intelligence is contrasted to "crystallized intelligence" in which automatic behaviors based on education and cultural learning is acquired and tends to remain stable throughout life. Certain aspects of these "fluid" cognitive domains have proven to be malleable and plastic, open to cognitive treatment.

For the most part, studies confirm one another that the ability to perform memory tasks is a key loss with normal aging (Petersen et al., 1992; Craik et al., 1990). This declining performance is thought to be true for primary (immediate) recall as well as secondary (delayed) recall. But even so, the decline is difficult to pin to age alone. Studies that correlate performance with age find many fewer age-related correlates than do those studies that contrast cohorts of young adults with cohorts of old adults. This is because the very wide variation of cognitive performance within any given age cohort lowers the effect of age alone upon performance (Petersen et al., 1992). Howieson and others (1993) and Perls and others (1993), who studied the healthy oldest of old, noted that many cognitive functions were well preserved in this group of individuals aged 85 years and older. Contrary to the belief that those who are healthy and who have lived a life span beyond 80 years will show significantly declining cognitive functioning. Howieson and others (1993) found that the substantial decline was not inevitable. At least 47 percent of the young-old (age between 58 and 65 years) declined at the same rate as that found in the old-old group. Visuospatial and construction skills, probably due to incapacities of motor function, showed the greatest decline, even though memory loss or benign senescent forgetfulness is the complaint most often expressed by many elders. Also accompanying the older ages are such problems as declining vision, hearing acuity, and motor function interfering with task performance on cognitive tests (Duke, Haley, & Bergquist, 1991).

Is Senior Poor Memory Due in Part to a Self-Belief?

In the early 1990s, Levy and Langer (1994) began a series of studies investigating short-term memory in elders. They found that in China, a society that respected elders, there was significantly less short-term memory dysfunction than in the United States. Their hypothesis that this might be related to a self-belief system created by the subtle influence of a prevailing societal belief was confirmed when they found that deaf-from-birth elderly Americans had significantly less memory dysfunction than hearing American elders. Stereotypes, whether cultural or self-subscribed, may have critical effects on both cognitive and physical factors, even influencing longevity and the will to live. It became obvious to Levy and associates that these self-stereotype about aging operate below the level of awareness, starting early in childhood and becoming stronger throughout adulthood (Levy, 2003; Levy & Myers, 2004; Levy, Slade, & Kasl, 2002).

One study was particularly interesting in demonstrating the influence of self-perceptions on longevity. In that study, the researchers examined the survival rates of participants of the Ohio Longitudinal Study of Aging and Retirement (OLSAR). The effect on survival of positive self-perceptions of aging was significant even after a univariate Cox proportional-hazards regression model was applied using age at baseline, race, gender, socioeconomic status (SES), functional health, self-rated health, and loneliness as covariates. The risk ratio for positive self-perception of aging alone was 0.78 ($p < .001$). Adding the significant variables of age, sex, SES, functional health, and loneliness led to a 0.87 risk ratio ($p < .001$), a similar level of significance. By dichotomizing the positive-negative self-perception, the median survival of the positive self-perception group was 22.6 years, whereas the negative group median survival was 15 years. This effect of a positive self-perception of aging is a psychological mechanism of critical importance.

Priming Positive Self-Esteem?

The plasticity of self-stereotyping in aging was demonstrated in a study (Levy, 1996) in which positive priming (subliminally presented phrases on a computer screen) was used to increase self-esteem and scores on pre and post memory tests. Neutral and negative priming phrases did not produce positive changes. The subliminal presentation appears to bypass the defense mechanisms, which ordinarily block the absorption of such positive affirmations. This result suggests the possibility of using priming phrase software to produce positive changes in elderly users.

The Stress Response and Cognitive Functioning in the Elderly

The stressors of old age are particularly noxious. Typically stressors can be multiple, chronic, and severe. A few examples of daily stressors of the elderly include pain, loss-related grief, chronic illness, physical decline, physical and mental isolation, changes in social support, fewer coping options, changes in mobility, decreased financial security, nonprivate living situations, communication barriers, safety concerns, and societal prejudice against old age. Solutions to reduce stress or coping choices, such as medications, hearing aids, changes in living situation, etc. may offer only partial relief and often introduce a new set of stressors.

Chronic and repeated stressors have been shown to have a negative influence on cognitive functioning at the social, behavioral, and physiological levels. At the physiological level, chronic glucocorticoid secretion can reduce hippocampal volume and produce reversible atrophy of dendritic processes in the hippocampus where memory and declarative learning is active (Sapolsky, 1996a). Furthermore, glucocorticoids induce metabolic vulnerability by disrupting neurotropic regulation of glutamate and calcium, leading to atrophy of the hippocampal dendrites. Sapolsky (1994) depicts this as the degenerative cascade shown in Figure 10.1.

Sapolsky's examination of data from persons suffering from Cushing's syndrome was instructive where overproduction of glucocorticoids was manifest as a result of pituitary and adrenal tumors. This study showed that the amount of hypersecretion of glucocorticoids was correlated with the extent of hippocampal atrophy, and also with the extent of impairment of hippocampal-dependent cognition (1996b). A study of persons who were suffering from depression by Sheline and others (1996) also verified the relation of levels of glucocorticoids with amounts of loss of hippocampal volume. The greater were the number of days of depression, the greater was the loss of hippocampal volume.

Over 50 years of research has shown that the deleterious effects of uncontrolled and unpredictable stress events have produced a substantial variety of negative physiologic consequences. Inescapable stress in rats increased the susceptibility to tumor growth and ulcer

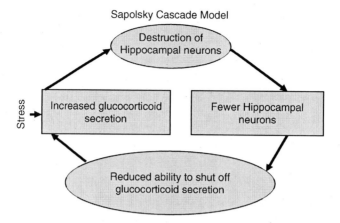

FIGURE 10.1. A degenerative cascade linking the ability of glucocorticoids to damage the hippocampus resulting in enhanced secretion of glucocorticoids *Source:* Adapted from Sapolsky, 1994.

development, decreased aggression, lowered dominant status, and suppressed lymphocyte proliferation (Shors et al., 1990). A chronic physical crisis, such as hypoglycemia in diabetes, oxygen deficit from sudden cardiac arrest, or blood circulation deficit in the brain as a result of epilepsy seizures, each create an energy crisis for the neurons in the hippocampus leading to their demise (Sapolsky, 1994). This interaction of the cognitive and physiological systems seems to indicate that improvement of one will improve the other.

Physical decline, illness, and communication barriers have been shown to foster infantilization, increased dependency, and additional social isolation—all factors which remove sources for mental stimulation and participation. The frustration of enduring chronic stressors with limited coping resources creates a sense of helplessness or hopelessness, turning a focus away from mental and social stimulation toward enduring the stressors. Cohen-Mansfield, Werner, and Reisberg, (1995) note that the impact of stress upon individuals can be better recognized by their perceptions of stressors rather than by examining the objective nature of stressors. These authors' measures of the perceptions of stress included the cognitive impact of global stress in terms of the degree to which individuals reported that it made their lives unpredictable, uncontrollable, and overloaded.

The impact of perceived stress on aging is nowhere more clearly demonstrated than in the work by Epel and associates (2004). While investigating the differences in telemere length (a DNA measure indicative of cellular aging), two samples were chosen, a healthy sample and one sample who were family caretakers (mothers) of young children who were seriously chronically ill. The significant difference was not between these two samples but within the sample where participants were under the daily stress of caretaking; the higher the report of perceived stress, the shorter the telemere structure and the lesser the telemerase activity, indicative of a higher rate of cell senescence. It was not simply the event of being the caretakers, which resulted in differences in cell aging. In the caretaker group, longer caretaking periods and greater levels of perceived stress also resulted in increased rates of cell aging.

COGNITIVE DECLINE AND PHYSICAL FACTORS

The dynamics of neural networks may account for the coexistence of cognitive decline and physical decline in older adults. In this view, cognitive decline is partially the product of the aging process resulting from deteriorating neurotransmitters, from poor cerebral blood flow, and from brain hypoxia. Research indicates that cognitive dysfunction is also related to increased hospital use, increased nursing home institutionalization, and mortality (Moritz, Kasl, & Berkman, 1989; Weiler et al., 1991; Branch & Jette, 1982; Kelman & Thomas, 1990; Kelman, Kennedy, & Cheng, 1994). Boaz (1994) reports that the more the cognitive impairment, the slower the recovery from long term disability. Although neural aging is an inevitable process in human life and affects cognitive function, the brain function also clearly influences the maintenance and/or decline of body systems. An examination of how these body systems interact, adapt, and maintain health is discussed in the following sections.

Flexibility and Balance of Body Systems in Healthy Functioning

Variability within physiologic activity of an organ, system, or complex of systems is associated with healthy functioning. Variability represents the capacity for systems to alter in adaptation to environmental living conditions. Giardino and others (2000) refer to these varying moment-to-moment actions of living systems as oscillations. Oscillations within single body systems and multiple interacting systems are self-regulatory, so as to be responsive when demands are made. Whereas, oscillations are rapid changes in body functioning, circadian rhythms are recognized as longer-term periodicities, allowing for body rest and repair (Giardino, Lehrer, & Feldman, 2000). However, these oscillations and rhythms operate within certain ranges. Operating beyond these ranges, body systems will produce negative reactions with other interacting systems. Disease susceptibility and ultimately, disease states, provide evidence that these oscillations and rhythms become less flexible and variable and after having persistently extended beyond the range of normal boundaries, set up a nonadaptive cycle.

An example is the cardiovascular system wherein heart rate, circulatory pressure and flow, and peripheral resistance make constant adaptations in response to neurochemical changes stimulating the sympathetic and parasympathetic systems. One can trace the pathology of hypertension to obtain an insight on how, after exceeding the normal oscillations of the cardiovascular and neurochemical system over an extended time, disease has developed. In the cardiovascular system, as in almost all other bodily systems, the autonomic system plays a major role in self-regulation. The two divisions, the sympathetic and parasympathetic, maintain the rate of blood flow through variability in heart rate control. Thus, flexibility in systems as measured by variability provides a depiction of healthy functioning. As noted in the cardiovascular example, an aspect of healthy cardiovascular status is in the balance of sympathetic and parasympathetic systems. Stated as a generality in this balance paradigm, hypertension is an overarousal of the sympathetic and underarousal of the parasympathetic branch. Increasingly, other disorders are showing evidence of failure of modulation of two or more normally integrated physiologic, mental, or skeletal systems—marked by lack of balance among them.

Plasticity of Cognitive Processes and Memory Functions

An important feature in changing the functioning of cognitive processes is the capacity for plasticity. Degree of plasticity indicates not only how readily humans can be trained for effective performance, but also how likely effective retraining will be to succeed (Baltes & Lindenberger, 1988; Kliegl, Smith, & Baltes, 1986). Some evidence for the way that cognitive plasticity occurs is seen in developmental studies of compensatory plasticity when deprivation in one sensory domain such as vision is compensated by hyperalertness in another domain such as hearing. Rauschecker (1995) suggests that at play are synaptic modifications, which probably employ a biochemical mechanism as well. There is a corollary in aging. Plasticity can be compromised by neuronal loss and change in synapses in the human hippocampal formation during normal aging (Geinisman et al., 1995; Coleman & Flood, 1987; Sapolsky, Krey, & McEwen, 1986), but there are also compensatory mechanisms at work here.

An emphasis placed on the functional neurophysiology may be especially fruitful in the light of the lack of strong correlates between neuroanatomical changes in the aging brain and cognitive deficits. Petit (1982) notes that most finite cellular changes are found as readily in the cognitively intact as found in those with senile dementia. An exception is the greater quantity of senile plaques found in senile dementia over the quantity found in normal aging persons; although, more recently, even the density of amyloid plaques has not consistently correlated with levels of cognitive deficit (Nagy et al., 1995). Nonetheless, a notable and consistent finding is that of density of dendritic branching, wherein significant differences in dendritic density are noted in the pathology of demented and normal aged individuals, and also between professional and nonprofessional postmortem brains (Buell & Coleman, 1979; Coleman & Flood, 1987; Jacobs, 1991; Peters, 1994). Related to this, the implication of the differences in dendritic growth found by Diamond (1988) between untrained and trained elderly rats poses the possibility that training in cognitive functioning may retain and enhance dendritic growth. This seems to be an attractive hypothesis in forwarding the concept of plasticity.

EEG PATTERNS AND THE ELDERLY

Experience with applying neurofeedback to elderly is slow to emerge. A problem is the lack of consistent deterioration of EEG patterns due to age. However, some of the EEG spectral patterns and frequency band power levels seen in elderly do tend to differ as a function of age. When compared to 30-year olds, adults aged 65 years and older typically exhibit EEG frequencies shifting toward lower values. There is a decrease in the magnitude of the dominant alpha frequency band (within the 8-12 Hz band), an increase in magnitude of theta rhythm (4-7 Hz), and a decrease in the magnitude of beta-1 (12.5-17.5 Hz) and beta-2 (17.5-25 Hz) (Duffy et al., 1984; Obrist, 1979; Matousek et al., 1967; Matejcek, 1980 (see Figure 10.2); Brenner et al., 1986; Nakano et al., 1992; Williamson et al., 1990). The visually assessed records of 420 normals showed the increased magnitude in slow waves with increasing age (Hughes & Cayaffa, 1977).

Also, the dominant alpha frequency generally declines in relation to physical decline and longevity (Obrist, 1979; Cahan & Yaeger, 1966). Dyro (1989) noted that in patients over the age of 75 years, it is common to find rhythmic posterior dominant frequencies in the 7-7.5 Hz range and an increase in bitemporal theta. The average frequency decline in a group of mentally normal elderly persons who survived in contrast to a group of 28 persons who died has also been reported. Obrist shows the average decline in the dominant alpha frequency of those remaining alive to be 0.3 Hz over a span of 7.3 years as contrasted to a significantly greater decline of 0.6 Hz over a span of only 5.1 years in those who died (Obrist, 1979).

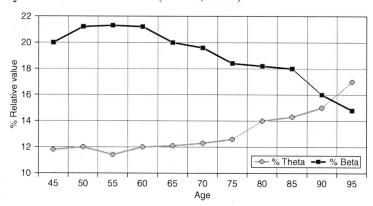

FIGURE 10.2. EEG changes with age in normals. *Note:* N = 619. *Source:* Reprinted from *Clinical Neurophysiology*, 10, Matejcek, "Some relationships between occipital EEG activity and age," pp. 122-130, 1980, with permission from Elsevier.

Niedermeyer, however, suggests that, "EEG changes ascribed to old age are essentially the result of a variety of pathological developments; there is only a small niche left for old age as such to be the causative agent" (1981). This thesis is further supported by Duffy and associates (1984) who found that neither power nor frequency changes demonstrated a high age correlation in normal adults. Furthermore, changes appear to be a nonlinear process and not wholly symmetrical across the cerebral hemispheres. Right hemisphere changes appear more prominent than left brain wave changes. High alpha band (10-12 Hz) power remains the hallmark of good memory performance, despite age level.

Some researchers report that among older adults who have cognitive decline,. the most pathognomonic characteristic in the quantitative EEG patterns is a generalized increase in diffuse slow activity, rather than the appearance of focal disturbances (Obrist, 1979; Nakano et al., 1992; Prichep et al., 1994; Hartikainen et al., 1992; Breslau et al., 1989). Increase in diffuse slow activity has been found in anterior as well as posterior temporal, frontal, and occipital areas. In persons suffering from dementia, the brain wave activity is characterized by a generalized significantly increased magnitude in theta and delta activity with decreased blood flow and cerebral metabolic rate. This may indicate that metabolic/circulatory activities are significant factors in cognitive decline (Kwa et al., 1993; Waldemar, 1995; Rockwood, 2002). Magnitude of theta and delta appear to be early prognostic indicators of cognitive decline and life expectancy. Williamson and others (1990) found significant correlations of beta 1 with performance on cognitive testing at frontal and central locations bilaterally. Also, reduction of alpha frequency was significantly related to decreased cognitive functioning.

Evoked Potentials

Evoked potentials (EPs) are defined as the electrical activity of the brain that is triggered by the presentation of a particular stimulus. The stimulation of the sensory system (visual, auditory, or tactile) is signaled by the appearance of a waveform at the cortex. One of the most useful waves is the P300, which occurs approximately 300 msec after the presentation of the stimulus. P300 latency increases with age (Verleger et al., 1991) but cognitive deficits can slow it even further.

The absence, diminution, or delay of the P300 wave can indicate the presence of cognitive impairment. With most demented patients, the P300 is delayed. Other types of head trauma may produce reduced amplitude P300s but the latency can be normal.

Moore and others (1996) found that a delayed P2 (P200) visual flash evoked response may be a marker of cognitive dysfunction in healthy elderly volunteers. Nine of the putatively healthy participants had a delayed P2. Although unaware of any memory deficits, 5 of the 27 had WMS-R (Wechsler Memory Scale-Revised) Visual Memory Span percentile scores 1 or more standard deviations less than age-matched controls. Four of the five had the delayed P2. The authors concluded that the delayed P2 in putatively healthy subjects is indicative of a visuospatial deficit, which might be a precursor of dementia later.

Keller (1988) found that a limited EEG band (36-44 Hz) showed increased magnitude as normal subjects were engaged in problem-solving, however, SDAT (Senile Dementia of the Alzheimer's Type) patients showed no significant increase. Could reduced 40 Hz latency under task serve as a warning of possible cognitive decline?

Coherence Changes in the Elderly

Coherence is one of the parameters that helps define the efficiency of the brain's information processing capability. It is calculated in various ways but it generally involves a mathematical calculation such as cross correlation. Essentially, coherence is a measure of how closely in morphology or shape EEG signals from one site agree with those from a second site. An essential condition for appropriate responses to external stimuli and higher nervous system processing is an optimal level of coherence throughout the cortex. However, Duffy and associates (1995) found that coherence tends to decrease with age. The neural connections between sites most likely become less efficient in communicating due to atherosclerosis, stress, plaques, and tangles, as well as a number of brain insults that accrue with daily living. Can coherence dysfunctions be remedied? Dillbeck and Bronson (1981) found that transcendental meditation of only two weeks duration could *increase* frontal coherence. Coherence also can be increased or decreased through neurofeedback training.

SUMMARY THUS FAR ON EEG AND AGING

At this point, several assumptions may be put forth:

1. Older individuals may be limited in their cognitive abilities by the belief fostered by our culture that the elderly do indeed suffer from these deficits and are therefore regarded less highly by the younger generations;
2. Older individuals normally show nonlinear changes in the EEG and cortical evoked response related to decreasing brain alertness. Only a portion of the changes are attributed to aging;
3. Older individuals normally show some decrease in cerebral blood flow;
4. Theta band power increases as individuals age;
5. The EEG typically shows some loss of power in the alpha band as one ages but not systematically in beta frequency power;
6. Reduced 40 Hz band power may serve as a marker of aging;
7. The evoked response shows that delayed P200 and P300 often occur as people age;
8. Coherence decreases are often seen as individuals age;
9. However, a proportion of the elderly show no significant decline in cognitive functioning and appear to have maintained the cerebral blood flow and the EEG of much younger individuals.

POTENTIAL PROTOCOLS FOR NEUROFEEDBACK WITH ELDERLY

Based upon the wide variation of EEG patterns in elderly with mild cognitive impairment (but with no other chronic brain pathology), diverse approaches rather than established protocols are being pursued by neurotherapists. Not unlike the approach for mild head injury, a combination of treatment of sites showing abnormalities (often-increased slow waveforms of delta and theta) and observed symptoms of impaired cognitive functioning are used. Coherence training may be the protocol of initial interest when the QEEG comparison with the database indicates significant deviations in coherence from norm. The following protocols are frequently useful:

1. Coherence training is typically done in segments of five sessions for the largest deviation (sites and band) first before proceeding to the second largest Z-score deviation sites, etc. Since coherence training can be easily "over-trained," clinical experience has evolved a five- session maximum before sequencing to another pair of sites.
2. Narrow frequency band deviations from norm (based on QEEG) can be addressed through neurofeedback protocols, which inhibit and enhance at these locations and bands. In most cases, the elderly require reduction in the theta and delta bands with enhancement of beta and sometimes, alpha band magnitudes.
3. If protocols allow, peak alpha frequency enhancement will often be required.
4. Enhancement of high alpha bands, for example, 11-13 Hz, from Pz is helpful.
5. A number of neurofeedback systems now employ AVS (audio-visual stimulation) as a part of the protocol. The AVS frequency can be controlled by the EEG. Besides entraining the EEG, the AVS also increases cerebral blood flow.
6. Home training can be accomplished through inexpensive neurofeedback devices, AVS units, or special purpose CDs (for improved memory, relaxation, and stress).

THE PONCE DE LEON PROJECT

In the early nineties, at the University of West Florida, a colleague and the first author developed an extensive program of training for the elderly. The start of the "Decade of the Brain" spurred our efforts. We used a number of techniques, including neurofeedback, light/sound stimulation, the Revitalizer and Brain Brightener cassette tapes, hand temperature biofeedback, and blood pressure measurements. One group received lectures on stress management and practiced together with the hand temperature feedback. Those who stayed in the group did indeed lower their pressures significantly. Surprisingly, the number of volunteers that came forward for this unique program was relatively mall. The potential subject pool came from a high-income independent living community that bordered the campus. Although we gave three 4-hour lecture demonstrations, the attitude of the potential participants was generally one of a high degree of skepticism about these alternative nonmedical interventions. However, two 80 year-old individuals, a man and a woman, volunteered for the neurofeedback package, which included not only the neurofeedback training but also the Brain Brightener, Neurobics and Revitalizer cassette tapes, and light/sound machines donated from Robert Austin and Synetic Systems in Seattle. The Revitalizer and Brain Brightener tapes were developed by Budzynski and incorporated below threshold (priming) binaural tones and multiple voice tracks to enhance the effect (see Figure 10.3) of change in peak alpha frequency. The original subliminal alpha binaural tone technique was developed by Swingle (1996).

The neurofeedback part of the Ponce de Leon Project was called the "Brain Brightener" program. Participants would receive neurofeedback from the scalp site, Cz, twice a week. A Focus 1,000 system was used with a reward bandpass of 15-18 Hz and inhibit of 2-8 Hz. Homework consisted of daily AVS (light/sound) sessions and listening to the various cassette tapes (the Revitalizer is only 12.5 minutes in duration).

Results for the two participants were gratifying although both scored above average on the Wechsler Memory Scale-Revised even before training began. Both participants however, decreased their 2-8 Hz

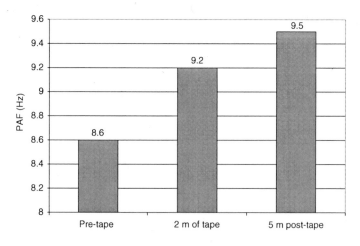

FIGURE 10.3. Peak alpha frequency change with sub A tape. *Note:* RH 80.

delta-theta EEG levels as they progressed through the training (Figure 10.4).

The female (DM) completed 20 sessions that included the first practice session. She was able to participate in the Pre-Post and Follow-up testing on the Wechsler Memory Scale. Her scores showed improvement as can be seen in Figure 10.5, even though her pre-scores were average for her age and education.

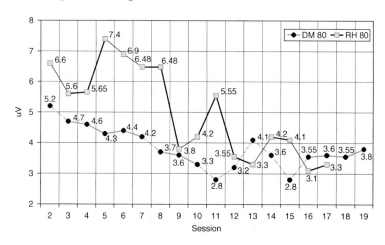

FIGURE 10.4. Delta-theta (2-8 Hz) across sessions.

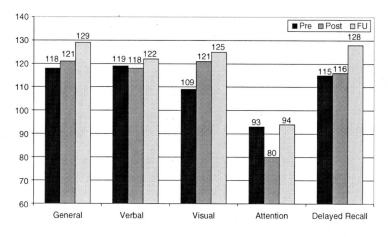

FIGURE 10.5. Wechsler memory scale. *Note:* Subject: DM 80.

Unfortunately the male (RH) developed a cancerous tumor on his thigh and had to drop out after 18 sessions. Two comments by the participants are noteworthy: DM commented that she was remembering small things again, like the names of friends and where she left items, and she was multitasking again. On the other hand, 80-year old RH was reluctant to voice any statements of progress. However, in his tenth session, he remarked that in the past two weeks he was once again playing bridge like the master he had been at 45. (He stated that he had no idea why this was occurring.)

A growing number of elderly clients reporting cognitive deficits have been trained by us since then. Elsa and Rufus Baehr (personal communication) are using combinations of "Brain Brightening" protocols, using the Microcog for evaluation before and after training. During or following training, the clients often report a resurgence of abilities in relevant areas of their lives, for example, recovering writing skills, card playing, short- and long-term memory, and sound, restful sleep.

THE EFFECTS OF STIMULATION ON COGNITIVE FUNCTIONING

The animal research of Diamond (1988) and others demonstrated the effects of stimulation on structural changes in the brain. Rats placed in a stimulating environment showed increased learning ability. There was unmistakable evidence of increased dendritic growth and other neuronal changes resulting in a heavier, denser, and larger brain than those rats left as unstimulated controls. Moreover, older rats equivalent to 70 to 80-year old humans, also exhibited the same structural and learning changes when given stimulating conditions.

Does increased stimulation of elderly humans help to preserve and even improve cognitive ability? The art of applying this kind of stimulation to older humans, producing an effective positive change is the challenge of today. A number of studies in various cultures (China, France, and the United States) have shown a consistent pattern—the greater the educational level and/or the intellectual challenge of the job, the greater the cognitive health in old age (Katzman, 1993; Datiques, 1993; Snowdon, 2001).

Enhancement of cognitive activity has a long history. Attempts to correct specific cognitive deficits such as information finding, speed of performance, memory span, encoding, recall, and spatial orientation have been made through cognitive/behavioral training (Willis, 1982; Duke, Haley, & Bergquist, 1991). Newer approaches in the way of neurologic stimulation are the use of audio-visual (AVS) stimulation and neurofeedback. The essence of work with neurofeedback is to attempt to lower the magnitude of slower frequency EEG bands and increase that of high alpha or beta bands (Budzynski, 1996; Budzynski & Budzynski, 2000).

Audio-Visual Stimulation

The use of photic stimulation can be traced as far back as Adrian and Matthews who elaborated on the Berger rhythm effect found in the occipital lobe (Adrian & Matthews, 1934). However, the work of Walter and Walter (1949) remains the classic in recognizing that photic stimulation can cause EEG patterns to match the frequency of the flickering lights. Extensive reviews of the phenomenon of light stimulation on brain activity have been published by Budzynski (1992) and Siever (1997). Audio-visual entrainment is accomplished through a natural phenomenon of visual evoked responses. When a stimulus reaches the visual cortex, a visual evoked response is produced, a response that follows the frequency characteristics of the stimulus. For example, a commonly used flash frequency band is 9-11 Hz. This flash stimulus tends to evoke a brain response of 9-11 Hz cortically. Entrainment to a higher frequency can be achieved in a slowed brain by flashing at a rate slightly higher than the desired alpha frequency. Entraining to a slightly higher frequency than the participant's mean alpha may allow at least a temporary stabilization of the brain at that level of frequency following a series of entrainment sessions.

Although variety of lightsets (light-emitting diodes or LEDs) patterns are possible, the usual approach in audio-visual stimulation treatment is to set the lights centrally over both eyes, with instructions to the participant to keep his or her eyes closed. Some lightsets are of clear plastic with the LEDs set around the periphery. The user can thus see through them in order to read, watch TV or a computer screen. Differing light patterns, colors, frequencies, and waveforms generate varying visual color patterns. The evidence indicates that blue and green colors seem to be calming, whereas red, orange, and yellow increase arousal. White light contains all the colors of the spectrum and thus may provide the most generalized effect upon participants by eliciting a variety of perceptions of color from users. Varying frequencies and waveforms can also be key factors in producing change. Programming the photic stimulation can guide the outcome in very specific ways. The frequency level of the light stimulus can influence mood and alertness. Budzynski designed the "pseudo-random" program, which ramps the light frequencies and sounds up and down at intervals within a range of 9-22 Hz.

Changing programs at intervals as the brain becomes habituated to one program can further activate the brain. If the changes occur very rapidly and in a pseudorandom fashion, the brain is unable to habituate and thus will maintain a higher rate of blood flow in certain regions. The Paradise XL (produced by David Siever) uses a semisquare waveform, a compromise between the pure square wave and the sine wave. The effect of the square wave is to stimulate the brain at a greater rate by employing the effect of harmonics, whereas sine waves produce relaxation by producing the single frequency response. These photic stimulation techniques provide a sound basis for audio-visual intervention (Siever, 1997).

Fox and Raichle (1985) studied the effect of photic stimulation on cerebral blood flow. They found blood flow to be increased by approximately 28 percent over baseline following stimulation (see Figure 10.6).

Mentis and others (1997) used PET scans with elderly subjects to show how photic stimulation can activate frontal areas of the brain. A report by Cady and others (1988) showed that exposure to self-selected photic stimulation frequencies produced increases of approximately 21 percent in serum serotonin and 24 percent in betaendorphins. These changes should decrease the effects of depression when it is characterized by lower than normal serotonin.

Auditory stimulation is also transformed into bioelectrical signals, which impact brain wave activity. The auditory projection centers are in the temporal lobes adjacent to the frontal area. Using auditory tones as an augmentation to photic stimulation, sound, particularly binaural beats, contributes to the entrainment effect of the photic stimulation.

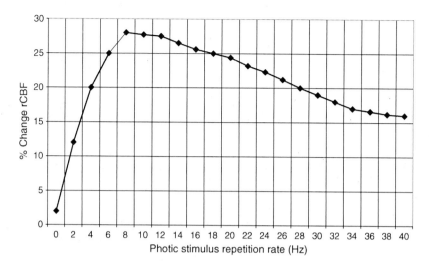

FIGURE 10.6. Photic stimulus rate and cerebral blood flow. *Source:* Adapted from Fox and Raichle, 1985. *Note:* Percent change from baseline.

Low frequency sounds are discerned more anteriorally and high frequency sounds, more posteriorally.

While much is known about the mechanisms of change following audio-visual stimulation, the data are uneven and unintegrated. However, there is enough evidence to suggest the considerable influence achieved by stimulating the brain in this manner.

The University of Washington Audio-Visual Stimulation Study with the Elderly

After we completed a study showing that audio-visual stimulation (AVS) could increase academic performance in university students (Budzynski, Jordy, Budzynski, Tang, & Claypoole, 1999), we wondered if we could apply this technology to elderly persons. This study involved the application of photic and auditory (light/sound) stimulation to the elderly, ages 53 to 87 years. These elderly persons showed wide individual variations in performance, thus leading to speculation as to how various characteristics of participants possibly affected the outcome. The group, which completed training, was composed of 31 men and women attending two senior centers who were living independently either in the community or in an independent living facility. All had been participants in a controlled research study, the results of which will be presented in the next section. These persons attended 20-minute sessions of light/sound therapy for three days a week over a three-month period. They could choose to come at any half-hour interval throughout the morning on any three of four days a week. Space was available for 10 subjects to obtain training at any one time. They could talk among themselves or with the investigator during those sessions as they wished. The light/sound stimulation sequence for this study was composed of a program computerized to drive EEG frequencies pseudo-randomly between 9 and 22 Hz. This method did not allow the brain to stay at static frequencies, but required it to make continual adaptations to the changing light and sound stimuli thus increasing brain activity and cerebral blood flow. Auditory stimulation also included left and right binaural tones and pulses of various frequencies to further activate the brain. Each participant had his or her own station consisting of a lightset and headphones and two controllers, one for light intensity and one for volume. All stations were driven off the master unit, which controlled the pseudorandom stimulation.

The purpose of the study was to discover if this light/sound stimulation over a period of time would result in positive changes in cognitive ability as measured by the Microcog and the Buschke Remembering Test. The study also examined changes in EEG patterns as a result of the treatment. The EEG placements for measuring changes in EEG patterns were at F7 and F8, obtaining three minutes of eyes open and eyes closed data with the Biograph Procomp for both the pre- and posttesting. Data were also collected on medications, chronic disorders, living arrangements, and daily activities.

Microcog Results

Thirty-one participants (N = 31) were able to complete AVS training and the pre-post testing. This group included 18 from the original experimental group and thirteen from the original waiting list control group who took the 30 session AVS training after completing the control period. Most subjects increased their scores in eight of the nine parameters of the Microcog as shown in Figure 10.7. Only in

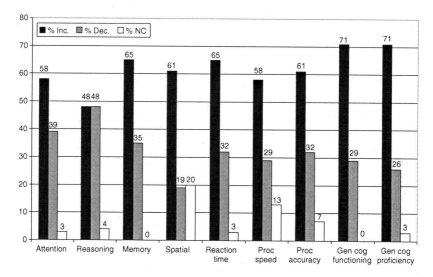

FIGURE 10.7. Percentage of Ss who increased, decreased, or remained the same after AVS.

the parameter, Reasoning, there was not a larger proportion who increased their scores.

Comparing AVS and Control Groups

A few of the participants experienced a worsening of their physical disorders during the study. Typically, they had been placed on new medications or had their existing prescriptions increased by their physicians. These individuals were eliminated from the final AVS and control group study, leaving an N = 13 in the AVS and 11 in the C group. Post- and pre-Buschke and Microcog scores for these two groups are shown in Figure 10.8.

The AVS group did better than the control group on the Buschke Remembering test and the AVS group did score at higher post-pre difference levels on seven of the nine Microcog scales, however, the control group had higher mean scores on Reasoning and General Cognitive Proficiency. Possibly the AVS group simply performed faster and with less caution on the posttesting. Moreover, experience with light/sound stimulation shows that after a session the participant

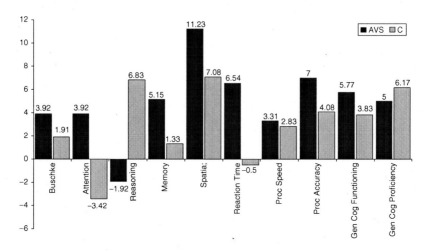

FIGURE 10.8. Mean post/pre differences in Buschke and Microcog standard scores.

may go through a period of 15 to 30 minutes in which he or she feels mild confusion. Considering that such stimulation would increase cerebral blood flow in a general way, both inhibitory and excitatory neural networks would be activated. Some individuals seem particularly sensitive to this change and although it seems to be of benefit for most cognitive abilities, it may temporarily hinder more complex functioning such as those required in the reasoning tasks. In fact, the losses in scores on both of these scales could be attributed to seven subjects. An examination of the characteristics that these seven held in common revealed that all had some degree of pathophysiology present, either cardiovascular or a hormonally linked problem such as Type II diabetes. Overall, all of the participants that completed the study expressed the belief that the training had helped them. It is not yet known if a different protocol of AVS training would have been more effective.

NUTRITION AND COGNITIVE HEALTH

A topic, which is a related discussion, is that of nutrition. The critical nutritional elements are hotly debated and somewhat unresolved as to how the dietary supplemental elements participate in reversing cognitive impairment.

Much is yet to be learned about what supplements such as antioxidants are necessitated by elderly in added amounts. The literature is frequently changing, but a short review here consolidates that which is accepted at the present time about nutritional recommendations.

One important and well-researched finding in elderly is that of the detrimental effects of glutathione deficiency. Glutathione is the master antioxidant produced in the liver which is the main protective cofactor against neurodegenerative diseases such as Parkinson's disease, Alzheimer's disease and multiple other major chronic disorders. The synthesis of glutathione depends upon adequate protein nutrition as precursors of cysteine development. Glutathione plays important roles in antioxidant defense, cell metabolism and regulation of cellular events such as cell proliferation and apoptosis, immune response and signal transduction. Interference with glutathione metabolism results in oxidative stress and ultimately, neurogenesis (nerve cell death) (Schulz et al., 2000; Jhat et al., 2000; Prasad et al., 1999).

For maintenance of the synthesis of glutathione metabolism, critical factors are N-acetyl cysteine and cofactors vitamins A, C and E and alpha-lipoic acid. Supplements of glutathione itself are not bioavailable by mouth. The various forms of glutathione are developed in the liver and travel to the brain to counter toxins such as metals and free radicals. In addition, free oxygen radicals, while being formed by mitochondria as a byproduct of producing the nutrient ATP, need to be countered by antioxidants to prevent the neurodegeneration of the brain cells. Glutathione and its cofactors, as well as vitamins such as biotin (B1, B2, B6, B9 [Folate], and B12) are critical to the health of the nervous system and have been determined to be the significant components protecting against neurodegeneration as found in Parkinson's disease, Alzheimer's disease and other neurologic degenerative diseases such as multiple sclerosis. There appears to be a correlation between glutathione depletion and poor health in the elderly.

Singly, many of these antioxidants are studied for brain health. A number of studies indicated that men and women who had higher levels of folate were able to remember more of the main details of a short story that had been read to them than did those with low folate.

Higher levels of B6 and B12 in subjects appear to be correlated with better memory skills. The damage from free radicals is known to be a result of high homocysteine levels in the blood, and these radicals are found in elevated amounts in Alzheimers and other chronic diseases. Folic acid, along with B12, is believed to counter high levels of homocysteine. Vitamin A, and its precursor, beta-carotene also are being studied because of the low levels found in persons suffering from Alzheimer's disease.

Intake of omega-3 fatty acids found in cold-water fish is suggested in order to maintain brain cell integrity, to stabilize arterial walls, and provide anti-inflammatory protection. Interestingly, this addition to the diet also appears to enhance cognition in learning dysfunctions.

Minerals such as calcium, magnesium, and zinc are highly recommended as supplements, as are two naturally occurring compounds, S-adenosylmethionine (SAMe), which helps to increase the body's levels of serotonin, melatonin, and dopamine; and phosphatidylserine, which promotes cell health and boosts the activity of acetylcholine and other brain chemicals (for more details see Kurzweil & Grossman, 2004).

A BRAIN BRIGHTENING PROGRAM FOR OPTIMAL AGING

Considering the aforementioned information, one could suggest a reasonably effective program that would enhance healthy aging. Although maintaining a normal bodyweight and engaging in a regular exercise program were not emphasized in this chapter, these two factors are of obvious importance. Moreover, a nutritional regime such as suggested earlier and detailed in Kurzweil and Grossman's Fantastic Voyage should certainly be included a brain-brightening program. Neurofeedback has been shown, at least in numerous anecdotal case studies, to enhance cognitive abilities in the elderly. AVS is showing more and more application to the problems of the elderly such as balance and memory. Stress and pain relief, and memory enhancement techniques using audio and computer software of a self-help nature, including priming, are available. Those seniors who have tried and regularly used yoga and/or meditation know how well these practices alleviate daily stress. Keeping occupied with cognitively challenging activities, from bridge to crossword puzzles and even taking courses at nearby institutions of higher learning help keep the brain young. Maintaining a pleasant social life with a cadre of good friends helps decrease stress and quite probably strengthens immune functioning. Research on telomeres and stem cells will one day, possibly surprisingly soon, allow scientists to extend lifetimes.

Nonetheless, there are individual concerns that demand treatments beyond the aforementioned treatment foci. Individuals are impacted by traumatic and emotionally damaging experiences, which cause chemical, electromagnetic, immunological, and hormonal imbalances in their bodies and brains. During those periods, when brain wave patterns go awry, neurotherapists can do much to restore the balance by first pinpointing the problem areas and then remediating these with neurofeedback and augmenting techniques. This field is broadening, not simply because of the increased population who are living longer and growing in numbers. It is broadening because more and more knowledge and technology is becoming available to counter the chronic symptoms that emerge, and consumers are ever more alert to the possibilities of a more symptom-free lifestyle.

REFERENCES

Adrian, E., & Matthews, B. (1934). The Berger rhythm: Potential changes from the occipital lobes of man. *Brain, 57,* 355-385.

Anokhin, A., & Vogel, F. (1996). EEG alpha rhythm frequency and intelligence in normal adults. *Intelligence, 23,* 1-14.

Baltes, P. B., & Lindenberger, U. (1997). Emergence of a powerful connection between sensory and cognitive functions across the adult life span: A new window to the study of cognitive aging? *Psychology and Aging, 12*(1), 12-21.

Boaz, R. F. (1994). Improved versus deteriorated physical functioning among long-term disabled elderly. *Medical Care, 32*(6), 588-602.

Branch, L. G., & Jette, A. M. (1982). A prospective study of long-term care institutionalization among the aged. *American Journal of Public Health, 72*(12), 1373-1379.

Brenner, R. P., Ulrich, R. F., Spiker, D. G., Sclabassi, R. J., Reynolds, C. F., 3rd, Marin, R. S., et al. (1986). Computerized EEG spectral analysis in elderly normal, demented, and depressed subjects. *Electroencephalography and Clinical Neurophysiology, 64*(6), 483-492.

Breslau, J., Starr, A., Sicotte, N., Higa, J., & Buchsbaum, M. S. (1989). Topographic EEG changes with normal aging and SDAT. *Electroencephalography and Clinical Neurophysiology, 72*(4), 281-289.

Budzynski, T. (1992). *Clinical considerations of sound/light*. Seattle, WA: Synetics.

Budzynski, T. (1996). Brain brightening: Can neurofeedback improve cognitive process? *Biofeedback, 24*(2), 14-17.

Budzynski, T., & Andrasik, F. (1995). *The Ponce de Leon project: Brain brightening. Report on pilot study*. Pensacola, FL: Center for Behavioral Research, University of West Florida.

Budzynski, T., & Budzynski, H. (2000). Reversing age-related cognitive decline: Use of neurofeedback and audio-visual stimulation. *Biofeedback, 28*, 19-21.

Budzynski, T., Jordy, J., Kogan Budzynski, H., Tang, J., & Claypoole, K. (1999). Academic performance enhancement with photic stimulation and EDR feedback. *Journal of Neurotherapy, 3*, 11-21.

Buell, S. J., & Coleman, P. D. (1979). Dendritic growth in the aged human brain and failure of growth in senile dementia. *Science, 206*(4420), 854-856.

Cady, R., Shealy, C., Veehoff, D., Liss, S., Closson, W., & Cox, R. (1983). *Neurochemical responses to cranial electrical stimulation, and photo-stimulation brain wave synchronization*. Unpublished manuscript, Springfield, MO.

Cahan, R. B., & Yeager, C. L. (1966). Admission EEG as a predictor of mortality and discharge for aged state hospital patients. *Journal of Gerontology, 21*(2), 248-256.

Cohen-Mansfield, J., Werner, P., & Reisberg, B. (1995). Temporal order of cognitive and functional loss in a nursing home population. *Journal of American Geriatric Society, 43*, 974-978.

Coleman, P. D., & Flood, D. G. (1987). Neuron numbers and dendritic extent in normal aging and Alzheimer's disease. *Neurobiology of Aging, 8*(6), 521-545.

Craik, F. I., Morris, L. W., Morris, R. G., & Loewen, E. R. (1990). Relations between source amnesia and frontal lobe functioning in older adults. *Psychology and Aging, 5*(1), 148-151.

Datiques, J. F. (1993). *Brain plasticity: A lifetime perspective*. Bristol-Myers Squibb Sumposium.

Diamond, M. C. (1998). *Enhancing heredity: The impact of the environment on the anatomy of the brain*. New York: The Free Press.

Diamond, M. C., Johnson, R. E., Protti, A. M., Ott, C. & Kajisa, L. (1985). Plasticity in the 904-day-old male rat cerebral cortex. *Experimental Neurology, 87*(2), 309-317.

Dillbeck, M. C., & Bronson, E. C. (1981). Short-term longitudinal effects of the transcedental meditation technique on EEG power and coherence. *International Journal of Neuroscience, 14*(3-4), 147-151.

Duffy, F. H., Albert, M. S., McAnulty, G., & Garvey, A. J. (1984). Age-related differences in brain electrical activity of healthy subjects. *Annals of Neurology, 16*, 430-438.

Duffy, F. H., Jones, K. J., McAnulty, G. B., & Albert, M. S. (1995). Spectral coherence in normal adults: Unrestricted principal components analysis; relation of factors to age, gender, and neuropsychological data. *Clinical Electroencephalography, 26*, 30-46.

Duke, L., Haley, W., & Bergquist, T. (1991). *Handbook of clinical behavior therapy with the elderly client (applied clinical psychology)*. New York: Plenum Press.

Dyro, F. M. (1989). *The EEG handbook.* Boston: Little, Brown and Company.

Ebly, E. M., Hogan, D. B., & Parhad, I. M. (1995). Cognitive impairment in the nondemented elderly. Results from the Canadian Study of Health and Aging. *Archives of Neurology, 52*(6), 612-619.

Elkins, R. (2002). *The new class of missing nutrients: Miracle sugars.* Pleasant Grove: Woodland Publishing.

Epel, E. S., Blackburn, E. H., Lin, J., Dhabhar, F. S., Adler, N. E., Morrow, J. D. et al. (2004). Accelerated telomere shortening in response to life stress. *Proceedings of the National Academy Sciences of the United States of America, 101*(49), 17312-17315. Epub 12004 Dec 17311.

Fox, P. T., & Raichle, M. E. (1985). Stimulus rate determines regional brain blood flow in striate cortex. *Annual Report of Neurology, 17*(3), 303-305.

Gage, F. H. (2002). Neurogenesis in the adult brain. *The Journal of Neuroscience, 22*(3), 612-613.

Geinisman, Y., Detoledo-Morrell, L., Morrell, F., & Heller, R. E. (1995). Hippocampal markers of age-related memory dysfunction: Behavioral, electrophysiological and morphological perspectives. *Progress in Neurobiology, 45*(3), 223-252.

Giannitrapani, D. (1969). EEG average frequency and intelligence. *Electroencephalography and Clinical Neurophyiology, 27,* 480-486.

Giannitrapani, D., & Murri, L. (Eds.). (1988). *The EEG of mental activities.* Basel, Switzerland: S. Karger AG.

Giardino, N. D., Lehrer, P. M., & Feldman, J. M. (1999). *Cardiovascular resonant frequency biofeedback.* Wheat Ridge, CO: Association of Applied Psychophyiology and Biofeedback.

Gilad, M. G., & Gilad V. H. (1995). Strain, stress, neurodegeneration and longevity. *Mechanisms of Aging and Development, 78,* 75-83.

Hanninen, T., Hallikainen, M., Koivisto, K., Helkala, E. L., Reinikainen, K. J., Soininen, H., Mykkanen, L., Laakso, M. & Riekkinen, P.J. (1995). A follow-up study of age-associated memory impairment: Neuropsychological predictors of dementia. *Journal of the American Geriatrics Society, 43*(9), 1007-1015.

Hartikainen, P., Soininen, H., Partanen, J., Helkala, E. L., Riekkinen, P. (1992). Aging and spectral analysis of EEG in normal subjects: A link to memory and CSF AChE. *Acta Neurology Scandivania, 86,* 148-155.

Horn, J. (1982). The theory of fluid and crystallized intelligence in relation to concepts of cognitive psychology and aging in adulthood. In F. I. M. C. S. Trehub (Ed.), *Aging and cognitive processes* (pp. 237-278). New York: Plenum.

Howieson, D. B., Holm, L. A., Kaye, J. A., Oken, B. S., & Howieson, J. (1993). Neurologic function in the optimally healthy oldest old. Neuropsychological evaluation. *Neurology, 43*(10), 1882-1886.

Hughes, J. R. C., & Cayaffa, J. J. (1977). The EEG in patients at different ages without organic cerebral disease. *Electroencephalography and Clinical Neurophysiology, 42,* 776-784.

Jacobs, R. G. (1991). *A quantitative dendritic analysis of Wernicke's area.* Unpublished Dissertation, University of California, Los Angeles, CA, Los Angeles.

Jagger, C., Clarke, M., & Clarke, S. J. (1991). Getting older—Feeling younger: The changing health profile of the elderly. *International Journal of Epidemiology, 20*(1), 234-238.

Jausovec, N. (1996). Differences in EEG alpha activity related to giftedness. *Intelligence, 23,* 159-173.

Jhat, N., Jurma, O., Lalli, G., Liu, Y., Pettus, E. H., Greenamyre, J. T., Liu, R., Forman, H. J., & Andersen (2000). Glutathione depletion in PC12 results in selective inhibition of mitochrondrial complex activity. *The Journal of Biological Chemistry, 275*(34), 26096-26101.

Katzman, R. (1993). Education and the prevalence of dementia and Alzheimer's disease. *Neurology, 43*(1), 13-20.

Keller, W. J. (1988). *Forty hertz EEG in elderly patients with mild dementia of the Alzheimer's type.* Paper presented at the 16th Annual meeting of the International Neuropsychological Society, New Orleans.

Kelman, H. R., & Thomas, C. (1990). Transitions between community and nursing home residence in an urban elderly population. *Journal of Community Health, 15,* 105-122.

Kelman, H. R., Thomas, C., Kennedy, G. J., & Cheng, J. (1994). Cognitive impairment and mortality in older community residents. *American Journal of Public Health, 84*(8), 1255-1260.

Kempermann, G., Jessberger, S., Steiner, B., & Kronenberg, G. (2004). Milestones of neuronal development in the adult hippocampus. *Trends in Neurosciences, 27*(8), 447-452.

Kirsch, D. L. (2002). *The science behind cranial electrotherapy stimulation* (2nd ed.). Edmonton: Medical Scope Publishing Corporation.

Kliegl, R., Smith, H., & Baltes, P. (1986). Testing the limits, expertise and memory in adulthood and old age. In Klix, F. & Hagendorf, H. (Eds). *Human memory and cognitive capabilities: Mechanisms and performances* (pp. 395-407). Amsterdam: North Holland.

Kokaia, Z., & Lindvall, O. (2003). Neurogenesis after ischaemic brain insults. *Current Opinion in Neurobiology, 13*(1), 127-132.

Kurzweil, R., & Grossman, T. (2004). *Fantastic voyage: Live long enough to live forever.* New York: Rodale, Inc.

Kwa, V. I., Weinstein, H. C., Posthumus-Meyjes, E. F., Van Royen, E. A., Bour, L. J., Verhoeff, P. N., & Ongerboer de Visser, B. W. (1993). Spectral analysis of the EEG and 99m-Tc-HMPAO-SPECT-scan in Alzheimer's disease. *Biological Psychiatry, 33*(2), 100-107.

Levy, B. R. (1996). Improving memory in old age by implicit self stereotyping. *Journal of Personality and Social Pscyhology, 71,* 1092-1107.

Levy, B. R. (2003). Mind matters: Cognitive and physical effects of aging self-stereotypes. *The Journals of Gerontology. Series B, Psychological Sciences and Social Sciences, 58*(4), P203-P211.

Levy, B. R., & Langer, E. (1994). Aging free from negative stereotypes: Successful memory in China and among the American Deaf. *Journal of Personality and Social Psychology, 66*(6), 989-998.

Levy, B. R., & Myers, L. M. (2004). Preventive health behaviors influenced by self-perceptions of aging. *Preventive Medicine, 39*(3), 625-629.

Levy, B. R., Slade, M. D., & Kasl, S. V. (2002). Longitudinal benefit of positive self-perceptions of aging on functional health. *The Journals of Gerontology. Series B, Psychological Sciences and Social Sciences, 57*(5), P409-P417.

Lindenberger, U., Kliegl, R., & Baltes, P. B. (1992). Professional expertise does not eliminate age differences in imagery-based memory performance during adulthood. *Psychology and Aging, 7*(4), 585-593.

Maeder, T. (2002). Sweet medicines. *Scientific American, 291*(7), 40-47.

Matejcek, M. (1980). [Some relationships between occipital E.E.G. activity and age. A spectral analytic study (author's transl)]. *Revue délectroencéphalographie et de Neurophysiologie Clinique, 10*(2), 122-130.

Matousek, M., Volavka, J., Roubicek, J., & Roth, Z. (1967). EEG frequency analysis related to age in normal adults. *Electroencephalography and Clinical Neurophysiology, 23*(2), 162-167.

Mentis, M. J., Alexander, G. E., Grady, C. L., Horwitz, B., Krasuski, J., Pietrini, P. et al. (1997). Frequency variation of a pattern-flash visual stimulus during PET differentially activates brain from striate through frontal cortex. *NeuroImage, 5*(2), 116-128.

Moore, N. C., Vogel, R. L., Tucker, K. A., Khairy, N. M., & Coburn, K. L. (1996). P2 flash visual evoked response delay may be a marker of cognitive dysfunction in healthy elderly volunteers. *International Psychogeriatrics, 8*(4), 549-559.

Moritz, D. J., Kasl, S. V., & Berkman, L. F. (1989). The health impact of living with a cognitively impaired elderly spouse: Depressive symptoms and social functioning. *Journals of Gerontology, 44*(1), S17-S27.

Nagy, Z., Esiri, M. M., Jobst, K. A., Morris, J. H., King, E. M., McDonald, B. et al. (1995). Relative roles of plaques and tangles in the dementia of Alzheimer's disease: Correlations using three sets of neuropathological criteria. *Dementia, 6*(1), 21-31.

Nakano, T., Miyasaka, M., Ohtaka, T., & Ohomori, K. I. (1992). Longitudinal changes in computerized EEG and mental function of the aged: A nine-year follow-up study. *International Psychogeriatrics, 4*(1), 9-23.

Niedermeyer, E. (Ed.). (1981). *EEG and old age.* Baltimore: Urban & Schqarzenberg.

Nottebohm, F. (2002). Neuronal replacement in adult brain. *Brain Research Bulletin, 57*(6), 737-749.

Obrist, W. D. (1979). Electroencephalographc changes in normal aging and dementia. *Brain Function in Old Age,* 102-111.

Ornstein, R., & Sobel, D. (1987). *The healing brain: Breakthrough discoveries about how the brain keeps us healthy.* New York: Simon & Schuster.

Orrell, M. W., & O'Dwyer, A. M. (1995). Dementia, ageing, and the stress control system. *Lancet, 345*(8951), 666-667.

Oschman, J. L. (2000). *Energy medicine: The scientific basis.* Edinburgh: Churchill Livingstone.

Parent, J. M. (2003). Injury-induced neurogenesis in the adult mammalian brain. *Neuroscientist, 9*(4), 261-272.

Perls, T. T., Morris, J. N., Ooi, W. L., & Lipsitz, L. A. (1993). The relationship between age, gender and cognitive performance in the very old: The effect of selective survival. *Journal of the American Geriatrics Society, 41*(11), 1193-1201.

Peters, A. (1993). The absence of significant neuronal loss from cerebral cortex with age. *Neurobiology of Aging, 14*(6), 657-658.

Petersen, R. C., Smith, G., Kokmen, E., Ivnik, R. J., & Tangalos, E. G. (1992). Memory function in normal aging. *Neurology, 42*(2), 396-401.

Peterson, D. A. (2002). Stem cells in brain plasticity and repair. *Current Opinion in Pharmacology, 2*, 34-42.

Petit, T. L. (1982). Neuroanatomical and clinical neuropsychological. Changes in aging and senile dementia. In F. I. M. Craik & S. Trehub (Eds.), *Aging and Cognitive Processes* (pp. 1-21). New York: Plenum.

Prasad, K.N., Cole, W.C., Hovland, A. R., Prasad, K. C., Nahreini, P., Kumar, B., Edwards-Prasad, J., & Adreatta, C. P. (1999). Multiple antioxidants in the prevention and treatment of neurodegenerative disease: Analysis of biologic rationale, *Current Opinions in Neurology, 12*(6), 761-770.

Prichep, L. S., John, E. R., Ferris, S. H., Reisberg, B., Almas, M., Alper, K. et al. (1994). Quantitative EEG correlates of cognitive deterioration in the elderly. *Neurobiol Aging, 15*(1), 85-90.

Rapp, P. R., & Heindel, W. C. (1994). Memory systems in normal and pathological aging. *Current Opinion in Neurology, 7*(4), 294-298.

Rauschecker, J. P. (1995). Developmental plasticity and memory. *Behavioural Brain Research, 66*(1-2), 7-12.

Reh, T. A. (2002). Neural stem cells: Form and function. *Nature Neuroscience, 5*(5), 392-394.

Rockwood, K. (2002). Vascular cognitive impairment and vascular dementia. *J Neurol Sci, 203-204*, 23-27.

Rudd, P. M., Elliott, T., Cresswell, P., Wilson, I, A., & Raymond, A. D. (2001, March 23, 2001). Glycosylantion and the immune system. *Science, 291*, 2370-2375.

Sapolsky, R. M. (1992). Do glucocorticoid concentrations rise with age in the rat? *Neurobiology of Aging, 13*(1), 171-174.

Sapolsky, R. M. (1994a). The physiological relevance of glucocorticoid endangerment of the hippocampus. *Annals of the New York Academy of Sciences, 746*, 294-304; discussion 304-297.

Sapolsky, R. M. (1994b). *Why Zebras don't get ulcers*. New York: W.H. Freeman and Co.

Sapolsky, R. M. (1996a). Stress, glucocorticoids, and damage to the nervous system: The current state of confusion. *Stress, 1*(1), 1-19.

Sapolsky, R. M. (1996b). Why stress is bad for your brain. *Science, 273*(5276), 749-750.

Sapolsky, R. M. (2004). Organismal stress and telomeric aging: An unexpected connection. *Proceedings of the National Academy of Sciences of the United States of America, 101*(50), 17323-17324. Epub 12004 Dec 17323.

Sapolsky, R. M., Krey, L. C., & McEwen, B. S. (1986). The adrenocortical axis in the aged rat: Impaired sensitivity to both fast and delayed feedback inhibition. *Neurobiology Aging, 7*(5), 331-335.

Schulz, J.B., Lindenau, J., Seyfried, J., & Dichgans J. (2000). Glutathione, oxidative stress and neurodegeneration. *European Journal of Biochemistry, 267,* 4904-4911.

Sheline, Y. I., Wang, P. W., Gado, M. H., Csernansky, J. G., & Vannier, M. W. (1996). Hippocampal atrophy in recurrent major depression. *Proceedings of the National Academy of Sciences of the United States of America, 93*(9), 3908-3913.

Shors, T. J., Foy, M. R., Levine, S., & Thompson, R. F. (1990). Unpredictable and uncontrollable stress impairs neuronal plasticity in the rat hippocampus. *Brain Research Bulletin, 24*(5), 663-667.

Siever, D. (1997). *The rediscovery of light and sound stimulation.* Edmonton, Alberta, Canada: Comptronics Devices Limited.

Snowdon, D. (2001). *Aging with grace.* New York: Bantam Books, Random House.

Swan, G. E., Carmelli, D., & LaRue, A. (1995). Performance on the digit symbol substitution test and 5-year mortality in the Western Collaborative Group Study. *American Journal of Epidemiology, 141*(1), 32-40.

Swingle, P. G. (1996). Sub threshold 10-Hz sound suppresses EEG theta: Clinical application for the potentiation of neurotherapeutic treatment of ADD/ADHD. *Journal of Neurotherapy, 2*(1), 15-22.

Verleger, R., Neukater, W., Kompf, D., & Vieregge, P. (1991). On the reasons for the delay of P3 latency in healthy elderly subjects. *Electroencephalography and Clinical Neurophysiology, 79*(6), 488-502.

Waldemar, G. (1995). Functional brain imaging with SPECT in normal aging and dementia. Methodological, pathophysiological, and diagnostic aspects. *Cerebrovascular and Brain Metabolism Review, 7*(2), 89-130.

Walter, P. G., & Walter, W. (1949). The central effects of rhythmic sensory stimulation. *Electroencephalography and Clinical Neurophysiology, 1,* 57-86.

Weiler, P. G., Lubben, J. E., Chi, I., Rodriguez, G., Nobili, F., Rocca, G. et al. (1991). Cognitive impairment and hospital use. *American Journal of Public Health, 81*(9), 1153-1157.

Williamson, P. C., Harold, M., Morrison, S., Rabheru, K., Fox, H., Wands, K., Wong, C., & Hachinski, V. (1990). Quantitative electroencephalograhic correlates of cognitive decline in normal elderly subjects. *Archives of Neurology, 47,* 1185-1188.

Willis, S. (1982). Cognitive training and everyday competence. In F. I. M. T. Craik, S. (Ed.), *Aging and cognitive processes* (pp. 159-188). New York: Plenum Press.

Wisocki, P. A. (1991). *Handbook of clinical behavior therapy with the elderly client (applied clinical psychology).* New York: Plenum Publishing Corporation.

Youngjohn, J. R., & Crook, T. H., 3rd. (1993). Learning, forgetting, and retrieval of everyday material across the adult life span. *Journal of Clinical Experimental Neuropsychology, 15*(4), 447-460.

Chapter 11

Neurofeedback Protocols for Subtypes of Attention Deficit/ Hyperactivity Disorder

Lynda Kirk

INTRODUCTION

In the United States, it is estimated that more than two million children have Attention Deficit/Hyperactivity Disorder (ADHD). Epidemiological studies conducted by the American Academy of Pediatrics show that ADHD is the most common neurobehavioral disorder of childhood. Recent studies estimate that up to 70 percent of children with ADHD exhibit symptoms into their adult years, and that these symptoms continue to interfere significantly with academic, vocational, and social functioning (Barkley, Fischer, Fletcher, & Smallish, 2001).

One thing this means for EEG neurofeedback practitioners is that more people are actively seeking neurofeedback for ADHD. In addition, both the public and health care professionals are becoming increasingly concerned about recent FDA warnings, adverse side effects, and the reported ineffectiveness of ADHD medications for many patients. Nondrug alternatives are becoming more viable and increasingly sought by the public and health care professionals.

This chapter will review ADHD, touching on its historical definitions and treatments; differential diagnoses and comorbidities; current interventions and treatments for ADHD; populations for whom

Handbook of Neurofeedback
doi:10.1300/5889_11

neurofeedback is appropriate; the historical development of neuro-feedback protocols for ADHD; the "basic three" neurofeedback protocols that are supported by published controlled, group studies; neurofeedback protocol modifications developed from the "basic three"; the use of quantitative EEG (QEEG); the ADHD subtypes identified by neuroimaging; and some clinical issues related to the frequency and length of neurofeedback training for ADHD.

ADHD: THE DISORDER

Attention deficit hyperactivity disorder is a condition that becomes apparent in some children during their preschool and early school years. The most identifiable symptoms in these children are difficulty in paying attention and controlling their own behaviors. According to the most recent version of the *Diagnostic and Statistical Manual of Mental Disorders* (DSM-IV-TR), three patterns of behavior point to ADHD: (1) Individuals with ADHD may show signs of being consistently inattentive. (2) They may exhibit patterns of hyperactive behavior and/or impulsive behavior (more so than others of their age may). (3) Individuals may exhibit all three types of behavior—inattention, hyperactivity, and impulsivity (American Psychiatric Association, 2000).

ADHD has been recognized and treated in children for over a century. In 1902 in England, Sir George Still gave a series of lectures to the Royal College of Physicians in which he described a group of impulsive children with significant behavioral problems—symptoms that today would likely be recognized as ADHD (Still, 1902).

With ADHD rates estimated to be between 3 and 5 percent of children in the United States, child and adolescent psychiatrists in North America report that as high as 50 percent of their clinical populations have ADHD symptoms (Cantwell, 1996). The combined prevalence of adult and child ADHD in the United States is reported to be approximately 7 percent of the nation's population (Pelham et al., 1992; Wolraich et al., 1996; Gadow & Sprafkin, 1997). International prevalence rates of ADHD range from 2 to 29 percent (Barkley, 1998).

For many years, it was believed that children and adolescents would outgrow the symptoms of ADHD by puberty. However, several studies done in recent years estimate that up to 70 percent of children with ADHD continue to exhibit symptoms in their adult years.

These children will continue to have symptoms of the disorder that significantly interfere with academic, vocational, or social functioning in their adult lives (Barkley et al., 2001).

THE IMPORTANCE OF EARLY TREATMENT

Ever-increasing knowledge about the effects of ADHD over the lifespan makes a strong case for early diagnosis and treatment. Studies show that without treatment, children and adolescents with ADHD are more likely to have behavioral and academic problems in school, as well as to be at a greater risk for anxiety and mood disorders (Biederman et al., 1996). They also are statistically more likely to "self-medicate" and have a higher incidence of substance abuse disorders (Mannuzza et al., 1991).

Young adults not treated for ADHD in childhood demonstrate a higher prevalence of poor academic performance, behavioral problems, and greater school dropout rates (Weiss & Hechtman, 1993). In mature adulthood, they are more likely to show poor job performance, substance abuse problems, psychiatric disorders, and criminal behavior than their non-ADHD peers (Weiss & Hechtman, 1993; Murphy & Barkley, 1996).

The National Institute of Mental Health, the American Academy of Pediatrics, and the American Academy of Child and Adolescent Psychiatry suggest a multimodal approach for the treatment of ADHD in children. Recommended approaches include parent and child education programs that cover the diagnosis and treatment of ADHD, the use of relevant behavior management techniques, specific school programs designed for the ADHD child, and symptom management with appropriate ADHD medications. Unfortunately, among the aforementioned recommendations, there is no mention of EEG neurofeedback to directly address the core symptoms of ADHD.

With a clearly demonstrated need to increase public and professional awareness of the benefits and efficacy of biofeedback, the Association for Applied Psychophysiology and Biofeedback (AAPB) presented a series of briefings to the National Institutes of Health (NIH) in April 2005, as part of its advocacy and public information efforts. In one of these briefings delivered to key members and staff of the NIH, AAPB presented recent, scientific, controlled-group studies demonstrating the efficacy and lasting effects of biofeedback (including the efficacy of neurofeedback with ADHD). This effort was particularly timely considering the FDA's ongoing concerns about the safety of certain ADHD medications, including potential liver damage associated with the ADHD medication Strattera (FDA Talk Paper T04-60, 12/17/2004), as well as recent animal studies in which test subjects given methylphenidate (Ritalin) showed dysfunctional brain reward systems and depressive behaviors that lasted into adulthood, at significantly higher rates of incidence than their control counterparts (Carlezon, 2003).

BEHAVIORALLY IDENTIFIED SUBTYPES OF ADHD

As stated previously, the DSM-IV-TR lists three subtypes of ADHD: the predominantly inattentive type, the predominantly hyperactive-impulsive type, and the combined type. These types are identified by differing clusters of ADHD behavioral symptoms (American Psychiatric Association, 2000).

The predominantly inattentive type, sometimes called ADD (without the "H") does not exhibit significant hyperactive or impulsive behavior. The predominantly hyperactive-impulsive type does not exhibit significant signs of inattention. The combined type exhibits both inattentive and hyperactive-impulsive symptoms. These three subtypes are reviewed more specifically as follows:

1. Predominantly Inattentive Type ADHD is marked by the following behaviors of inattention. For inclusion in this type, six or more of the following behaviors must be exhibited:
   - Inattention to details and making careless mistakes at school, work, or other activities
   - Inability sustaining attention at work or play
   - Not paying attention when spoken to
   - Not following or finishing instructions
   - Not finishing work or tasks
   - Exhibiting poor organizational skills
   - Disliking or avoiding tasks requiring sustained attention
   - Frequently losing things
   - Being easily distracted
   - Forgetful or "zoned out" in activities of daily living

2. Predominantly Hyperactive-Impulsive Type ADHD is marked by the following behaviors of hyperactivity-impulsivity. For inclusion in this type, six or more of the following behaviors must be exhibited:
   - Fidgetiness
   - Inability to remain seated (may present as feelings of restlessness in adults or adolescents)
   - Excessive and/or inappropriate physical activity such as running, climbing, and jumping (may present as feelings of restlessness in adults or adolescents)
   - Inappropriately noisy while working or during leisure time
   - Frequently feeling "hyper" or "revved up"
   - Talking nonstop or excessively
   - Impulsively answering before hearing the entire question
   - Intruding or butting in on conversations
   - Difficulty taking turns with others or awaiting turn
   - Interrupting or intruding on others' activities
3. Combined Type ADHD is marked by behaviors of inattention as well as by behaviors of hyperactivity-impulsivity, as noted in Items 1 and 2 previously. In order for a diagnosis of ADHD to be given, the individual must:
   - Have experienced the behavioral markers of ADHD for six months or longer
   - Have exhibited inattentive and/or hyperactive-impulsive behaviors before the age of seven years
   - Exhibit impairment from ADHD behaviors in at least two or more settings, such as school, work, or home
   - Exhibit significant impairment in social, school, or work contexts
   - Exhibit ADHD behaviors that cannot be attributed to another disorder

Differential Diagnosis

Specialists such as psychiatrists, psychologists, pediatricians or family physicians, neurologists, clinical social workers, licensed professional counselors, and psychotherapists who are experienced with ADHD can legally diagnose the disorder, depending upon the licensing practice laws of the state (USA) in which they are licensed. That having been said, the case for a thorough work-up (including medical) before concluding that ADHD is the cause of the behaviors and symptoms in question is a strong one.

It is important to both the neurofeedback clinician and the client suspected of having ADHD that a thorough diagnostic work-up includes a full medical evaluation. There are medical conditions that can mimic ADHD symptoms, such as thyroid or other medical disorders affecting metabolism or brain function. These should be ruled out as factors before ADHD is diagnosed and treated. Vision and hearing disorders can impair attention. Sudden life changes, learning disabilities, mood disorders, anxiety, depression, traumatic brain injury, and seizure disorders can all cause symptoms that imitate ADHD. To further challenge the diagnostic presentation, these same conditions can be comorbid with ADHD. In certain cases, autistic spectrum symptoms can resemble ADHD, and some autistic symptoms may also be comorbid with ADHD.

Common Comorbidities That May Accompany ADHD

It is important to be aware of comorbidities that frequently accompany ADHD because neurofeedback training may be tailored to address both ADHD as well as specific comorbid symptoms. Some of the most common comorbidities that may be present with ADHD include learning disabilities (LD).

Learning Disabilities (LD)

Approximately 20 to 30 percent of children with ADHD also have a specific learning disability (Wender, 2002). Preschool children may have learning disabilities that include difficulty understanding certain words or sounds and/or difficulty with verbal expression. School age children may exhibit reading, spelling, writing, and/or math disorders. Dyslexia, a specific type of reading disorder, is relatively common.

Oppositional Defiant Disorder (ODD)

An estimated one-third to one-half of children with ADHD, mostly males, meet criteria for oppositional defiant disorder. These children argue excessively with adults and refuse to obey rules. They are often noncompliant, stubborn, defiant, belligerent, and may have angry outbursts or "short fuses."

Conduct Disorder (CD)

Conduct disorder is considered a more serious behavioral disorder than ODD. Conduct disorder children and adolescents demonstrate a pattern of more overtly antisocial behavior such as lying, stealing, bullying, fighting, vandalizing, and destroying property, being aggressive and cruel to humans and animals, starting fires, carrying and using weapons, and violating the rights of others. They are at higher risk for substance abuse and getting into serious trouble both at school and with the law. About 20 to 40 percent of ADHD children eventually develop CD (CHADD ADHD Fact Sheet #3, 2004).

Tourette's Syndrome (TS)

Although the prevalence of Tourette's syndrome is low, many people with Tourette's syndrome also have ADHD. Symptoms of TS include nervous tics and repetitive mannerisms such as facial twitches or grimaces, eye blinks, throat clearing, sniffing, snorting, or barking out words (including cursing and other socially inappropriate words). Some ADHD medications may increase symptoms of Tourette's syndrome.

Anxiety and Depression

Many individuals with ADHD present with comorbid anxiety and/ or depression. In general, anxiety is considered to be an expression of cortical "irritability" or hyperarousal, while depression is considered to be an expression of cortical hypoarousal. Both these disorders can often be addressed successfully with neurofeedback simultaneously with the ADHD symptoms.

Bipolar Disorder

Classic bipolar disorder in adults is characterized by mood cycling between periods of intense emotional highs and lows. Often, one of these two emotional extremes will dominate. In children, it may be difficult to distinguish between ADHD and bipolar disorder. Child-hood bipolar disorder may present as chronic moodiness with alter-nating periods of elation and excitement, or depression, and anger or irritability. There are some symptoms that are present in both bipolar disorder and ADHD, including excess energy and reduced sleep. Symptoms that should particularly alert the clinician to possible bipolar disorder are elevated expressions of elation or grandiosity (Geller et al., 1998).

A BRIEF HISTORY OF ADHD DEFINITIONS AND TREATMENT

In 1902, Dr. George Still, a British doctor, lectured at the Royal College of Physicians about cases of impulsive children behaving badly. He deemed this a medical diagnosis and labeled it a "Defect of Moral Control" (Still, 1902).

In 1922, after the influenza pandemic in the early twentieth century, ADHD symptoms were described as "Post-Encephalitic Behavior Disorder" (or encephalitis lethargica) in an early attempt to ascribe a neurological basis for the symptoms in cases described by Hohman (Hohman, 1922) and others.

In 1937, Dr. Charles Bradley, Medical Director of the Emma Pendleton Bradley Home, in East Providence, R.I., was the first to use stimulants to treat hyperactive children (Gainetdinov & Caron, 2001).

In 1956, Ritalin (methylphenidate) was first introduced to treat hyperactivity in children (Attention Deficit Help Center, 2003).

In the early 1960s, the term "Minimal Brain Dysfunction" was used to characterize ADHD symptoms. In the late 1960s, the term was changed to "Hyperkinetic Disorder of Childhood." Stimulant medi-cation became more widely prescribed to treat the symptoms (Atten-tion Deficit Help Center, 2003).

In 1967, Dr. Barry Sterman published his ground-breaking EEG studies in which he identified and named the EEG "sensorimotor rhythm" (SMR) and described the ability to operantly condition, or up-train SMR in cats and humans (Roth, Sterman, & Clemente, 1967; Sterman & Wyrwicka, 1967; Wyrwicka & Sterman, 1968).

In 1976, Dr. Joel Lubar published his preliminary work using EEG SMR training with a hyperkinetic child (Lubar & Shouse, 1976).

In 1980, The American Psychiatric Association used the term "Attention Deficit Disorder +/−" in the *Diagnostic and Statistical Manual of Mental Disorders, Third Edition,* to describe what was earlier called "Hyperkinetic Disorder of Childhood." ADD and ADHD were considered separate diagnoses (APA, 1980), with the plus ("+") and minus ("−") designations indicating the presence or absence of hyperactivity. Attention Deficit Disorder +/− was classified as an official disorder by the National Institutes of Mental Health (Attention Deficit Help Center, 2003).

In 1987, The American Psychiatric Association changed the name "Attention Deficit Disorder +/−" to "Attention Deficit Hyperactivity Disorder" and categorized it as a medical condition that could cause behavioral problems, different from those caused by stress or major life changes such as divorce or death of a loved one (Attention Deficit Help Center, 2003).

In 1996, after Ritalin, a second medication, Adderall was approved by the FDA for treatment of ADHD (Attention Deficit Help Center, 2003).

In 1998, The American Medical Association stated that ADHD was "one of the best researched disorders" (Attention Deficit Help Center, 2003).

From 1999 to present, several additional medications, such as Concerta, Metadate, Focalin, and Strattera were approved for the treatment of ADHD (Attention Deficit Help Center, 2003).

In 2004, Dr. Vince Monastra published his study showing that neurofeedback was as effective as Ritalin in treating ADHD symptoms. His study demonstrated that improvements in ADHD symptoms continued after cessation of pharmacological treatment in the group receiving both Ritalin and neurofeedback. In contrast, the group receiving Ritalin alone (without neurofeedback) lost any gains that occurred while they were on medication after cessation of medication treatment (Monastra, 2004). The FDA issued a warning that Strattera could cause liver damage (FDA, 2004). Dr. Thomas Rossiter replicated earlier studies demonstrating the equivalence of neurofeedback to stimulant medication (Rossiter, 2004). In this year alone, sales of ADHD medications soared from $759 million in 2000 to $3.1 billion in 2004 (Associated Press, 2006).

In 2005, Methylphenidate hydrochloride (Ritalin) treatment induced cytogenetic abnormalities in pediatric patients at therapeutic dosages (El-Zein et al., 2005).

In 2006, an FDA committee tied 25 deaths to medications used to treat ADHD and urged the use of warning labels (Harris, 2006).

Current Interventions and Treatments for ADHD

Historically, the most common treatments for ADHD have been medication, behavioral therapy, and psychotherapy, either alone or in combination. Medication is by far the most frequent treatment of choice in North America, and it can help alleviate some ADHD symptoms when the medication is well matched to the ADHD subtype.

Although controlled, group studies show that medications are effective in treating some ADHD symptoms, about 25 percent of ADHD patients show either no response or an adverse response to medication (Swanson et al., 1995). Neurofeedback is often an attractive alternative for individuals who do not respond to ADHD medications, who cannot tolerate the side effects associated with medications, or those who are concerned about the safety and long-term physiological or psychological effects of using such medications. At the author's Austin Biofeedback and EEG Neurofeedback Center, many adult clients and parents of young clients with ADHD who are already being treated with medications, choose neurofeedback because they do not want pharmacological treatment to continue indefinitely. Neurofeedback is the one treatment modality that offers durable improvement posttreatment (Monastra, 2004).

As with medication, neurofeedback may also be an effective option for ADHD clients when behavioral therapy, or psychotherapy alone are not sufficient to meet their clinical needs. Neurofeedback therapy can be especially valuable in many cases when provided in combination with any or all of these other therapeutic alternatives.

THE CASE FOR NEUROFEEDBACK

Over the past 30 years, since Lubar's preliminary study (Lubar & Shouse, 1976), a number of case studies and controlled, group studies investigating the efficacy of neurofeedback with ADHD have been conducted. These studies reported improvements in attention and other problem behaviors. Quantitative electroencephalographic (QEEG) data often showed increased cortical activation after neurofeedback training, and improvements in intelligence test scores and academic achievement have been documented (Monastra, Monastra, & George, 2002; Fuchs et al., 2003).

In *Evidence-Based Practice in Biofeedback and Neurofeedback* (Yucha & Gilbert, 2003), the authors note four controlled group studiesr eported in peer-reviewed journals (Rossiter & LaVaque, 1995; Linden, Habib, & Radojevic, 1996; Monastra, Monastra, & George, 2002; Fuchs et al., 2003). These studies examined the effects of neurofeedback with patients diagnosed with ADHD and controlled for factors such as age, intelligence, and severity of ADHD symptoms before beginning treatment. Each of these studies demonstrated consistent beneficial effects of neurofeedback on measures of intelligence, ADHD behavior ratings scales, QEEG measures of cortical arousal, and on computerized continuous performance tests of variables of attention.

Numerous additional case studies, which demonstrate the clinical benefits of neurofeedback in patients diagnosed with ADHD, are also cited by Yucha and Gilbert (2003). Since Lubar's initial case study, there have been many impressive case reports such as those that follow.

In Thompson and Thompson's study of 111 patients diagnosed with ADHD, gains of 12 points on the Wechsler full-scale intelligence quotient were reported (Thompson & Thompson, 1998). Kaiser and Othmer also investigated neurofeedback in 1,089 patients, among whom 186 were diagnosed with ADHD (Kaiser & Othmer, 2000). In both of these multiple-case studies, clinical gains included improvements in scores on tests of attention and impulse control. Neurofeedback training for ADHD students within a school setting was associated with gains in attention on both continuous performance tests and behavioral measures (Carmody et al., 2001).

Long-term and lasting effects of neurofeedback training with ADHD clients are reported by both Tansey and Lubar. Tansey reported on a ten-year follow-up study showing that a fourth-grade child trained with neurofeedback was able to maintain improvements in hyperactivity during adolescence and early adulthood (Tansey, 1998). Lubar's retrospective study of 52 clients seen over a ten-year period, who had completed EEG neurofeedback treatment for ADHD, showed continuing control in sixteen targeted ADHD symptoms. Primary improvements included sustained control over symptoms of hyperactivity, emotional reactivity, homework completion, and satisfactory or improved grades on report cards (Lubar, 2003). The body of research has increased dramatically in recent years, but Yucha and Gilbert (2003) rightfully note that still more randomized, controlled, group studies on the effects of neurofeedback therapy for ADHD are needed.

Development of Neurofeedback Protocols for ADHD

Neurofeedback protocols in controlled, group, and case studies to date have targeted the cortical regions primarily involved in attention and behavioral inhibition. Both neuroimaging (Hynd et al., 1990, 1993; Mostofsky et al., 1998) and quantitative electroencephalography (QEEG) research show underarousal in frontal and central, midline cortical regions in approximately 85 to 90 percent of individuals with ADHD (Mann et al., 1992; Chabot et al., 1996; Monastra et al., 1999; Clarke et al., 2001; Monastra, Lubar, & Linden, 2001). Individuals with ADHD who do not respond favorably to stimulant medications also show a secondary pattern of hyperarousal in the frontal cortical regions (Chabot et al., 1999; Clarke, Barry, McCarthy, & Selikowitz, 2002).

The ADHD neurofeedback protocols used in the studies cited, demonstrated efficacy for the three behaviorally defined DSM-IV ADHD subtypes (inattentive, hyperactive-impulsive, or combined types) on standardized tests of intelligence, attention, and behavior following EEG neurofeedback. In addition, QEEG data of patients treated with neurofeedback show increased levels of cortical arousal.

Potential Exclusion Criteria

Due to exclusion criteria involved in the previously referenced controlled case and group studies using neurofeedback with ADHD, positive outcomes were not specifically obtained with individuals such as the following:

- Less than six years of age
- Mental retardation or the presence of a medical or mental health condition with potential attention or behavior components (e.g.,

thyroid, anemia, hypoglycemia, diabetes, psychosis, severe depression, or bipolar disorder)
- History of neurological disease (including seizure and traumatic brain injury)
- Substance abuse
- Families with significant dysfunction that interfered with participation in the treatment process

Despite the aforementioned criteria, many clinicians anecdotally report positive outcomes with clients who fall within the exclusionary criteria listed earlier. For example, our own experience at Austin Biofeedback and EEG Neurofeedback Center includes successfully working with ADHD clients significantly younger than six years of age, as well as with clients exhibiting symptoms of ADHD along with all of the exclusionary criteria listed earlier except mental retardation or diagnosed psychosis.

Nevertheless, external social factors, personality or behavioral factors, or comorbid conditions can impact successful outcomes with neurofeedback for ADHD. These factors should be addressed prior to or concurrent with neurofeedback training. For example, noncompliant individuals with serious substance abuse or chemical dependence should first address these issues before starting neurofeedback for ADHD. Likewise, in order to optimize success, families with significant family dysfunction should address family dynamics issues during or prior to starting neurofeedback for a family member with ADHD.

Physiological issues may also need to be identified and addressed before neurofeedback training is initiated. These may include such serious concerns as the diagnosis and treatment of suspected brain lesions or metabolic disorders. They may also include simple, but significant, factors such as the need for glasses or hearing aids.

The "Tried and True Trio"

There are three basic neurofeedback protocols for ADHD subtypes supported by published controlled, group studies.

The following three protocols for neurofeedback training for ADHD are supported by four published controlled group studies (Rossiter & LaVaque, 1995; Linden, Habib, & Radojevic, 1996; Monastra, Monastra, & George, 2002; Fuchs et al., 2003).

Hyperactive/Impulsive Protocol Targeting Hypo-Arousal:
Increase Sensorimotor Rhythm (SMR)/Decrease Theta

In this EEG neurofeedback protocol, trainees were rewarded for increasing amplitude of 12-15 Hz sensorimotor rhythm (SMR) activity and simultaneously rewarded for decreasing amplitude of 4-7 Hz (theta) activity, recording from one of two active sites (C3 or C4) and referenced to linked ears (Figure 11.1). EEG feedback was provided based upon meeting any of the following conditions:

1. The trainee's success in controlling the amplitudes (microvoltage) of theta and/or SMR
2. The trainee's success in controlling the percentage of time that theta was below or SMR was above pre-treatment baselines
3. The trainee's success in controlling the ratio of theta amplitude to SMR amplitude

This protocol specifically targets hyperactive and impulsive behaviors in trainees who may be hypoaroused. Rossiter and LaVaque used this type of protocol in the first controlled group study of EEG biofeedback for ADHD (Rossiter & LaVaque, 1995). A list of the *Hyperactive/Impulsive Protocol Targeting Hypo-Arousal: Increase*

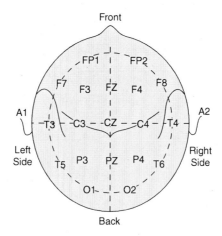

FIGURE 11.1. Electrode placement sites.

Sensorimotor Rhythm (SMR)/Decrease Theta (Electrode Placement: C3 or C4 active with linked ear lobe reference; see Figure 11.1) appears as follows:

Reward Frequency	12-15 Hz
Inhibit Frequency	4-7 Hz
Behavioral Duration	Minimum 0.5 second (1/2 second) to obtain reward
Sampling Rate	Minimum of 128 per second per Rossiter & LaVaque
Rate of Reward	Settings for Reward EEG and Inhibit EEG: Approximately 15-20 auditory/visual rewards per minute
Feedback Delivery	Depending on neurofeedback system: Auditory tones or music; visual counter displays; animations; video games; movie DVDs; tactile vibrating pillows or stuffed animals; vibrating video game controllers
Clinical Outcome	Reduce behavioral symptoms of hyperactivity and impulsivity

A QEEG topograph from a client seen at Austin Biofeedback and EEG Neurofeedback Center with this subtype showing excessive relative theta is pictured in Figure 11.2. Note the yellow and red coloring in the first two rows at all sites, indicating absolute and relative power in the theta frequency band.

Hyperactive/Impulsive Protocol Targeting Hyper-Arousal: Increase Sensorimotor Rhythm (SMR)/Decrease Beta-2 Protocol

In this EEG neurofeedback protocol, trainees were rewarded for increasing amplitude of 12-15 Hz sensorimotor rhythm (SMR) activity and simultaneously rewarded for decreasing amplitude of 22-30 Hz beta-2 activity at one central site (C4). EEG activity was recorded from the C4 active site and referenced to linked ears. EEG feedback was provided based upon meeting either of the following criteria:

1. The trainee's success in appropriately controlling the amplitudes (microvoltage) of SMR and/or beta-2
2. The percent time that beta-2 was below, or SMR was above pretreatment baselines.

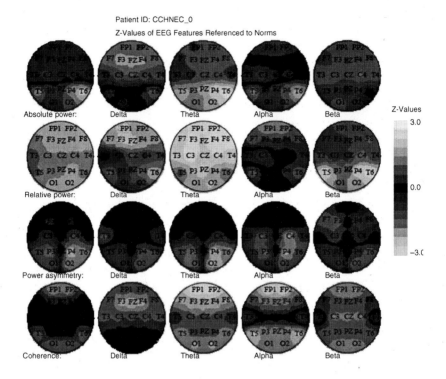

FIGURE 11.2. QEEG hyperactive/impulsive type ADHD protocol (Hypo-aroused). (See also color gallery.)

This protocol specifically targets hyperactive and impulsive behaviors in trainees who may be hyperaroused. SMR training with a fast beta (beta-2) inhibit has been examined in a controlled, group study (Fuchs et al., 2003). In Fuchs and others', patients with a Combined Type of ADHD received a split-session training, increasing 12-15 Hz SMR at C4 while simultaneously decreasing 22-30 Hz beta-2 with a linked ear reference in the first half of each session as shown in the following table (Electrode Placement: C4 with linked ear lobe reference; see Figure 11.1). During the second half of each session, trainees switched to a left hemisphere protocol of increasing 16-20 Hz beta-1 at C3, while simultaneously decreasing 4-8 Hz theta (see Enhance Beta-1/Decrease Theta Protocol description). In this (Fuch's protocol), feedback was provided based upon meeting either of the following conditions:

1. The trainee's success in controlling the amplitudes (microvoltage) of theta, SMR, beta-1, and/or beta-2
2. The percent time that the targeted frequencies were above or below pretreatment baselines.

Reward Frequency*	12-15 Hz
Inhibit Frequency	22-30 Hz
Behavioral Duration	Minimum 0.5 second (1/2 second) to obtain reward
Sampling Rate	Minimum of 128 per second
Rate of Reward	Settings for Reward EEG and Inhibit EEG: Approximately 15-20 auditory/visual rewards/minute
Feedback Delivery	Depending on neurofeedback system: Auditory tones or music; visual counter displays; animations; video games; movie DVDs; tactile vibrating pillows or stuffed animals; vibrating video game controllers
Clinical Outcome	Reduce behavioral symptoms of hyperactivity and impulsivity

*First Half of Fuchs Inattentive Split Protocol for Combined ADHD.

A QEEG topograph from a client seen at Austin Biofeedback and EEG Neurofeedback Center with this subtype showing excessive relative beta as seen in Figure 11.3. Note excessive absolute and relative power at all sites in the beta frequency bands (top two rows).

This protocol, with its four variations in electrode placement, specifically targeted inattentive behaviors in trainees who were hypoaroused. In this EEG neurofeedback protocol, trainees were rewarded for increasing amplitude of 16-20 Hz beta-1 activity and simultaneously rewarded for decreasing amplitude of 4-8 Hz theta activity over one of three central midline sites. In three of the four controlled, group ADHD neurofeedback studies cited in the literature to date, EEG activity was recorded from one of the following three central midline sites (see Figure 11.1): (1) Cz or C3 (referential montage) with linked ear reference; (2) FCz (half-way between Fz and Cz), and PCz (half-way between Pz and Cz), in a bipolar montage with ear lobe reference;

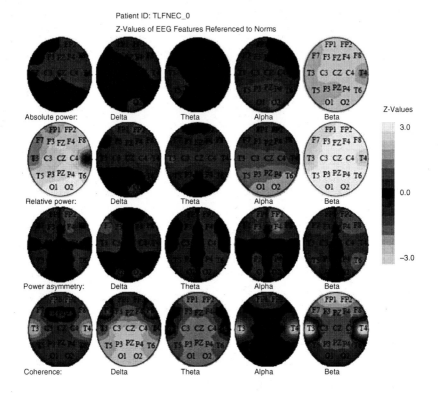

FIGURE 11.3. QEEG hyperactive/impulsive type ADHD protocol hyper-aroused inattentive protocol targeting hypo-arousal: increase beta-1/decrease theta. (See also color gallery.)

(3) Cz-Pz (bipolar montage) with ear lobe reference (Rossiter & LaVaque, 1995; Linden, Habib, & Radojevic, 1996; Monastra, Monastra, & George, 2002).

In the fourth study, EEG activity was recorded from a C3 active site and referenced to linked ears (Fuchs et al., 2003). In each of the four studies, EEG feedback was provided based upon meeting either of the following conditions:

1. The trainee's success in appropriately controlling the amplitudes (microvoltage) of theta and/or beta-1
2. The percent time that theta was below, or beta-1 was above pretreatment baselines.

Reward Frequency*	16-20 Hz
Inhibit Frequency	4-8 Hz
Behavioral Duration	Minimum 0.5 second (1/2 second) to obtain reward
Sampling Rate	Minimum of 128 per second
Rate of Reward	Settings for Reward EEG and Inhibit EEG: Approximately 15-20 auditory/visual rewards/minute
Feedback Delivery	Depending on neurofeedback system: Auditory tones or music; visual counter displays; animations; video games; movie DVDs; tactile vibrating pillows or stuffed animals; vibrating video game controllers
Clinical Goal	Reduce behavioral symptoms of inattention, hypo-arousal

*Second Half of Fuchs Inattentive Split Protocol for Combined ADHD.

A QEEG topograph from a client seen at Austin Biofeedback and EEG Neurofeedback Center with this subtype showing excessive relative theta (and posterior relative delta) is shown in Figure 11.4. Note excessive absolute and relative power at nearly all sites in the theta frequency bands (top two rows).

The author has chosen to first outline the "Basic Three" ADHD protocols presented earlier because they are based on controlled, group studies with peer-reviewed published literature to support the efficacy reported. These protocols also specifically target the behaviorally defined DSM-IV ADHD subtypes. There are also many experienced and respected clinicians in the United States and abroad who have reported success anecdotally or in case studies using modifications of the "basic" ADHD protocols. Lubar (2003), for example, reports successful outcomes using a protocol suppressing a combination of theta and alpha or "thalpha" (6-10 Hz) with both adolescents and adults, using the original "Increase Beta/Decrease Theta (with "thalpha" substituted for theta) Protocol."

Other multiple-case studies include Thompson and Thompson's (1998) study of 111 patients diagnosed with ADHD, and Kaiser and Othmer's (2000) study with 186 patients diagnosed with ADHD. Both Thompson and Thompson (1998) and Kaiser and Othmer (2000) showed participant improvements on tests of attention and impulse control after neurofeedback training, using their own protocol modi-

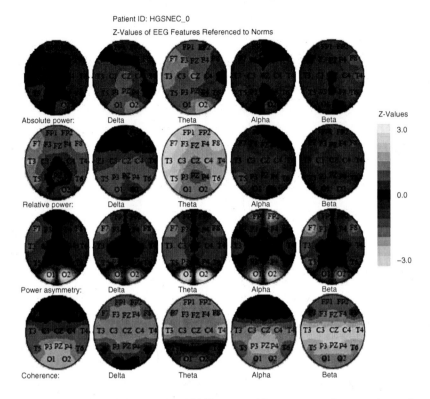

FIGURE 11.4. QEEG inattentive ADHD protocol hypo-aroused protocols modified from the three basic "Tried and True Trio." (See also color gallery.)

fications. Thompson and Thompson's trainees also showed increases on a standard measure of intelligence.

Using various modifications of the "basic" ADHD protocols, a neurofeedback project for students with ADHD in a school setting reported gains in attention on behavioral measures and on a continuous performance test (Carmody et al., 2001). Siegfried and Sue Othmer currently report success with a series of interhemispheric neurofeedback protocols using bipolar montages at primarily homologous sites, with varying reward and inhibit bandwidths selected according to the client's subjective response to the locations and bandwidths chosen (Othmer & Othmer, 2005).

The clinicians cited previously provide a few examples of the many throughout the world who are continuing to search for the most efficacious neurofeedback protocols to help their clients remediate ADHD behaviors and symptoms. Based on the continual evaluation of over 900 ADHD cases seen since 1991 at Austin Biofeedback and EEG Neurofeedback Center, we determine client-specific neurofeedback protocols on the basis of each individual's clinical history and clinical intake assessments, as well as an initial EEG assessment of several cortical sites. In many cases, we also require a full-head QEEG using normative database comparisons, including challenge states such as listening, reading, math, and others specific to the client's needs and desired outcomes. Clinical protocols used may range from any of the protocols discussed previously in this chapter, to protocols developed directly from information based on the client's history, from behavioral and neuropsychological assessment data, from computerized continuous performance tests, from the client's QEEG, and from other assessments.

To "Q" or Not to "Q"—That Is the Question

There is significant disagreement in the field about the necessity of having full-head computerized quantitative EEG (QEEG) data prior to beginning neurofeedback with a client. Some clinicians insist on a QEEG before ever starting neurofeedback. Some clinicians rely on behavioral checklists and clinical interviews to determine the apparent ADHD subtype and the appropriate neurofeedback protocols. Still other clinicians may start neurofeedback training based on interview and assessment data without a QEEG, but switch to QEEG-based neurofeedback if the client is not making progress as expected. A number of clinicians who do not routinely do QEEGs on every ADHD client will insist on a QEEG if the client has had a history of traumatic brain injury, stroke, seizures, or multiple comorbidities with ADHD. Adding validity to the pro-QEEG camp, there is evidence that matching specific neurofeedback protocols with QEEG types has been associated with an improved treatment response rate (Monastra, et al., 2002; Fuchs et al., 2003).

QEEG appears to be one of the few assessment procedures capable of providing an independent physiological marker for ADHD. Two studies (Monastra et al., 1999; Monastra, Lubar, & Linden, 2001) correlated EEG markers (elevated theta/beta ratios) with diagnostic criteria for ADHD with sensitivity figures of 90 percent and specificity figures of 94 percent.

It is clearly important to do some type initial EEG assessment before starting any neurofeedback training. For example, patently assuming that decreasing theta and/or increasing beta is a "standard protocol" for a typical ADHD client, may not only be incorrect, it may be potentially detrimental and clinically counterproductive. Some ADHD clients do not have excessive theta and some already produce excessive beta in their EEGs.

Optimal clinical outcomes are likely to be realized by conducting a pretraining assessment looking at the EEG in multiple locations and assessing the EEG in multiple states (eyes open, eyes closed, and under various cognitive challenges). Whether one uses a full-cap QEEG or measures several sites along the midline and across hemispheres (e.g., Fz, Cz, Pz, F3, F4, C3, C4, P3, P4, etc.), it is important to assess the EEG relative to the client's clinical presentation. It then becomes easier to determine the potential ADHD subtype and to construct appropriate neurofeedback protocols specific to the client's neurophysiological and behavioral presentation and their desired outcomes.

Neuroimaging Studies Reveal Evidence of Core Symptoms of ADHD

There is evidence from a number of neuroimaging studies that the core symptoms of ADHD can be associated with the following:

- brain metabolic abnormalities (Zametkin et al., 1990; Zametkin & Rapoport, 1987);
- brain circulatory or perfusion abnormalities (Amen, Paldi, & Thisted, 1993);
- brain neuroanatomical abnormalities (Casey et al., 1997; Hynd et al., 1993); and
- brain electrophysiological abnormalities (Chabot et al., 1996; Chabot & Serfontein, 1996; Mann et al., 1992; Monastra et al., 1999; Clarke et al., 2001; Monastra, Lubar, & Linden, 2001).

Neuroimaging studies utilizing PET (positron emission tomography), SPECT (single photon emission computed tomography), fMRI (functional magnetic resonance imaging), and QEEG (quantitative electroencephalography) identify brain regions of hypoarousal and/or hyperarousal that have been helpful in selecting both medications and specific neurofeedback protocols that target certain ADHD symptoms. For example, Daniel Amen (Amen, 1997) demonstrated with SPECT imaging that 65 percent of his ADHD group showed decreased perfusion in the prefrontal cortex with intellectual stress, compared to only 5 percent of the control group. These findings are consistent with both PET and QEEG findings.

ADHD Subtypes Identified by QEEG Neuroimaging

QEEG evaluation before neurofeedback training may prove especially useful in clinical practice, since it can detect both hypoarousal and hyperarousal, which have often been noted in the frontal and central midline cortical regions of patients diagnosed with ADHD. As previously noted, there is evidence that matching specific neurofeedback protocols with QEEG subtypes has been associated with an improved treatment response rate (Monastra, Monastra, & George, 2002; Fuchs et al., 2003).

The ability of QEEG neuroimaging to map the exact locations of brain abnormalities associated with the core symptoms of ADHD is proving to be very useful in creating individualized EEG neurofeedback protocols. These protocols target the client's specific symptoms. For example, Clarke and others (1998, 2001) identified a subtype of ADHD-Combined-Type children that showed an elevated level of beta EEG activity in both frontal and posterior brain regions. Children with this elevated beta profile exhibited "short-fuse" and moody behaviors in addition to the typical DSM-IV behaviors of ADHD-Combined Type. The subtype identified by this study is similar to one of the "basic three" subtypes in the controlled, group study by Fuchs (Fuchs et al., 2003) which responded to the hyperactive/ impulsive neurofeedback protocol targeting hyper-arousal protocol that addresses elevated frontal beta.

Expanding on their investigation of potential ADHD subtypes, (Clarke et al., 2001) used cluster analysis to identify three QEEG-defined ADHD subtypes. All study participants presented with ADHD behaviors, but they showed different EEG profiles.

The first cluster, suggesting cortical hypoarousal, showed increased relative theta amplitude and theta/beta ratio, as well as decreased relative beta and delta amplitudes at all sites. An example of this QEEG-defined subtype is illustrated by the following QEEG topograph (Figure 11.5) from one of our clients at Austin Biofeedback and EEG Neurofeedback Center, which shows increased relative theta amplitudes and decreased relative beta and delta amplitudes globally.

The second cluster, which suggests maturational lag, showed increased delta and theta amplitudes and decreased alpha and beta amplitudes (Clarke et al., 2001). An example of this QEEG-defined subtype is illustrated by the following QEEG topograph (Figure 11.6) from one of our clients at Austin Biofeedback and EEG Neurofeedback

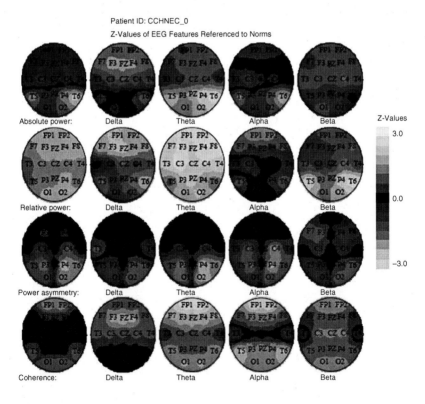

FIGURE 11.5. QEEG cortical hypo-arousal. (See also color gallery.)

Patient ID: CHPEECA_0

Z-Values of EEG Features Referenced to Norms

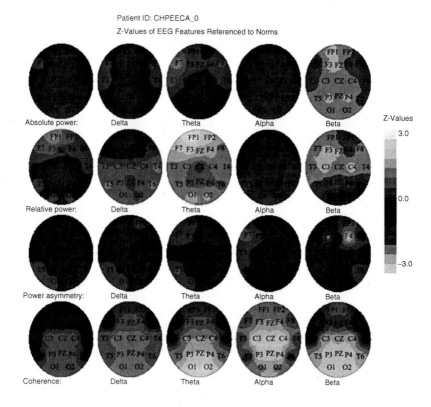

FIGURE 11.6. QEEG Maturational Lag. (See also color gallery.)

Center. Note the increased relative delta and theta amplitudes and decreased relative beta and alpha amplitudes.

The third cluster, suggesting hyperarousal, showed the excessive beta "short-fuse" subtype with excess beta amplitudes in both frontal and posterior regions. An example of this QEEG-defined subtype is illustrated by the following QEEG topograph (Figure 11.7) from one of our clients at Austin Biofeedback and EEG Neurofeedback Center showing excessive relative beta amplitudes globally.

ADHD Subtypes Identified by SPECT Neuroimaging

Amen (Amen et al., 1993) identified six subtypes of ADHD using single proton emission cerebral tomography imaging. SPECT imaging

Patient ID: TLPNEC_0

Z-Values of EEG Features Referenced to Norms

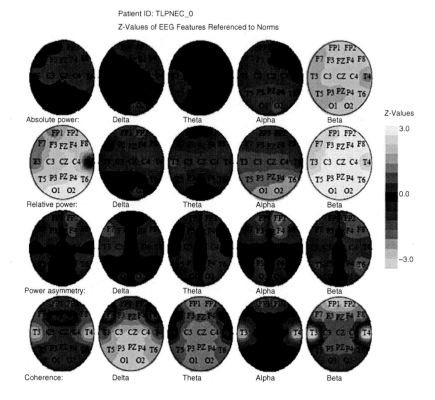

FIGURE 11.7. QEEG hyper-arousal, "short-fuse" subtype. (See also color gallery.)

measures cerebral blood flow and thereby provides information regarding brain metabolism. Amen (2001) used SPECT imaging plus his clinical experience to determine neurotransmitter abnormalities and how to medicate for his six ADHD subtypes. He also suggests neurofeedback protocols for five of his identified subtypes (Amen, 2001).

Following are the descriptions of the six subtypes, the medications, and neurofeedback protocols that Amen has found helpful:

1. *"Classic" ADHD with SPECT showing normal brain activity at rest and prefrontal cortex hypoarousal during a concentration task.* Key behavioral symptoms include hyperactivity, impulsivity, inattention, distractibility, forgetfulness, and disorganization. Amen sees a

correlation with this subtype of ADHD and dopamine deficiency, and finds that this subtype responds to stimulant pharmacotherapy.

Per Amen, neurofeedback for this subtype consists of rewarding prefrontal beta and decreasing theta (Amen, 2001).

2. *"Inattentive" ADHD with SPECT showing normal brain activity at rest and prefrontal cortex hypoarousal during a concentration task.* Key behavioral symptoms include inattention, daydreaming, distractibility, forgetfulness, and procrastination. Amen also sees a dopamine deficiency in this subtype, and like "Classic" ADHD, he finds that this subtype responds to stimulant pharmacotherapy.

Per Amen, neurofeedback for this subtype consists of rewarding prefrontal beta and decreasing theta (Amen, 2001).

3. *"Over focused" ADHD with SPECT showing hyperarousal in the anterior cingulate gyrus.* Key behavioral symptoms include the core ADHD symptoms plus difficulty shifting attention, obsessive-compulsive behaviors, rumination/worrying, inflexibility, and oppositional/argumentative tendencies. Amen sees a deficiency of both dopamine and serotonin, and finds that this subtype responds to either venlafaxine (Effexor) or a combination of stimulant and SSRI (selective serotonin reuptake inhibitor) if pharmacotherapy is used.

Per Amen, neurofeedback for this subtype consists of rewarding high alpha over the anterior cingulate gyrus (Amen, 2001).

4. *"Temporal Lobe" ADHD with SPECT showing decreased temporal lobe activity at rest (one or both lobes) plus reduced blood flow to the prefrontal cortex during concentration tasks.* Key behavioral symptoms include irritability, quick temper, explosive rages, panic/fear, mild paranoia, "dark" or violent thoughts, head or stomach pain of uncertain origin, and emotional instability. Amen finds that this subtype responds to anticonvulsant medication.

Per Amen, neurofeedback for this subtype consists of rewarding SMR and inhibiting theta over the affected temporal lobe(s) (Amen, 2001).

5. *"Limbic" ADHD with SPECT showing hypoarousal in the prefrontal cortex both at rest and during a concentration task, as well as hyperarousal in the deep limbic (emotional centers) of the brain.* Key behavioral symptoms include symptoms of both depression and ADHD (without hyperactivity) such as inattention, poor memory, disorganization, procrastination, negativity, sleep disturbances, feelings

of hopelessness and guilt, low energy/low libido, social isolation, and low self-esteem. Amen sees a deficiency of norepinephrine and dopamine in this subtype, and finds that amino acid supplements DL-phenylalanine and L-tyrosine (precursors to norepinephrine and dopamine) are beneficial. If antidepressant medication is indicated, Amen finds that stimulating antidepressants such as Wellbutrin or Norpramin may be helpful.

Per Amen, neurofeedback for this subtype consists of rewarding beta and inhibiting theta over the left prefrontal cortex (Amen, 2001).

6. *"Ring of Fire" ADHD with SPECT showing diffuse cortical hyperarousal in the prefrontal cortex, the cingulate gyrus, the temporal lobes, and the parietal lobes, indicating global cortical disinhibition.* Key behavioral symptoms include high impulsivity and core ADHD symptoms, anger and aggression, inflexibility and rigid thinking, cyclical moodiness, fast excessive talking, multiple sensitivities (tactile, auditory, visual, olfactory, etc.).

Amen cites no neurofeedback protocols for this ADHD subtype, but finds that an antipsychotic or anticonvulsant medication combined with a psychostimulant or stimulating antidepressant helps moderate the symptoms (Amen, 2001).

Our clinical experience shows neurofeedback to also be very helpful in these cases. At Austin Biofeedback and EEG Neurofeedback Center, we always do a QEEG evaluation when a client presents with symptoms similar to those included in Amen's "Ring of Fire" subtype. Tailoring neurofeedback to fit both the specific behavioral symptoms and the QEEG-defined abnormalities can help to increase psychophysiological calm and to reduce impulsivity and oppositional, manipulative behavior in this subtype. It may be difficult to distinguish this subtype from bipolar disorder (which can also be comorbid with ADHD). In adults who have bipolar disorder but not ADHD, periods of manic behavior and the relative absence of core ADHD symptoms are clues to the diagnosis. In children, it may be harder to distinguish bipolar disorder from severe ADHD. If children are bipolar but not ADHD, their symptoms will tend to be more cyclic.

Although there is an understandable need for more corroborative research on Amen's subtypes, the author often finds his descriptions helpful in fleshing out the overall clinical picture of ADHD clients' presentations. The author finds Amen's subtype descriptions particularly useful when asking clients which medications, if any, have helped their specific symptoms, which medications have not helped, and which have made their symptoms worse. Comparing a client's medication data and behavioral symptoms within the framework of subtypes identified by QEEG, SPECT, and other research, can add valuable information to an understanding of the etiology of their symptoms. I evaluate this information in the light of client-specific EEG assessments, QEEG assessment if used, and other relevant check-lists and assessments, to get the most comprehensive picture possible before developing neurofeedback protocols specific to the client's presentation and needs.

Frequency and Length of Neurofeedback Training for ADHD

In 2004, an ADHD White Paper was written as a joint effort of the Association for Applied Psychophysiology (AAPB) and Biofeed-back and the International Society for Neuronal Regulation (ISNR) (Monastra, Lynn, Linden, Lubar, Gruzelier, & Lavaque, 2005). Among the many relevant issues addressed in the ADHD White Paper, treat-ment schedules based on published, peer-reviewed literature were identified. Positive outcomes were noted with a wide variance in the frequency of training, ranging from one session per week to five ses-sions per week. The duration of actual EEG neurofeedback training within a session (after a 2-5 minute no-feedback baseline) varied, de-pending on the clinical response and learning curve of the client. Studies showed that early in training, the client might have been able to do only five minutes of training. As the brain learned to respond, training time could be gradually increased, with most sessions even-tually consisting of approximately 30 minutes of neurofeedback training time.

The courses of treatment varied between 20 and 50 or more ses-sions. Progress was determined by calculating and reviewing quantita-tive markers of client progress after each session (e.g., microvoltages of theta, beta-1, beta-2, or SMR; percent of time above or below thresholds). Progress was also assessed by continuous performance tests and behavioral rating scales.

Based on 15 years of the author's experience using neurofeedback with ADHD clients at Austin Austin Biofeedback and EEG Neurofeedback Center, the author finds that approximately 40 sessions are needed for the training effects to "hold" longitudinally. If the client has multiple comorbidities or is on medication, it is likely that more than 40 sessions of neurofeedback will be needed.

SUMMARY AND CONCLUSIONS

The historical foundations laid down in both neurofeedback research facilities and clinics across the United States (and now, increasingly, around the world) have brought us to a time of great hope and anticipation in our field. Evidence of efficacy and the general acceptance of neurofeedback as a therapeutic modality for the treatment of ADHD are increasing along with a steadily growing body of favorable research.

Many factors increasingly are providing us more powerful tools for delivering this safe, effective nonpharmacological therapeutic alternative for the treatment of ADHD. These include the research-validated effectiveness of the "basic three" neurofeedback protocols, along with many, rapidly evolving newer variations and approaches; the increasing capabilities we have at our fingertips through the continued development of QEEG and other neuroimaging technologies; a growing technical knowledge base that is expanding our understanding of the functional mechanisms of therapeutic neurofeedback, as well as the biological, behavioral processes that we recognize as ADHD; and the continued refinement of our clinical delivery systems, including enhanced computing capabilities coupled with more sophisticated therapeutic EEG hardware and software.

As EEG neurofeedback has matured as a therapy, we have been afforded the ability and the opportunity to train the human brain in increasingly more complex and precise ways. And this is fitting, because the world of ADHD with its many faces, its variable symptom sets, its differential diagnoses, and potential comorbidities is indeed a complex world in its own right.

REFERENCES

Amen, D.G. (2001). *Healing ADD*. New York: Berkley Publishing Group.

Amen, D.G. & Carmichael, B.D. (1997). High-resolution brain SPECT imaging in ADHD. *Ann Clin Psychiatry, 9*(2), 81-86.

Amen, D.G., Paldi, J.H., & Thisted, R.A. (1993). Evaluating ADHD with brain SPECT imaging. *Journal of the American Academy of Child and Adolescent Psychiatry, 32*(5), 1080-1081.

American Psychiatric Association (1980). *Diagnostic and statistical manual of mental disorders,* (3rd ed. Text Revision). American Psychiatric Association, Washington, D.C.

American Psychiatric Association (2000). *Diagnostic and statistical manual of mental disorders,* (4th ed. Text Revision). American Psychiatric Association, Washington, D.C.

Attention Deficit Help Center (2003). The history of ADHD and attention deficit disorder. http://www.add-adhd-help-center.com/newsletters/newsletter_15 Accessed on July 2003.

Barkley, R.A. (1998). *Attention-deficit hyperactivity disorder: A handbook for diagnosis and treatment* (2nd ed.). New York: Guilford Press.

Barkley, R.A., Fischer, M., Fletcher, K., & Smallish, L. (Submitted for publication) Young adult outcome of hyperactive children as a function of severity of childhood conduct problems, *I: Psychiatric Status and Mental Health Treatment.*

Biederman, J., Faraone, S., Milberger, S., Guite, J., Mick, E., Chen, L., Mennin, D., Ouellette, C., Moore, P., Spencer, T., Norman, D., Wilens, T., Kraus, I., & Perrin, J. (1996). A prospective four-year follow-up study of attention-deficithyperactivity and related disorders. *Archives of General Psychiatry, 53,* 437-446.

Cantwell, D. (1996). Attention deficit disorder: A review of the past 10 years. *Journal of the American Academy of Child and Adolescent Psychiatry, 35,* 978-987.

Carlezon, W.A. Jr. (2003). Preteen Ritalin may increase depression. *Biological Psychiatry, 54,* 1330-1337.

Carmody, D.P., Radvanski, D.C., Wadhwani, S., Sabo, M.J., & Vergara, L. (2001). EEG biofeedback training and attention-deficit/hyperactivity disorder in an elementary school setting. *Journal of Neurotherapy, 43*(3), 5-27.

Casey, B.J., Castellanos, F.X., Geidd, J.N., Marsh, W.L., Hamburger, S.D., Schubert, A.B. et al. (1997). Implication of right frontostriatal circuitry in response inhibition and attention-deficit hyperactivity disorder. *Journal of the American Academy of Child and Adolescent Psychiatry, 36,* 374-383.

Chabot, R.A., Merkin, H., Wood, L.M., Davenport, T.L., & Serfontein, G. (1996). Sensitivity and specificity of QEEG in children with attention deficit or specific developmental learning disorders. *Clinical Electroencephalography, 27,* 26-34.

Chabot, R.A., Orgill, A.A., Crawford, G., Harris, M.J., & Serfontein, G. (1999). Behavioral and electrophysiologic predictors of treatment response to stimulants in children with attention disorders. *Journal of Child Neurology, 14*(6), 343-351.

Chabot, R.A. & Serfontein, G. (1996). Quantitative electroencephalographic profiles of children with attention deficit disorder. *Biological Psychiatry, 40,* 951-963.

CHADD Fact Sheet #3. (2003). *Children and adults with attention-deficit/hyperactivity disorder: Evidence-based medication management for children and adolescents with AD/HD,* Retrieved October 1, 2004, from http://www.chadd.org/fs/fs3.htm.

Clarke, A.R., Barry, R.J., McCarthy, R., & Selikowitz, M. (2001). Electroencephalogram differences in two subtypes of attention-deficit/hyperactivity disorder. *Psychophysiology, 38,* 212-221.

Clarke, A.R., Barry, R.J., McCarthy, R., & Selikowitz, M. (2002). EEG differences between good and poor responders to methylphenidate and dexamphetamine in children with attention-deficit/hyperactivity disorder. *Clinical Neurophysiology, 113,* 194-205.

El-Zein, R.A., Abdel-Rahman, S., Hay, M., Lopez, Bondy, M., Morris, D., & Legator, M. (2005). Cytogenetic effects in children treated with methylphenidate. *Cancer Letters, In Press, Corrected Proof, Elsevier Ireland, Ltd.*

Food and Drug Administration (2004). Talk Paper T04-60.

Fuchs, T., Birbaumer, N., Lutzenberger, W., Gruzelier, J.H., & Kaiser, J. (2003). Neurofeedback treatment for attention-deficit/hyperactivity disorder in children: A comparison with methylphenidate. *Applied Psychophysiology and Biofeedback, 28,* 1-12.

Gadow, K.D. & Sprafkin, J. (1997). *Child symptom inventory 4: Norms manual.* Stony Brook, NY: Checkmate Plus.

Gainetdinov, Raul R. & Caron, Marc G. (2001). Genetics of childhood disorders: XXIV. ADHD, part 8: Hyperdopaminergic mice as an animal model of ADHD. *Journal of the American Academy of Child and Adolescent Psychiatry, 40*(3), 380-382.

Geller, B., Williams, M., Zimerman, B., Frazier, J., Beringer, L., Warner, K.L. (1998). Prepubertal and early adolescent bipolarity differentiate from ADHD by manic symptoms, grandiose delusions, ultra-rapid or ultradian cycling. *Journal of Affective Disorders, 51,* 81-91.

Harris, G. (2006). Warning urged on stimulants like Ritalin. *New York Times,* Feb. 10, 2006.

Hohman, L.B. (1922). Post-encephalitic behavior disorders in children. *Bulletin of the John Hopkins Hospital, 33,* 372.

Hynd, G.W., Hern, K.L., Novey, E.S., & Eliopulos, D. (1993). Attention deficit-hyperactivity disorder and asymmetry of the caudate nucleus. *Journal of Child Neurology, 8,* 339-343.

Hynd, G.W., Semrud-Clikeman, M., Lorys, A.R. et al. (1990). Brain morphology in developmental dyslexia and attention deficit disorder/hyperactivity. *Archives of Neurology, 47,* 919-926.

Kaiser, D.A. & Othmer, S. (2000). Effect of neurofeedback on variables of attention in a large multicenter trial. *Journal of Neurotherapy, 4*(1), 5-28.

Linden, M., Habib, T., & Radojevic, V. (1996). A controlled study of the effects of EEG biofeedback on cognition and behavior of children with attention deficit disorder and learning disabilities. *Biofeedback and Self-Regulation, 21*(1), 35-49.

Lubar, J.F. (2003). Neurofeedback for the management of attention deficit disorders. In M.S. Schwartz & F. Andrasik (Eds.), *Biofeedback: A practitioner's guide* (3rd ed., pp. 409-437). New York: Guilford Press.

Lubar, J.F. & Shouse, M.N. (1976). EEG and behavioral changes in a hyperkinetic child concurrent with training of the sensorimotor rhythm (SMR): A preliminary report. *Biofeedback and Self Regulation, 1,* 293-306.

Mann, C., Lubar, J., Zimmerman, A., Miller, C., & Nuenchen, R. (1992). Quantitative analysis of EEG in boys with attention-deficit-hyperactivity disorder: Controlled study with clinical implications. *Pediatric Neurology, 8,* 30-36.

Mannuzza, S., Klein, R.G., Bonagura, N., Malloy, P., Giampino, H., & Addalli, K.A. (1991). Hyperactive boys almost grown up: Replication of psychiatric status. *Archives of General Psychiatry, 48,* 77-83.

Monastra, Lynn; Linden, Lubar, Gruzelier, & Lavaque (2005). Electroencephalographic biofeedback in the treatment of attention-deficit hyperactivity disorder. *Applied Psychophysiology and Biofeedback, 30*(2), 95-114.

Monastra, V.J. (2005). *Parenting children with ADHD: 10 lessons that medicine cannot teach.* Washington, DC: American Psychological Association.

Monastra, V.J., Lubar, J.F., & Linden, M. (2001). The development of a quantitative electroencephalographic scanning process for attention deficit-hyperactivity disorder: Reliability and validity studies. *Neuropsychology, 15,* 136-144.

Monastra, V.J., Lubar, J.F., Linden, M., VanDeusen, P., Green, G., Wing, W., Phillips, A., & Fenger, T.N. (1999). Assessing attention deficit hyperactivity disorder via quantitative electroencephalography: An initial validation study. *Neuropsychology, 13*(3), 424-433.

Monastra, V.J., Monastra, D.M., & George, S. (2002). The effects of stimulant therapy, EEG biofeedback, and parenting style on the primary symptoms of attention-deficit/hyperactivity disorder. *Applied Psychophysiology and Biofeedback, 27*(4), 231-249.

Mostofsky, S.H., Reiss, A.L., Lockhart, P., & Denckla, M.B. (1998). Evaluation of cerebellar size in attention-deficit hyperactivity disorder. *Journal of Child Neurology, 13,* 434-439.

Murphy, K. & Barkley, R.A. (1996). Attention deficit hyperactivity disorder adults: Comorbidities and adaptive impairments. *Comprehensive Psychiatry, 37,* 393-401.

Othmer, Othmer, & Putman (2005). TOVA results for interhemispheric training, a historical comparison and model implications. Presented at the 13th International Society for Neuronal Regulation meeting, Denver, CO.

Pelham, W.E., Gnagy, E.M., Greenslade, K.E., & Milich, R. (1992). Teacher ratings of DSM-III-R symptoms for the disruptive behavior disorders. *Journal of the American Academy of Child and Adolescent Psychiatry, 31,* 210-218.

Rossiter, T.R. (2004). The effectiveness of neurofeedback and stimulant drugs in treating ADHD. Part II. Replication. *Applied Psychophysiology and Biofeedback, 29,* 233-243.

Rossiter, T.R. & LaVaque, T.J. (1995). A comparison of EEG biofeedback and psycho-stimulants in treating attention deficit/hyperactivity disorders. *Journal of Neurotherapy, 1*(1), 48-59.

Roth, S.R., Sterman, M.B., & Clemente, C.C. (1967). Comparison of EEG correlates of reinforcement, internal inhibition, and sleep. *Electroencephalography and Clinical Neurophysiology, 23,* 509-520.

Sterman, M.B. & Wyrwicka, W. (1967). EEG correlates of sleep: Evidence for separate forebrain substrates. *Brain Research, 6,* 143-163.

Still, G.F. (1902). Some abnormal psychical conditions in children. *Lancet, 1,* 1008-1012, 1077-1082, 1163-1168.

Swanson, J.M., McBurnett, K., Christian, D.L., & Wigel, T. (1995). Stimulant medication and treatment of children with ADHD. In T.H. Ollendick & R.J. Prinz (Eds.), *Advances in clinical child psychology* (Vol. 17, pp. 265-322). New York: Plenum Press.

Tansey, M. (1993). Ten-year stability of EEG biofeedback results for a hyperactive boy who failed the fourth grade perceptually impaired class. *Biofeedback and Self-Regulation, 18*(1), 33-38.

Thompson, L. & Thompson, M. (1998). Neurofeedback combined with training in metacognitive strategies: Effectiveness in students with ADD. *Applied Psychophysiology and Biofeedback, 23*(4), 243-263.

Weiss, G. & Hechtman, L. (1993). *Hyperactive children grown up,* (2nd ed.). New York: Guilford Press.

Wender, P.H. (2002). ADHD: *Attention-deficit hyperactivity disorder in children and adults.* London: Oxford University Press.

Wolraich, M.L., Hannah, J.N., Pinnock, T.Y., Baumgaertel, A., & Brown, J. (1996). Comparison of diagnostic criteria for attention-deficit hyperactivity disorder in a countrywide sample. *Journal of the American Academy of Child and Adolescent Psychiatry, 35,* 319-324.

Wyrwicka, W. & Sterman, M.B. (1968). Instrumental conditioning of sensorimotor cortex EEG spindles in the waking cat. *Physiology and Behavior, 3,* 703-707.

Yucha, C. & Gilbert, C. (2003). *Evidence-based practice in biofeedback and neurofeedback.* Association for Applied Psychophysiology and Biofeedback, Wheat Ridge, CO.

Zametkin, A.J., Nordahl, T.E., Gross, M., King, A.C., Semple, W.E., Rumsey, J. et al. (1990). Cerebral glucose metabolism in adults with hyperactivity of childhood onset. *New England Journal of Medicine, 323,* 1361-1366.

Zametkin, A.J., & Rapoport, J.L. (1987). Noradrenergic hypothesis of attention deficit disorder with hyperactivity: A critical review. In H.V. Metsler (Ed.), *Psychopharmacology: The Third Generation of Progress* (pp. 837-842). New York: Raven Press.

Chapter 12

Multichannel EEG Phase Synchrony Training and Verbally Guided Attention Training for Disorders of Attention

Lester G. Fehmi

INTRODUCTION

Significance of Synchrony

Experiments (Fehmi, Lindsley, & Adkins, 1965; Fehmi, Adkins, & Lindsley, 1969) at the Brain Research Institute at UCLA in the early 1960s led to an interesting discovery: synchrony in the visual system of primates is crucial for information processing. The data showed that just the leading narrow sliver of a visual evoked response activity and less than 10 msec of activity is sufficient for accurately communicating shape information to the brain. What is special about this initial brief section of the evoked response is that it is composed of synchronous activity on parallel neurons, such that the synchronous activity that follows is apparently redundant and unnecessary for perception in most situations. In other words, there exists a direct link between certain forms of brain synchrony and perception. This relationship of synchrony to shape or form information directly supports the fundamental role of synchrony for information processing in the nervous system. Simultaneous or synchronous activity, that is, any "bump" in ongoing electroencephalography (EEG) activity, has the potential of

Handbook of Neurofeedback
© 2007 by The Haworth Press, Inc. All rights reserved.
doi:10.1300/5889_12

communicating information. Various forms of attention described later are also considered concomitants of parallel information processing. This supports the fundamental role of synchrony in attention.

Phase, Coherence, Correlation, and Synchrony

These are fundamental concepts and phenomena in electroencephalography, and it is useful to understand similarities and differences among them. Phase synchrony is depicted in Figure 12.1 by comparison of the middle two waves where peaks and troughs occur at the same times, that is, synchronously.

Peaks and troughs occur oppositely in the top two waves and are considered perfectly (180 degrees) out-of-phase. The bottom two

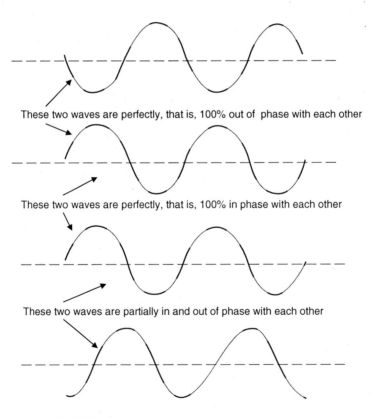

These two waves are perfectly, that is, 100% out of phase with each other

These two waves are perfectly, that is, 100% in phase with each other

These two waves are partially in and out of phase with each other

FIGURE 12.1. Examples of sine wave phase relations.

waves are less in or out of phase with each other than are any other comparison of waves.

Figure 12.2 depicts relationships among coherence, correlation, and synchrony. The major feature of coherence is that any fixed phase relationship between two waves of equal frequency would yield a 100 percent coherence score, that is, a coherence of 1.0. That is, it does not matter whether the two waves were exactly in phase, partially out of phase, or completely (180 degrees) out of phase, as long as this relationship is fixed (consistent), coherence is 100 percent.

Each example of fixed phase relations (shown in the left column) yields a coherence of 1.0 (shown in the next column from the left). This is not so in case of correlation (shown in the third column). The correlation score varies from +1.0 (in-phase) through 0.0 (an intermediate phase) to minus 1.0 (180 degrees out-of-phase). Thus, in contrast to the way many think of coherence, it is not the same as correlation. The synchrony score (shown in the fourth column) varies from 1.0 to 0.5 to 0.0 as phase relations vary. In the example for which synchrony is 1.0 (100 percent), the coherence and the correlation are also 1.0 (100 percent). However, when coherence is 1.0, synchrony is not necessarily 1.0 and could even be zero. When we train for 100 percent in-phase synchrony, we are training for a special case of 100 percent coherence and of 100 percent correlation.

Attention

In order to further understand phase synchrony training for disorders of attention, it is necessary to define attention. Few would argue against the notion that attention is *a*, and perhaps *the*, most im-

Fixed phase relations	Coherence	Correlation	Synchrony
0°	1	1	1
90°	1	0	0.5
180°	1	−1	0
270°	1	0	0.5

FIGURE 12.2. The effects of various phase relations upon coherence, correlation, and synchrony scores.

portant skill, and the most fundamental behavior in which we humans engage (Lindsley, 1961; Fehmi, 2003). Research and personal experience of the author led to the delineation of four independent types of attention, which may occur individually or in many combinations as illustrated in Figure 12.3 (Fehmi & Fritz, 1980).

Any optimization of performance must include being able to employ, direct, sequence, and maintain types, or configurations of types, of attention (Fehmi, 1970). Figure 12.3 illustrates a model used by the author of separate types of attention and possible configurations or combinations of these (Fehmi, 1978; Fehmi, 1986). The inner and outer circles shown in Figure 12.3 include equal elements of all the four attention types, simultaneously, and will be later referred to as Open Focus* attention. However, it must be considered that preeminent among attention skills is a sort of "meta-attention," that is, attention to attention, making possible the voluntary control of flexibility and stability of any single type or combination of attention types. Each of the attention types that are depicted will be discussed in what follows.

Focused (narrow, pointed) attention is directed toward a limited field of experience, excluding all else, while diffused (wide; broad,

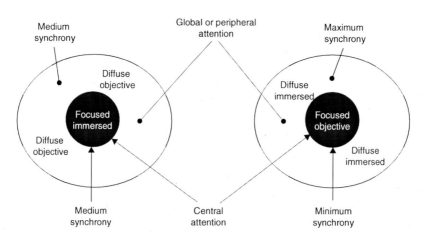

FIGURE 12.3. Individual attention types.

---

*Open Focus® is a registered trademark of Biofeedback Computers, Inc.

multisensory) attention, conversely, includes all available experience simultaneously and more or less equally. Objective (remote, separate) attention refers to one's conscious awareness of subject and object, of time and space, and the multisensory contents thereof, that is, of sensations (objects). Immersed (engaged; absorbed) attention can engage experience partially or completely to the point where all awareness is lost. Considered generally, attention might be defined as the behavior that controls awareness and meta-awareness.

To help clarify this model, examples of each of the individual types of attention will be provided here. Of course, it must be realized that in real life, the different types will interact and all or several may be present during even short time periods. An example where focused attention is dominant would be the reader's present and ongoing effort to read and understand this chapter. Diffused attention might appropriately occur while witnessing a nature scene, for example, a panoramic sunset with sounds (e.g., crickets), feelings (e.g., breeze), and smells, etc. Objective attention is most appropriate during the conscious learning phase of skill training, while perfected skills are often associated with immersed attention and unconscious execution. Playing a musical instrument is an example that comes to mind: at first, learning is self-conscious, but then it becomes less rigidly conscious and more automatic and effortless as skill level increases.

One combination of attention types used by most people most of the time is the combination of focused/objective (quadrant "A" of Figure 12.3). Such chronic, narrow/objective attention is a major vehicle of acculturation, that is, learning to name objects (objectifying) and the skills, rules, and mores of our time and place. Table 12.1 depicts various combinations of attention (quadrants "A" "B" "C" "D") and corresponding examples, the impact of their use, and associated EEG parameters, all positioned upon an arousal continuum. Immersed combined with diffused (quadrant "C") and/or immersed combined with narrow (quadrant "D") attention also is often emphasized in the visual and performing arts as well as in sports. This is, because connectedness with one's body, this moment, and/or with teammates can bring with it optimization of function and performance.

Figure 12.4 shows examples of what will be referred to here as Open Focus combinations of attention types (Fehmi, 1975, 1977). Development of an ability to flexibly move among these types is a goal

TABLE 12.1. Combinations of styles of attention, examples, and their effects and associated EEG characteristics.

	Example	Effects	EEG
Quadrant "C" diffuse-immersed	Meditation with mind unself-conscious and body at rest. Most rapid normaliza-tion. Sleep. Most relaxed.	Parasympathetic nervous system dominance. Low arousal. Right brain dominant drifting into sleep.	Low frequencies dominant at high amplitude. Most whole brain synchrony.
Quadrant "B" diffuse-objective	Panoramic view in a "symphony of sensory experi-ence." Objective sensations hang suspended in the midst of a diffuse awareness of space, Playing in a band.	Relative sympa-thetic and para-sympathetic balance. Moderate arousal. Relative left-right hemi-sphere balance. Relaxed alert.	Middle frequencies dominant in amplitude. Moder-ate whole brain synchrony.
Quadrant "D" narrow-immersed	Immersed in enjoy-ment, amplified by a narrow focus to intensify and savor experience. Enrap-tured thinker. Deep massage recipient.	Relative sym-pathetic-para-sympathetic balance. Left-right hemisphere bal-ance. Alert relaxed.	Middle frequencies dominant in ampli-tude. Moderate whole brain syn-chrony.
Quadrant "A" narrow-objective	Lion stalking prey. Emergency. College exam. Obsessing on work to narrow focus away from (deny) an emotional prob-lem. Self-conscious mind and body highly toned.	Sympathetic nervous system dominance. High arousal and adren-aline. Left brain dominant. Flight or fight.	High frequencies dominant at low amplitude over all. Least whole brain synchrony.

of the multichannel EEG phase synchrony training and related Open Focus training activities described later in this chapter. This figure also introduces the terms "peripheral" or "global" and "central" atten-tion, which is not to be confused with the attention types mentioned earlier. Here, they refer to a type of figure-ground situation wherein, for example, an Open Focus combination of focused/immersed atten-tion is the central "figure" surrounded by a more global level "back-

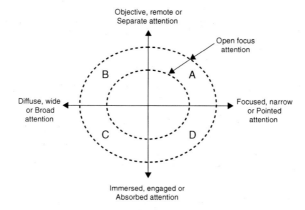

FIGURE 12.4. Examples of open focus combinations of attention types.

ground" of diffuse/objective attention (see left side of illustration in Figure 12.4). Figure 12.4 also depicts a more common Open Focus configuration, that is, central focused/objective attention surrounded by diffuse/immersed attention (right side illustration) (Fehmi & Robbins, 2001; Fehmi, 2003).

EVOLUTION OF THE EEG SYNCHRONY/ ATTENTION CONNECTION

Serendipity and informal experiments by the author and associates led to the observation that certain conscious experiences regarding attention and awareness strongly relate to the presence of greater synchrony in the EEG, perhaps especially synchrony within the alpha frequency band. When whole head alpha synchrony was abundant, it was very often reported to be associated with a subjective sense of lightness, clarity, spaciousness, effortlessness of attention, and immersion of awareness in the sensations or objects of experience. Release of tension also frequently was reported to accompany such whole brain alpha frequency synchrony.

One day in 1968, out of curiosity, the paper speed of EEG equipment being used to simultaneously record five channels of EEG activity from a research participant was increased, allowing a visual comparison of the phase relations among the five samples. The author observed that when the participant was just sitting with eyes closed, then four of the five samples were virtually in phase, while one was close to 180 degrees out of phase with the others. This same relationship was noted frequently in three subsequent participants. In all cases, the trace out-of-phase with the other four was reflecting activity from the occipital lobe (Oz). This serendipitous finding led to the thought that brain function may, in some manner, use phase relations to support attention. It was further speculated that this thought might be supported if it could be demonstrated that persons could learn to control phase relationships. Subsequently, results of a controlled experiment (Fehmi & Osborne, 1971) showed that, with appropriate feedback, participants could respond accurately to commands to alternately produce more and then less phase synchrony. Feedback was given only when waves recorded from the left and right occipital lobes were within 15 degrees of being perfectly in phase. Experimental participants were significantly better at controlling phase synchrony than control participants who received sham feedback.

Clinical practice and informal research with the four types of attention noted previously led to the following hypothesis: Conscious subject/object attention exists when the activity elicited by an object of sensation in a cortical projection area of the brain is out of phase with the rest of the brain. It also was hypothesized that, conversely, immersed attention is represented by whole head synchrony. Later, research with clients engaged in five-channel EEG synchrony training supported the latter hypothesis. Specifically, increases in whole head EEG wave synchrony were associated with reports of a disappearance of the witnessing of self. In order for reestablishment of the "witness" with sensory contents (objective attention), whole head synchrony had to give way to partially out-of-phase activity in the cortical area associated with the sensations. The specific brain locus of out-of-phase activity was noted to vary with shifts in specific sensory awareness. Thus, the separation of the "witness" from its sensory contents of attention apparently was achieved by the mechanism of phase shift.

In an attempt to further explain these phenomena, various synchrony relationships were hypothesized (see Figure 12.5). Specifically, it was hypothesized that when brain waves associated with simple awareness, "A1," interact with waves stimulated by the contents

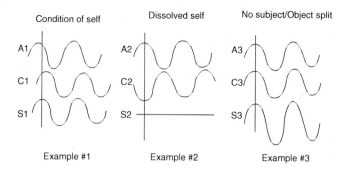

FIGURE 12.5. The proposed phase mechanism for flexible creation, maintenance and dissolution of the functional separation between three processes: the
contents of attention (the object wave "C"), *awareness* of the contents (the subject wave "A"), and their phase disparity, which gives rise to a sense of *self* or *witness,* (reflected by the interference wave "S"), created by the interaction of
waves "A" and "C."

of awareness, "C1," with which the former waves are less than 100 percent in phase and less than 100 percent out-of-phase, then a resultant
third wave, "S1," an interference wave is produced, which is phase
shifted from both the other waves (see Example #1 in Figure 12.5).
This interference wave (the sum of its components) represents "witnessing" or self-awareness. When waves "A2" and "C2" of Figure
12.5 are 100 percent out-of-phase and of equal amplitude, then the
interference wave, "S2," is completely cancelled, resulting in the
total dissolution of self-awareness (see Example #2 in Figure 12.5).
When "A3" and "C3" are 100 percent in-phase then the third interference wave, "S3," which is the in-phase sum of "A3" and "C3," results
in a merged self, not distinguishable from subject/object (see Example #3 in Figure 12.5). These "A" and "C" interactions may take place
at more than one brain loci simultaneously.

To this point, background information on combinations of types of
attention (including Open Focus types of combinations) has been
given, and their hypothesized relationships to brain wave synchrony/
and asynchrony have been discussed. This chapter now proceeds to
descriptions of how EEG synchrony training and various attention-
training exercises are being used by the author to enable clients to
voluntarily enhance and be more flexible with various types of attention in order to optimally adapt to changing life situations.

PRACTICAL APPLICATIONS
OF PHASE SYNCHRONY TRAINING

In traditional talk therapy, a common goal is to bring into consciousness unprocessed noxious material, which requires the suspension of certain chronic maladaptive attention strategies. Such catharsis, when fully processed, supports the diffusion of emotional experience and can result in a temporary sense of well being, even euphoria. However, attention habits created by the use of chronic attention strategies remain as powerful forces in opposition to permanent normalization of function. Attention flexibility training can break any remaining grip of attention habits or rigidities upon system function.

A common example is that of avoidance of attention from unpleasant experience (Fehmi and Selzer, 1980). This resistance is an ongoing process for most, if not all, of us. We attend narrowly, and direct our narrow exclusive attention away from noxious experience to objectify, and to fixate upon other experience. Thus, by choosing and maintaining control over narrow-objective attention, and by shutting down immersed-diffuse attention, we can escape unpleasant personal experience. There are other examples of using attention types to manage personal and transpersonal experience (Fehmi & Selzer, 1978, 1980), for example, a positive strategic use of attention styles can lead to the dissolution of experience.

Dissolving Pain and Other Sensations

A significant component of the attention-training program used in the author's clinic is devoted to the learned dissolution of pain (Fehmi & Selzer, 1978). By expanding one's scope of attention and centering one's attention upon the pain, and by engaging increasingly with pain, and finally immersing the witness into the experience of pain and the space in which it exists, the pain dissolves. These attention processes when applied to pain, or any other object of attention, bring about the dissolution of any central experience. The repeated practice of dissolving experience followed by the reestablishment of it provides an excellent opportunity to practice flexibility by changing attention types from diffuse/immersed to focused/objective and back again.

Attention Disorders

A wide array of attention disorders and many other symptoms of disregulation, both physical and mental, are the result of chronic avoidance and the rigid maintenance of otherwise adaptive combinations of attention. Excessive use of certain types of attention (especially focused/objective attention) ultimately manifests as attentional rigidity, and many neurotransmitters and chemical-nutritional deficits may result from chronic exhaustion of underlying systems.

Training flexibility of EEG activity by, for example, learning to increase and decrease EEG wave synchrony across a range of frequencies and sites, teaches adaptive volitional attentional flexibility (and stability). Here, bipolar and referential recording are used to train out-of-phase and in-phase activity respectively (see Fehmi & Sundor, 1989). Successful flexibility training requires the daily practice of synchrony and asynchrony for many days to give rise to an ongoing thirst for normalization and optimization of neural and somatic function.

Appropriate attentional flexibility is at the heart of optimum performance. The continuum from autism, to ADD and ADHD, to high-level performance is directly related to the degree of attention rigidity. Learning to alternately enhance and reduce individual and combinations of attention types is necessary in order to break up attention fixations. Chronic fixations such as extremes of objective/focused attention prevent the release of stress and tension and in doing so, support their accumulation and can maintain and exacerbate one's pain. Diffuse/immersed attention also can have a downside when it becomes chronic, by making it so that one cannot readily grasp objects of sensation, or experience witnessing awareness. Only the autonomic balance that results from ideal attention choices and flexibility supports general improved performance. Members of civilized cultures everywhere can benefit from attention flexibility training via recorded training exercises and neurofeedback. Attention training can modify the rigid attention biases inculcated by every society, which lead to attention disorders.

Details of the synchrony training procedures presently used by the author will be presented next.

INSTRUMENTATION FOR INDIVIDUAL
AND MULTIPERSON SYNCHRONY TRAINING

A standalone five-channel analog feedback device filters for variable training frequencies and produces delayed "beeps" and flashes when the channel sum exceeds a preset threshold of phase synchrony. A second device, a five-channel neurosynchrony trainer with phase delay, integrates input activity and produces an output whose amplitude reflects degree of synchrony. Either device can also serve as a unity gain preamplifier to any existing neurofeedback instrumentation.

With the addition of one device per person, each may learn to share a common synchrony with the others in the group. Figure 12.6 shows a schematic diagram of equipment for training couples synchrony, within individuals, and between them.

Since the 1960s, the effort expended to accomplish whole head monitoring has been reduced by minimizing the number of samples of EEG activity and by using saline sensors. For whole head synchrony, we simultaneously monitor FPz, Cz, Oz, T4, and T3 (Jasper, 1958), which samples the four major brain lobes bilaterally. A referential sensor configuration to one or both ears is always used. Using the ubiquitous differential amplifier, bipolar configurations cancel in-phase activity through common mode rejection. Thus, it is not possible to engage in whole head in-phase synchrony training using bipolar sensor placements (Fehmi & Sundor, 1989). Only multiple site referential recording and integration of these samples can accurately reflect the presence of in-phase synchrony between brain loci.

Saline sensors have certain advantages over paste electrodes. They can be placed easily and quickly by sliding them under a velcro band or cross-piece. Seldom is any skin preparation necessary. The sensors are kept in a super-saturated salt solution and are always ready. No cleaning of hair, scalp, or sensors is usually necessary before or after training.

Phase synchrony is measured by integrating the five referentially recorded signals simultaneously. When, through the production of synchrony, the algebraic average of these waves exceeds threshold, a delayed flash and beep are produced. The feedback delay is adjusted so that the excitation produced by the flash and beep arrives at the cortex at a time when the next cycle of synchronous activity is beginning its

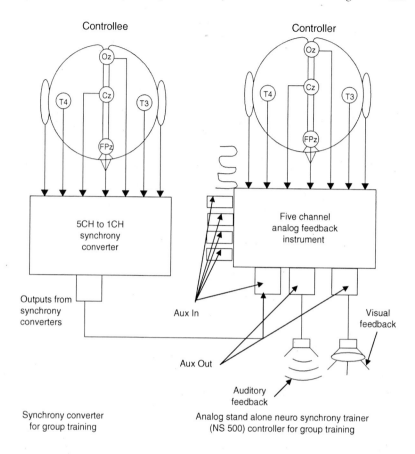

FIGURE 12.6. Equipment diagram for multi-person five channel synchrony training (only couples training shown).

excitatory climb. Thus, this recruitment of excitement facilitates the continued production of synchrony. This delay of feedback is most effective with an analog neurofeedback system, which is fast enough to augment the excitement of the next excitatory cycle, which for 10 Hz activity, is a delay between 50 and 75 msec, depending on the person.

Synchrony and asynchrony can be trained at any frequency. As noted earlier, synchrony can be defined as in-phase activity between waves of identical frequency. On the contrary, there are many forms of asynchrony. Any degree of out-of-phase activity would qualify and any differential change in frequency between waves would also qualify. Also qualifying would be any cancellation of activity that occurs when two waves of equal amplitude and frequency are 180 degrees out-of-phase and nullify each other. Any lapse of synchronous activity as might occur during brain desynchronization in response to sympathetic autonomic activation, would also qualify. Learning to move quickly and effortlessly between phase synchrony and desynchronization represents a particularly valuable form of flexibility training in our work, often associated with the effortless back and forth movement between diffuse/immersed attention and focused/objective attention.

BEHAVIORAL PERFORMANCE, ATTENTION, AND BRAIN ACTIVITY

The suggested relationship of attention to performance and their relationship to both brain wave peak frequency and arousal are shown in Figure 12.7.

In this model, performance improves up to a certain EEG frequency or level of arousal, and then declines. Peak performance occurs when the effects of focused-objective and diffuse-immersed

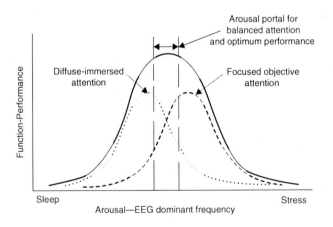

FGB 2ﬁ proposed relationslp betœen arousal,EEG dominant fre quency,and attention style as tby impact function-performance.

attention sum, at mid EEG frequencies, that is, at middle levels of arousal. Focused/objective attention operates at higher frequencies and with less synchrony, and diffuse/immersed attention operates at low frequencies with greater synchrony. The former relates more to sympathetic activation and the latter to parasympathetic activation. The former is seen as object (figure or foreground) of experience and the latter as space (background or ground) of experience. These EEG/attention relationships can be observed directly by experiencing the four independent attention types, first one at a time, and then in combination, and noting the nature of resultant EEG activation.

The nature of the EEG is directly related to the types of attention employed and their weighting. When all four types of attention are present equally and simultaneously, there is presumed to be autonomic balance, for example, stress is rapidly diffused. The effects of EEG and attention upon each other are reciprocal. Training EEG impacts attention and training or employing attention impacts EEG.

In our work and that of others (Day, 1967), it has been found that hemispheric dominance is related to the production of alpha synchrony. Figure 12.8 shows that, before feedback, right hemisphere

	Dominant hemisphere	
Alpha	Right (RDH)	Left (LDH)
Initial average baseline	14.6 uv	6.4 uv
Asked to increase feedback	21%	−11%
Asked to decrease feedback	1%	−17%
	Positive alpha bias	Negative alpha bias

FIGURE 12.8. Alpha synchrony biases for dominant right and left hemisphere trainees.

dominant (RHD) clients generally have more than twice the base line alpha of left hemisphere dominant (LHD) clients. Dominance is defined here as related to a bias or tendency to engage one of the hemispheres more than the other to answer questions even though the chosen hemisphere is ill equipped to do so (Day, 1964). Examples of questions are, can you picture the last time you saw a man crying (RHD) versus, can you tell me the sum of 389 and 797 (LHD). When asked to increase feedback, signaling the production of alpha, RHD clients produce 21 percent above base line, while LHD clients actually decrease alpha by 11 percent. When asked to decrease feedback, RHD clients increase alpha by 1 percent while LHD clients decrease alpha below base line by 17 percent. These differences are statistically significant (unpublished). RHD clients have a positive bias and capacity to produce alpha while LHD clients have a negative bias. As previously described, synchrony is related to attention. So it follows that the increased alpha of RHD clients supports diffuse/immersed attention and the decreased alpha of LHD clients supports focused/objective attention.

Using a controlled research design, Fern Selzer (Selzer and Fehmi, 1974) found that LHD individuals learn to produce alpha with auditory feedback and not well or not at all using visual feedback. On the other hand, RHD individuals learn to produce alpha with visual feedback and not so well with auditory feedback. Thus, synchrony biases may relate to sensory learning variables, and the nature of the sensory feedback may impact the learning of synchrony control in a significant segment of the population.

It appears that diffuse and immersed attention is organized by the right hemisphere and is reflected by phase synchrony and high amplitudes. The functional characteristics emerging from these right hemisphere mechanisms include: letting or releasing (versus holding or controlling); the process of awareness (versus the content of awareness); diffuse inclusive awareness (versus narrow exclusive); awareness of figure and ground (versus figure only); all inclusive past, present, and future time (versus a narrow sense of time); medium levels of arousal (versus extremes); unselfconsciousness (versus self-consciousness); diffusion of stress (versus it's accumulation); space (versus the contents of space). The contrary characteristics are connected to narrow and objective types of attention and generally appear to be organized by the left hemisphere. It is important to remember that the left and right hemispheres can and do function simultaneously. As a result, the previous characterizing may be present simultaneously and equally, and, thus, may cancel each other's impact to some degree.

This chapter concludes with further comments and speculation on the dynamics of EEG synchrony and attention, and summarizes some research-based support for efficacy of synchrony training for alleviating symptoms of a variety of stress related disorders.

In the author's clinical work, EEG synchrony training commonly is used in conjunction with recorded attention training exercises collectively referred to as Open Focus training exercises. They are designed primarily to help clients attain the ability to flexibly enter and leave states of Open Focus attention, which was described earlier. However, use of these exercises alone, EEG synchrony training alone, and the combination of both have been demonstrated to be useful with a large variety of disorders and situations. Results of some controlled research illustrate this.

Fee and Sinoway (unpublished, see Attention to Attention, 2003)* demonstrated, first in a pilot study, then in a controlled experiment, that rehearsing a daily experience of Open Focus training, which guides one's attention to the experience of space, identical to one aspect of the attention training program used by the author, resulted in the improvement or maintenance of peripheral vertical and horizontal fields of visual awareness, over the course of one college semester. The members of the control group, who were not asked to practice experiencing space, found that their visual fields contracted at the end of the semester, presumably due to increasing stress, and culminating with upcoming final exams.

In a double-blind experiment investigating the effects of only neurofeedback on middle management executives (Fehmi, 1974), experimental participants learned to increase and decrease alpha both with and without feedback. Control participants, receiving yoked feedback, did not. In addition, baseline alpha increased in experimental participants and did not increase in control participants. Pre- versus postquestionnaires confirmed that the flexibility of attention types

---

*See details at www.openfocus.com.

increased, and was accompanied by general relaxation and wellness. Again, the control group did not respond similarly.

An engaged and open form of attending, coupled with the regular practice of multichannel alpha brain wave synchrony feedback, is a highly effective means of resolving many common stress related disorders. Analysis of 132 cases of persons with such disorders using a dual approach of systematic recorded attention training and brain wave synchrony training found that more than 90 percent of the clients reported an alleviation of symptoms (McKnight and Fehmi, 2001). These early (1980s) positive results with stress-induced headache, joint pain, and gastrointestinal diseases were subsequently extended to the treatment of diseases involving maladaptive immune responses, anxiety, depression, addictive behavior, attentional deficit problems, posttraumatic stress disorder, and epilepsy. It was also observed that levels of intellectual functioning and artistic and athletic performance were improved.

Maria Valdés engaged in a series of experiments (Valdés, 1985a,b, 1988) evaluating the benefits of home practice of *Open Focus* exercises along with a few sessions each of GSR, Thermal, EMG, and EEG biofeedback training. Of twenty independent variables, seventeen were significantly improved at the $P = 0.001$ level or better, two were at the $P = 0.003$ level and one was at the $P = 0.053$ level. Improved independent variables included heart rate, GSR, temperature, systolic blood pressure, diastolic blood pressure, EMG forehead, EMG temporal, EMG forearms, anger, performance anxiety, somatic anxiety, speaking anxiety, social anxiety, heart racing, memory, overeating, gastrointestinal symptoms, headaches, bruxism, and insomnia. In addition, a 0.66 difference score in grade point average between the experimental and control participants was observed; the former increased by 0.14 grade points and the latter decreased by 0.52 grade points.

It is further proposed that attentional flexibility leads to autonomic self-balancing and thus supports health and growth. To realize fully our human potential is to become consciously aware of, to choose flexibly, and to implement effortlessly an expanding, dynamic range of attentional types or styles for the optimal allocation of mental resources needed for any given task or situation. (For further details, see www.openfocus.com.)

REFERENCES

Day, M.E. (1964). An eye movement phenomenon relating to attention, thought, and anxiety. *Perceptual and Motor Skills, 19,* 443-446.

Day, M.E. (1967). An eye movement indicator of individual differences in the physiological organization of attentional processes and anxiety. *Journal of Psychology, 66,* 51-52.

Fehmi, L.G. (1970). Feedback and states of consciousness and meditation. In B. Brown (Ed.), *Proceedings of Biofeedback Research Society* (pp. 1-22), Los Angeles, California.

Fehmi, L.G. (1974). *Effects of biofeedback training on middle management executives.* Paper presented at the Annual Meeting of the Biofeedback Research Society, Colorado Springs, Colorado.

Fehmi, L.G. (1975). *Open focus™ training.* Paper presented at the Annual Meeting of the Biofeedback Research Society, Monterey, California.

Fehmi, L.G. (1977). *Open focus™ cassette training series.* Biofeedback Computers, Inc.

Fehmi, L.G. (1978). EEG biofeedback, multi channel synchrony training, and attention. In A. Sugerman (Ed.), *Expanding Dimensions of Consciousness* (pp. 155-182), New York: Springer Press.

Fehmi, L.G. (1986). Biofeedback—Assisted Attention Training: Open focus™ workshop. *Psychotherapy in Private Practice, 4*(4).

Fehmi, L.G. (2003). Attention to attention. www.openfocus.com.

Fehmi, L.G., Adkins, J.W., & Lindsley, D.B. (1969). The electrophysiological correlates of perceptual masking in monkeys. *Experimental Brain Research, 7,* 299-316.

Fehmi, L.G. & Fritz, G. (1980). Open focus™: The attentional foundation of health and well-Bring. *Somatics,* 24-30.

Fehmi, L.G., Lindsley, D.C., & Adkins, J.W. (1965). Electrophysiological correlates of visual perception in man and monkey. *Com 6th International Congress Electroencephalography and Clinical Neurophysiology, 6,* 237-238.

Fehmi, L.G. & Osborne, S. (1971). *Auto-regulation of occipital EEG phase relations.* Paper presented at the Annual Meeting of the Biofeedback Research Society, Los Angeles, California.

Fehmi, L.G. & Robbins, J. (2001). Mastering our brain's electrical rhythms. *Cerebrum, (The Dana Forum on Brain Science), 3*(3) 55-67.

Fehmi, L. & Robbins, J. (2007) *The open-focus brain-harnessing the power of attention to heal mind and body.* Boston, MA: Trumpter Books.

Fehmi, L.G. & Selzer, F.A. (1978). *Controlling the intensity of conscious experience: Dissolving pain.* Paper presented at the Annual Meeting of the Association for Humanistic Psychology, Toronto, Canada.

Fehmi, L.G. & Selzer, F.A. (1980). Biofeedback and attention training. Boorstein, H.D., Seymour (Eds.). *Transpersonal Psychotherapy* (pp. 314-337), Palo Alto, California: Science and Behavior Books, Inc.

Fehmi, L.G. & Sundor, A. (1989). The effects of electrode placement upon EEG biofeedback training: The monopolar-bipolar controversy. *International Journal of Psychosomatics, 36,* 23-33.

Fritz, G. & Fehmi, L.G. (1982). The open focus™ handbook: The self-regulation of attention in biofeedback training and everyday activities. New York: Biofeedback Computers, Inc.

Jasper, H.H. (1958). The ten twenty electrode system of the international federation. *Electroenceph. Clin. Neurophysiol., 10,* 371-375.

Lindsley, D.B. (1961). Attention, consciousness, sleep and wakefulness. J. Field, H.W. Majour & V.E. Hall (Eds.), *Handbook of physiology, 1: Neurophysiology,* (pp. 1553-1593), Washington, DC: American Physiology Society.

McKnight, J.T. & Fehmi, L.G. (2001). Attention and neurofeedback synchrony training: Clinical results and their significance. *Journal of Neurotherapy, 5*(1/2), 45-61.

Selzer, F.A. & Fehmi, L.G. (1974). *Auto-regulation of mid-frontal lobe EEG activity as a function of the direction of conjugate lateral eye movement.* Paper presented at the Annual Meeting of the Biofeedback Research Society in Colorado Springs, Colorado.

Valdés, M.R. (1985a). Biofeedback in private practice, and stress reduction in a college population using biofeedback and open focus technique. *Psychotherapy in Private Practice Journal, 3*(1), 43-55.

Valdés, M.R. (1985b). Effects of biofeedback-assisted attention training in a college population. *Biofeedback and Self-Regulation Journal, 10*(4), 315-324.

Valdés, M.R. (1988). A program of stress management in a college setting. *Psychotherapy in Private Practice Journal, 6*(2), 43-54.

Chapter 13

Use of Neurofeedback
with Autistic Spectrum Disorders

Betty Jarusiewicz

INTRODUCTION

The fastest growing population of individuals likely to profit from neurofeedback may be those on the autism spectrum. Recently it was estimated by the National Institutes of Health (NIH) that about one in 250 persons now are considered to be on this spectrum. This is up from one in 2,500 in the 1970s (NIMH, 2005). Twenty-three states have reported an increase of 1,000 percent or more among children between the ages of 6 and 21 years. For many years, and continuing today, there has been much misdiagnosis, and poor understanding of these conditions by physicians and other mental health workers. Often parents are told that there is very little that can be done for their child. Frequently they are told that if their child does not speak by the age of five, he or she will never do so. Sadly, physicians often quote what they heard in medical school, that is, that 70 percent of individuals in the autism spectrum are mentally retarded. Such reports and negative prognoses add to the difficulty of dealing with children in the autism spectrum. Other institutions such as school systems often help make life even more difficult for parents because of poor understanding of autism and lack of adequate financing for training programs. When this is combined with having to deal with their child's behavioral symptoms and his or her frequent inability to communicate distress and needs, it is not surprising that parents are frustrated, exhausted,

Handbook of Neurofeedback
© 2007 by The Haworth Press, Inc. All rights reserved.
doi:10.1300/5889_13

and downcast. They often have little to show for their efforts but expensive bills. Neurofeedback can be of great benefit to these children and their families. The children become calmer, more communicative, and better able to participate in family life. And, as therapy progresses, these families can be a joy to work with.

The following pages of this chapter will: (1) summarize symptoms of the various levels of the autism spectrum as given in the Diagnostic and Statistical Manual of Mental Disorders of the American Psychiatric Association-IV (DSM-IV) (American Psychiatric Association, 1994); (2) mention other symptoms and behaviors frequently reported; (3) briefly review some unpublished and published research on use of neurofeedback with autism spectrum disorders; (4) discuss specific diagnostic procedures, neurofeedback protocols, and overall treatment approaches the author has found useful for these individuals; (5) describe some successfully treated cases; (6) discuss the author's opinions regarding the role of neurofeedback in the future treatment of the autism spectrum disorders.

The author's clinical experience has been primarily with children with mild to severe levels of symptomatology. Although the emphasis is upon children, much of what is discussed in this chapter regarding assessment and treatment also is relevant to adult clients and those with more extreme symptoms.

DEFINITIONS OF AUTISM DISORDERS

According to the *Diagnostic and Statistical Manual of Mental Disorders-IV* (DSM-IV), a number of disorders are classified under pervasive developmental disorders. Clinicians and educators in the field often refer to them as being in the autism (or autistic) spectrum, and consider especially the more common ones, that is, autistic disorder, Asperger's disorder and pervasive developmental disorder, not otherwise specified. However, two other quite rare disorders are included in this DSM-IV category: childhood disintegrative disorder and Rett's disorder. Autism Disorder requires six or more impairments from 3 groups. At least 2 must come from social interaction issues, at least 1 from ability to communicate, and at least 1 from use of repetitive patterns. There is no requirement of any normal development. Rett's requires a deceleration of head growth between the ages of 4 and 5, loss of social engagement and hand skills and impaired language development, Childhood Disintegrative Disorder requires normal development until at least 2, and then loss of language, social and motor skills, play, and bowel or bladder control. Asperger's Disorders require; impairment in social interaction, restricted interests and no delay in language or cognitive development. Pervasive Developmental Disorder, Not Otherwise Specified requires that some of the impairments be present, but not in a pattern permitting diagnosis of any of the other specific Pervasive Developmental Disorders or DSM-IV diagnoses.

The author, in reviewing responses to detailed questionnaires from two groups very much involved with autism, classified the major specific symptoms and behaviors that were reported. The two groups were: (1) several hundred families with children diagnosed as being in the autism spectrum, and (2) a dozen adults who were diagnosed as being in the autism spectrum and who have written books about their own experiences. This was done in order to identify common life experiences and determine activities that might improve symptoms.

Based on the DSM-IV criteria and the questionnaire responses, the following general conclusions seem warranted regarding persons diagnosed as being on the autism spectrum:

(1) Speech, language, and communication are a major problem;
(2) Socialization is difficult;
(3) Eye contact is often restricted;
(4) Age appropriate playing is rare;
(5) They are often late in toilet training;
(6) They may experience major dietary difficulties, and may choose limited diets, particularly carbohydrate and sugar-based items;
(7) They often have many allergies, particularly to food, and taking the form of skin rashes;
(8) Anxiety is prevalent, and associated with headaches, muscle aches, and impatience; and
(9) Stress exacerbates all of the aforementioned factors.

Impaired socialization and vocalization are experienced almost 100 percent of the time by children on the autistic spectrum, and adults struggle with these issues their entire lives. Children often have difficulty in learning situations due to their need to find their own method after observing that the "required" method is less effective for them. Many schools attempt to force a method of learning, not allowing students to find their own. If forced to learn a certain way, individuals become frustrated and anxious; and, anxiety is prevalent in the majority of children in the autism spectrum. When children fail to learn under these forced and anxiety-provoking conditions, schools commonly, but erroneously, conclude that they have less than normal intelligence.

To date, the following general conclusions seem warranted regarding adults in the autism spectrum: (1) Most do not choose to socialize, sometimes even with their parents. They often have an aversion to using a telephone. However, some find a sibling or a person of the opposite sex to live or keep company with; (2) Many report specific coping mechanisms. Most require more rest that a typical person, some take calming baths, while others look at inane television shows to calm themselves. "Quick-rest" time is often taken during the day to help reduce anxiety and fatigue, and may include not looking directly at other persons or objects, and closing eyes from time to time to reduce continuous stimulation. Rhythmic activities are often used to reduce built-up tension and anxiety. These may include swimming, moving rhythmically by running, jumping on a trampoline, and getting regular exercise. Exercise is usually of the type where there is little interaction with others such as swimming, cycling, skating, skiing, walking, and running. Coping strategies can include music, and they may play an instrument and/or sing. Singing also often helps with verbalization as words come easier for many in a rote form. When confronted with overwhelming input, some cope by dissociating or "compartmentalizing" perceptions and thought; (3) Most prefer predictable domestic routines, and may try to maintain order and sameness in their lives by using filing systems and hoarding whatever seems to make them feel calm; (4) They often do not completely understand questions, and thus are not succinct or clear in their responses. During conversations with some individuals, they may "overtalk" to try to cover the subject; (5) Even though they sometimes may "act silly," they often do not comprehend or appropriately tell jokes; (6) These individuals often do not immediately comprehend, but prefer to think about what is asked of them, and then, in private, make their own "sense" of it. Many say they "think differently," as in pictures and/or nonverbal concepts rather than in words. Computers can have special learning value for many, since they permit impersonal, self-paced learning according to one's unique learning style and tempo; (7) Many individuals have, or have had difficulty with speech. Learning sign language and appropriate use of gestures often aids in the communication process. Some elect to limit their exposure to situations where they will not have to communicate, and often just observe or even choose to totally limit social interaction; (8) Many individuals mimic others in their learning process. This has led to suggestions that being grouped with academically gifted persons could be beneficial. Usually there is not a problem with learning by modeling if there is sufficient calmness, and sufficient time after watching to develop their methodology. This often leads to unique ways of learning and understanding concepts. As the author sees it, individuals with this type of brain almost always think "outside of the box," and may not even know what is "inside"; (9) Some report an aversion to fluorescent lights or bright rooms. Some mention a need for minimization of noise in their environments, while others claim to need to listen to radios or other sound sources to help provide a sound barrier to their constant vigilance.

RESEARCH ON NEUROFEEDBACK AND AUTISM SPECTRUM DISORDERS

When the author initially was trained in neurofeedback, there had not been a significant focus on these individuals, and even today, there is very little published research on use of neurofeedback with autistic spectrum disorders. The research by Sichel, Fehmi, and Goldstein (1995) is one of only two published reports found. They reported positive results using neurofeedback treatment with a case of mild autism. A personal interest in determining whether neurofeedback could be effective with the autism disorders, led the author to conduct a pilot research project (Jarusiewicz, 2002). Results indicated that neurofeedback could be efficacious in helping individuals on the autism spectrum obtain relief from most if not all of their major symptoms. The study consisted of an experimental group diagnosed with an autism spectrum disorder, and a control group similarly diagnosed who continued with more traditional treatments for the duration of the study. The control group participants later were given the opportunity to use neurofeedback, which all did. The experimental group averaged 36 neurofeedback training sessions over a 4.5-month period. Results indicated a 26 percent reduction in autism symptoms in the experimental group compared to a 3 percent reduction in the control group. Parents reported remarkable improvement in socialization, vocalization, schoolwork anxiety, tantrum frequency, and sleep. These reports were commensurate with score changes on the Autism Treatment Review Checklist (ATEC) (Rimland and Edelson, nd), which showed improvements in sociability of 33 percent, speech/language/communication of 29 percent, overall health of 26 percent, and sensory/cognitive awareness of 17 percent. Incidentally, in reviewing the family histories of the experimental group, it was found that in 56 percent of the families, there was evidence in other family members of one or more of the following: addiction, attention deficit/hyperactivity disorders, learning disabilities, delayed speech, anxiety disorders, and depression.

The author also conducted a small, unpublished pilot study with five children in a school for special needs children. One purpose of this study was to determine if and how neurofeedback could be integrated into a school program. A major concern was whether it would be possible to get the children to sit for neurofeedback training without their parents' assistance. And, of course, a main issue was whether neurofeedback training could make significant changes in the brain's regulation of electrical activity and be associated with improved behaviors in the children.

We were able to seat four of the children at computers. They were given something to play with to keep them occupied. We checked on them to be sure they would accept electrodes being placed on their scalps. The fifth child resisted having anything fitted to his head. Remembering that he tolerated a headset for his Walkman, we customized a headset using headphones that he was willing to use, and this prepared him for eventual acceptance of electrodes. Initial training attempts were not successful, but after a few sessions, the situation improved and actual neurofeedback training became possible. Spectral analyses of the EEGs of all five children showed significant improvement in terms of reduction of power in the delta and theta frequency bands. Their abilities to focus at school also reportedly improved. Unfortunately, the school was unable to obtain funds for equipment and staff training to continue the project, and it was stopped. However, the parent of one of the children became trained as a neurotherapy technician, and leased equipment in order to continue her child's treatment. That child reportedly showed dramatic changes, going from being nonverbal to verbal after several months of neurofeedback training.

ASSESSMENT

It is well known that this is a difficult population to assess. Symptoms may be present, absent, or different in nature, depending on hour-to-hour variations in stress levels related to psychological issues or to impact of home, school, and physical environmental factors. And, communication problems can make interactions with examiners very difficult. If there is any consistency to these individuals, it is that they are consistently inconsistent! Results of any single evaluation session are likely to be invalid, and indicative of only one moment or period of time.

Within the autism research and treatment community, the "gold standard" for evaluation has become the Autism Diagnostic Interview-Revised (ADI-R) (Lord, 2000). This instrument was designed particularly for research purposes and is used by many. When funds are available to use it, this tool increases the reliability of research data. However, for clinical use, the ATEC has been found to be very effective, as long as it is used consistently.

The ATEC is the assessment tool used most often by the author. It is available at www.ari-atec.com. Each family is given forms to complete prior to and during treatment. Data from completed forms is entered into the same forms online and the results are calculated. Assessments are repeated as necessary to ascertain improvement and provide feedback to parents. Another form often used by the author is the Autism Research Institute Treatment Effectiveness Survey (Rimland, nd) available at www.ari.com/treatrating. It enables a full picture of what a family has tried with their child, with or without success. In conjunction with this form, a summary of all data input by all users also is available, which shows statistically what has or has not been of benefit to these children according to their parents.

In addition, in the author's clinic, a family history is taken and behaviors needing modification are reviewed with parents. When possible, a 15-minute videotape of the child interacting with parents is recorded, and can be used for before-, during-, and after-treatment comparisons. During assessment, the author places emphasis on checking for behavioral indications of over, under, or unstable arousal, as shown by questioning of the parents as to the type of issues the client is experiencing. The questionnaire used for this process was developed by Othmer (1997). For example, symptoms of inattention, daydreaming, poor sustained attention, and lack of motivation are categorized as signs of underarousal, while impulsivity, distractibility, and stimulus seeking fall under overarousal. Symptoms of unstable arousal include, but are not limited to, seizures, manic-depressive cycles, panic attacks, asthma, and migraines.

Behaviors vary widely within the autistic disorder spectrum, and there is no universal agreement regarding specific brain disorders underlying symptoms or EEG abnormalities in this group. While some clinicians rely on a quantitative EEG (QEEG) evaluation to guide treatment, it has been the author's experience that they are not useful, particularly in the beginning of therapy. Individuals in the autistic spectrum show extreme variability over very short periods of time (seconds), and from day to day. Therefore, a reading taken on one date may not be indicative of the EEG activity of the client at another date. Furthermore, the normative databases commonly used with QEEG evaluations may not be relevant for this population. Although the author does not include QEEGs in her assessments, she does note the EEG microvoltage readings at least three times during each treatment session as a means of becoming acquainted with the client's unique brain activity. Spectrals for each session can be generated and trends evaluated.

TREATMENT

The major components of the author's treatment approach involve neurofeedback, parenting, and schooling. Speech and occupational therapies also often are involved and can be synergistic with our approach. In the author's opinion, disordered brain activity is the basic problem with persons in the autism spectrum. Therefore, neurofeedback plays an essential role in our treatment. In the following paragraph, the author presents a theoretical rationale for its use, and discusses specific training protocols.

The impact of calming to the disordered brain cannot be overstated. As Gruzelier and Egner (2005) report, there is a close association between EEG frequencies and one's state of arousal. Individuals with disordered brains often have far too much power in the delta and theta EEG frequencies (greater than 50 percent of total EEG power). To date, the author has noted and focused primarily on the ratio between delta power and total EEG power, and secondarily on delta-beta and delta-alpha ratios with her clients. This is in contrast to the often-used manipulation of beta and theta frequencies in studying efficacy of neurofeedback in AD/HD. We have found no absolute standard of "correct" theta-beta power ratio for our clients, and have been unable to predict an efficient ratio for any specific person's brain. Abarbanel (1999) describes several neural mechanisms, including the theta-beta ratio, which may help explain how neurofeedback works at the neurophysiological level, and which may be of special interest to readers. An explanation, which makes sense to the author, especially in regard to autistic spectrum disorders, is presented as follows.

The author has postulated that the excessive power in the delta frequency band, which often is associated with a sense of brain "sleepiness," causes the individual to cope by "revving-up" the brain. This, in turn, periodically causes him or her to get "stuck" at inappropriately aroused levels, which are associated with hyperactivity and sleep problems. Such fluctuations often occur very frequently. We have found that if the individual's brain can be calmed, he or she can then begin to deal with various life issues.

It is the author's belief that the simplest of clinical approaches often work best. These individuals' brains already are disordered, and there is no value in adding to the confusion by using complex training protocols. A unipolar (single) electrode placement (typically at site T4, referenced to A2) based on the International 10-20 Electrode Placement System works well. Training for reduction of relative power in lower frequency bands also works well, that is, lowering the ratio of low frequency microvoltage (power) to total EEG voltage. This is accomplished by setting the equipment to inhibit power in the delta and high beta ranges, and to reward a frequency range that is on average somewhat higher than the average delta range disorders. Generally speaking, the goal is to calm brain activity, yet ensure that the client remains awake.

Since consistency is considered very important, one should not make protocol changes lightly. In fact, a protocol usually is not changed by us even after the client's behavior improves. One hypothesis is that when an "efficient" reward is found, this may help the client over a number of developmental stages, if not for years. This may be because the brain seems to find a comfortable frequency pattern in which to work. Any attempt to change it could be confusing, especially before a calm demeanor is attained and stabilized. Almost all of the author's clients ask to continue treatment after a few sessions. This is true even for the very young, as they apparently begin to feel better and recognize the benefits of being calmer. However, in our experience, overly frequent sessions (more than two per week) may hinder the client's integration of results of neurofeedback training into his or her everyday life. Behavior is the result of the combination of how the person's brain reacts to a situation and how he or she has learned to cope with an experience. For example, a client came to the office nonverbal. With several neurofeedback sessions, he became significantly calmer, but had not yet learned how to behave with his new calmness. We suggested to the parents they require the child to sit at the dinner table with a parent, and the parent engage in a "conversation" with the child. This activity was totally new to the child so it took a little while to learn what was expected now that he was calm enough to sit with the family.

Dramatic changes happen when there is neurological readiness for social interaction, learning is added, and parental encouragement and support then make everything work synergistically. But this process works best when given some time, particularly early on in therapy. In fact, the author sometimes provides a break in therapy to allow the client to have the freedom of a more uncomplicated and less stressful life and to integrate his or her new abilities into daily life. Little or no regression has been noted, and growth often continues at a rapid rate even during these breaks. As stated earlier, stress has very strong effects on a disordered brain. Neurotherapists (as well as teachers and parents) must be careful not to add to stress levels by adding too many treatments or other sources of environmental stimulation too quickly.

Although most emphasis in the author's neurofeedback practice is on training the brain to modify the slower brain wave frequencies, at some point high beta level frequencies also are examined and modified as seems needed. This is done, in part, to determine whether they are excessive, and are having negative effects on behavior. Attempts also are made to determine whether they are in response to outside activities, or to psychological issues. As treatment proceeds and a state of stabilized calm is achieved, it becomes easier and more productive for the therapist to work on other concerns that may be present, for example, speech and communication skills. In conjunction with this, the author has found that a stimulating protocol with electrode placement at F7 (referenced top A1), used for a short period of time, and followed by a calming protocol, for example, electrode at T4 (referenced to A2) is useful. Training time with the stimulating protocol is increased when it becomes obvious the client is able to integrate this new information. The stimulating protocol usually involves rewarding increases in amplitude in the 15-18 Hz frequency range, while the calming protocol used would be one that formerly had been found effective for the specific client. During this phase of treatment, professional speech/language therapy and/or occupational therapy often can be especially helpful. It appears that as the brain's ability to function better develops, one must teach it to use that function beneficially. This combination of neurofeedback training and education is synergism at its best.

As noted earlier, the author's approach to treatment of individuals with autism spectrum disorders includes more than neurofeedback. This is true especially for the child client. The author works with parents to help them to understand their child. It is explained that the children may feel bored and must struggle to keep their brains awake or activated. Unless they are kept busy with positive activity, they will find ways to cope with boredom such as spinning or focusing on a single object. It may be suggested that parents move and talk faster in the child's presence. It also has been noted that many of the children in the autism spectrum work at a faster pace than most, and can successfully complete schoolwork a year or more above their actual grade placements. Helping the children move fast through their work also often results in reducing any boredom that may arise. Also, it is recommended for the child to become active in a sport, which can provide needed exercise as well as help to keep them calm. Swimming, running, skiing, biking, skateboarding, and use of a trampoline are examples. Usually a sport involving teamwork would not be recommended, especially early in therapy when it may be more difficult for the child to communicate and act in a socially appropriate manner with others. To help their child calm down during or after a stressful period, it may be suggested that parents allow quiet play in their own room, watching nonviolent televisions shows, reading and playing a musical instrument or computer game, which can facilitate needed learning. Parents are encouraged to use certain strategies to deal with various behavioral issues. Examples include maintaining consistent daily schedules, using music to trigger certain activities or transitions between activities, providing calming "assists" such as heavy blankets, and developing a "downtime" plan for periods of maximum stress, such as when getting ready for school in the morning, coming home after school, or preparing for a guest's arrival. If their child has difficulty transitioning upon morning awakening, it can be recommended that they arrange for a light to be turned on automatically about forty-five minutes before time to get up. This will allow a longer transition period.

In initial visits, the author never asks a parent to stop any medication, dietary supplements, or other type treatment being used with their child. However, during the course of treatment, progress is examined to ascertain what may be impeding expected new behaviors. It has been the author's experience that other treatment modalities can interfere with neurofeedback treatment. The approach has been to tell parents and clients that, if there is evidence that is occurring, we would selectively curtail or discontinue one or more of the treatments, including neurofeedback. This could help determine what might be causing lack of expected progress.

In some cases, it is beneficial for parents to provide neurofeedback training at home. This can be particularly usefully when the family resides a considerable distance away from a neurofeedback clinician. Another advantage is that a number of family members may be served. It often is noted that other family members of persons diagnosed with an autism spectrum disorder have symptoms similar to those of the client. In such cases, we have sometimes seen what appear to be synergistic effects from multiple use of neurofeedback. It seems that as other family members' symptoms improve, so do those of the primary client. However, there are some potential problems with home training. Individuals with autism spectrum disorders require swift computer response to their swift brain changes, thus making it a necessity to have equipment with fast response time. Some parents may have insufficient training or experience in the use of computers, be unable to learn the training techniques, and/or be lacking in the patience or consistency needed for this kind of work. In any event, a trained clinician must supervise all work, and require and regularly inspect written or computer-generated comments regarding progress. It is the author's practice not to sell the neurofeedback equipment, but to lease it, in order to provide more control. We spend as much time as needed training the parent or whoever will be providing the home training, and then go to their home to install the system and check out the technician's technique. The home trainer is encouraged to obtain further training and interact with others working under similar circumstances.

In the author's treatment approach, it is necessary to also consider the child's school environment. It is recommended that when schools are being chosen, the most productive environment is mainstreaming, with an aide available. This is true even if the child does not have many communications skills. Of course, not all such classrooms will be appropriate. Some may have too many students, and some teachers will be too rigid in their approaches for this to be effective with children with autism spectrum disorders. Generally, however, it has been my experience that these children are happier and more successful in such situations. They often pick up academic information and positive behaviors from typically learning and behaving children. The author has seen many of these children go into regular classrooms with minimal or no extra requirements. It has been noted that as their ability to be calm grows, they usually can learn as rapidly as or more rapidly than the general population of children. However, this does not mean that all, or even most, will become indistinguishable from the general population. Most will continue to seem somewhat lacking in social skills, and may require more rest and "downtime" during and after school.

The author's treatment approach often involves supplemental educational activities performed at home. For example, we may show parents how to work with their child during reading activities by sitting with him or her, placing a finger on the words being read and moving at a rapid pace. As noted earlier, these children usually learn better when material is presented at a fast pace, and this includes learning to read. We encourage the family to sing together, and to use music to learn new words. An example of the latter is to allow a spot in the song where the focus is on one word where everyone stops and the parent encourages the child to join in singing or saying that one word. This seems to help the child focus, remember, and feel part of the family sing-a-long. Currently, The Lighthouse Network, Inc., a nonprofit group sponsored by the author, is investigating computer programs that may be of special assistance both for more efficient learning of new material and better use of play time both at home and at school.

EXAMPLES OF SUCCESS

Nearly all persons with autism spectrum disorders the author has worked with have shown major improvements in school, at home, and in social situations. These improvements are seen as better communication, improved speech, and a generally calmer approach to all situations, leading to better integration into all phases of their lives. In this section, the author will describe two typical cases, including symptomatology before, during, and after treatment; details of treatment; and present status.

Casey came with his mother to our office at the age of five. His major symptoms included no speech, and very little social interaction with either his siblings or his schoolmates. He also appeared very depressed, and showed a number of other typical autism symptoms. According to the ATEC, Casey scored 74 (24 in speech/language/communication, 15 in sociability, 19 in sensory/cognitive awareness, 16 in health/physical/behavior), which is at about the 70th percentile for autism symptoms. The school had indicated that the child might never speak, and therefore, the parent should acquire a keyboard that would take the place of typical language. We requested that they wait until neurotherapy was begun in order to give the child a chance to learn to speak. There was a concern that he might not be motivated to learn if he used an assist such as the keyboard.

As Casey progressed with neurotherapy, coming in about twice a week, he calmed significantly. Working with us along with a speech therapist, he began to make sounds even though when initially assessed he was frequently mute. The speech therapist worked with Casey to make animal sounds. We noted that he loved to use the "Moo" sound. We encouraged Casey to see the similarity between "Moo" and "Mom," and it wasn't long before he could say "Mom." Needless to say, each time Casey said "Mom," we all cried. So many individuals had told the mother he would never be able to say this very important word. As Casey got more words, he communicated more with his siblings, and also with his mother. Later, he added school as a place to try out his words. Casey's progress was very quick: He went from a 74 ATEC score to 34 (second lowest autism ATEC level) within four months, and by eight months went to 28, which is within the mildest category in the ATEC model. This reflected the major overall changes he made in all parts of his life. It was, however, only after about 100 sessions that his speech became fluent.

The school district worked with his mother to get the best combination of mainstreaming and separate work he needed, and by the third grade, Casey needed very little additional help. He appears to have become extremely happy because he wanted to communicate, but was unable. Many autistic individuals appear not to care if they do or do not socialize, but Casey was not one of these. If one did not know that Casey initially had been significantly impaired, one could not tell today. He continues to progress in learning as a "gifted" child, and is blessed with excellent social behaviors. He requests to return to our offices when other members of the family come for treatment and asks to have some more neurotherapy experience. Once when he was having minor problems due to a family situation, he came for additional training and was helped with only a few sessions. This case represented an excellent outcome, with major changes occurring within a reasonably short period of time, and more extensive integration occurring in all life categories within significant period of time.

A second case, with a girl named Jamie, progressed somewhat slower even though she was integrated more quickly into school. The parents involved the author in picking out the kindergarten environment. We chose the local school that had a plan to integrate children with autism as soon as possible. Even though Jamie had almost no language skills, the school included her in a regular class with teacher aides available to help all children as needs arose. Jamie was sent to school by bus, and the children were encouraged to learn how to behave on the bus by singing one song to get on the bus, one to sit down in the bus, one to get off the bus, one to get to the classroom, and one to take off their coats etc. This singing mode helped the children, especially Jamie, to learn acceptable behaviors. This helped even at home because it was clear to Jamie that when a certain song was sung, toys were to be put away. Compliance was immediate. This is a case where a trait of individuals in the autistic spectrum can be used to facilitate calm and beneficial behaviors. Regular routines can help both the school and family function significantly more efficiently.

It was not practical for Jamie to come to our office frequently, so we provided once weekly neurotherapy sessions for one school year. She progressed regularly, including her language development. After the kindergarten year was complete, it was decided to stop neurotherapy for the summer. When school began again in the fall, Jamie had progressed so much that it was decided not to continue so long as she continued to develop well. Jamie's language is not perfect, but certainly is no longer an impediment to her growth. It continues to improve rapidly. Jamie went from a position where there was primary focus on her overall behavior and impediments to her learning in a regular school situation, to where she was seen as an intelligent girl with some issues, particularly speech, which could easily be handled in the regular schoolroom.

The author has found through her studies that there is no statistically significant correlation between age, gender, or recovery schedule and level of autism. While attempting to discover the "problems" causing longer recovery periods, we have noted that the variables to be discussed later are likely to be implicated. We had a case where a client named Michael got to a certain level and did not seem to improve. When this became clear, we asked the mother to see what was different in the child's life since the initial assessment. It was found that the mother wished to try another therapy, homeopathy, at the same time she was bringing in Michael for neurotherapy. After a few months of little improvement following neurofeedback, we suggested she stop either homeopathy or neurofeedback, because we could not find out what the problem was by considering two therapies at once. When it was decided to drop homeopathy, Michael's behavior improved significantly. He still has some problems with speech, perhaps because he does not feel motivated to communicate and socialize. Michael may always be a type person who does not wish to socialize much. He has always seemed to be a happy child although speech continues to be poor.

We also have had less than excellent success if the parent persists on keeping the child on major drugs. We then are working with a drugged brain. We have often been able to encourage the parent to work with the prescribing physician in reducing drug dosages. This has worked really well, probably in part because it was a gradual approach to change that benefited all. Finally, we have had difficulty when a client's family is in crisis. No matter how quickly we may be able to help the brain regulate itself better, if the family is very unstable, the child may not be able to cope.

CONCLUSIONS AND FUTURE CONSIDERATIONS

There has been a long history of misunderstanding of the disorders of the autism spectrum. In large part, this has been due to communication problems during evaluation, to day-to-day (even hour-to-hour) variability in symptoms, to the wide range in severity and nature of presenting symptoms, and to lack of agreement on underlying causes. The latter, especially, has led to a great many different treatment recommendations including use of aversive stimulation, dietary changes, administration of tranquilizing medication, and placement in residential facilities to remove autistic children from presumably "cold," uncaring parents. Reported long-term success rates generally have been low for all these approaches. Although exact mechanisms remain controversial, it now is almost universally agreed that these disorders have a biological basis (Akshoomoff, Pierce, & Courchesne, 2002).

Hirshberg, Chiu, and Frazier (2005) report that 70 to 80 percent of individuals in the autism spectrum benefit from neurofeedback, and there are few risks or contraindications. When costs of neurofeedback are compared with medication alone, a long-range view of each individual's situation must be taken, because medication only helps during its use, compared to neurotherapy, which has been found to endure long after treatment ends. Insurance companies need to be educated regarding this cost-benefit situation since they currently spend so much money on medications and other therapies that do not last.

Based on six years of clinical experience and research with more than several hundred persons diagnosed with autism spectrum disorder, the author has concluded that such persons rarely, if ever, are truly mentally retarded. To the contrary, the author believes they just learn differently. This different type learning may be due to disordered/dysregulated brains, which primarily need calming. There is much lack of understanding on the part of parents, peers, teachers, and other professionals with whom they come in contact. This lack, in the author's opinion, leads to disagreement regarding the best ways to assist individuals in the autism spectrum, with a resulting lack of appropriate education for most. Also, current medical and educational systems often require quick answers, which often results in ineffective or damaging medication or therapies given in haste and with little follow-up. This problem is exacerbated by parent's understandable fears that their children will not develop in a typical fashion. In the best of all worlds, it would be wise to have a professional who has knowledge of all beneficial therapies and assess training needs of each child. They then could assign them, one at a time, to different therapies, with continual assessment, until the most effective therapy would become the focus. It is also important to note that each person may require different therapies or levels of therapies and training. There have been some efforts to design computer programs to aid professionals in this process, but their success has not yet been proven. To date, the author has found that appropriate neurofeedback training provides the most effective means of positively modifying the aberrant brain activity of people with autism and other dysregulated brain disorders. However, as noted earlier, it is important not to use or recommend neurofeedback treatment in isolation. It is critical to consider home, school, and other environmental factors, and when needed, supplement treatment with speech/language training, occupational therapy, and other professional services.

Undoubtedly, there will be modifications to the author's views as experience and research findings accumulate. There is great need for controlled research on the role of neurofeedback in the treatment of autism spectrum disorders. If the efficacy of a neurofeedback-based treatment approach can be demonstrated through scientifically acceptable research, it should lead to greater professional acceptance, and therefore, to provide greater help for the rapidly growing numbers of persons suffering from these disorders. Topics that the author considers to be in special need of research include: (1) Consideration of most effective neurofeedback training protocols for specific subtypes of disorders, for example, Asperger's Disorder; (2) Exploration of whether optimal reward and inhibit EEG frequencies vary with age, gender, and/or severity and nature of symptoms; (3) Synergistic effect of combining other treatment or activities with neurofeedback, for example, use of educational computer programs, speech/language therapy, exercise, participation in art; (4) Effect of placing such children in "gifted child" classes to accommodate their tendency to mimic and their need for faster paced learning; (5) The special role neurofeedback might play in assisting extraordinarily talented (savant-type) persons from this general group to maximize their potential.

Although there is a strong need for research, use of neurofeedback with individuals in the autism disorder spectrum can become a very important part of the practice of professionals who work with this population. Using the author's treatment approach, which has evolved to date and is described in this chapter, professionals can provide very valuable service to the community at large and to many individuals in particular. This is especially true considering there is little else presently available that seems to work as well and as quickly.

REFERENCES

Abarbanel, A. (1999). The neural underpinnings of neurofeedback training. In Evans, J. R. & Abarbanel, A. (Eds.). *Introduction to quantitative EEG and neurofeedback*. San Diego: Academic Press.

Akshoomoff, N., Pierce, K., & Courchesne, E. (2002). The neurological basis of autism from a developmental perspective. *Development and Psychopathology* *14*(3), 613-634.

American Psychiatric Association. (1994). *Diagnostic and statistical manual of mental disorders, Fourth Edition* (DSM-IV).

Gruzelier, J. & Egner, T. (2005). Critical validation studies of neurofeedback. *Child & Adolescent Psychiatric Clinics of North America, 14*, 83-104.

Hirshberg, L. M., Chiu, S., & Frazier, J. A. (2005). Emerging brain-based interventions for children and adolescents: Overview and clinical perspective. In Hirshberg, L. M., Chiu, S. & Frazier, J. A. (Eds.). *Child and Adolescent Psychiatric Clinics of North America: Emerging Interventions, 14*(1), 1-20.

Jarusiewicz, B. (2002). Efficacy of neurotherapy in the autistic spectrum: A pilot study. *Journal of Neurotherapy, 4*(6), 39-49.

Lord, C. (2000). Commentary: Achievements and future direction for intervention research in autism spectrum disorders. *Journal of Autism and Developmental Disorder, 30*(5), 393-398.

NIMH. *Autism spectrum disorders.* Retrieved January 17, 2005, from National Institute of Mental Health Web site: http://www.nimh.nih.gov/healthinformation/autismmenu.cfm.

Othmer, S. (1997). *Assessment. EEG Spectrum biofeedback training manual.* Encino, CA: EEG Spectrum, Inc.

Rimland, B. (nd.). *Autism research institute treatment effectiveness survey.* http://www.autismwebsite.com/ari/treatment/treatrating.htm.

Rimland, B. & Edelson, S. M. (nd.). *Autism research institute autism treatment review checklist (ATEC).* http://www.ARI-ATEC.com.

Sichel, A. G., Fehmi, L. G. & Goldstein, D. M. (1995). Positive outcome with neurofeedback treatment in a case of mild autism. *Journal of Neurotherapy, 1-1*(8): 1-6.

Chapter 14

Current Status of QEEG
and Neurofeedback in the Treatment
of Clinical Depression

Jonathan E. Walker
Robert Lawson
Gerald Kozlowski

INTRODUCTION

Depression is an almost universal experience. Fortunately, it usually remits spontaneously after a period of time. Unfortunately, it does not spontaneously remit in many individuals, and they are diagnosed as being 'clinically' depressed, requiring treatment to be able to have an acceptable quality of life and be able to work. Several depression subtypes have been defined based on their semiology (Table 14.1). We have indicated the most common abnormalities found in our clinic for each type of depression, and indicated the type of neurofeedback training that, in our experience, most effectively remediates the depression and prevents further episodes. Note that one EEG abnormality, alpha asymmetry, appears in most cases to be a state marker rather than a trait marker, and is not seen with the linked ears reference used in all commercially available databases. One must use a Cz reference to identify the asymmetry and Cz is not an inactive reference. However, alpha asymmetry may represent a trait marker in some patients, and alpha asymmetry training may produce long-lasting remissions in some patients (Baehr & Baehr, 1997; Baehr, Rosenfeld, & Baehr, 1997; Rosenfeld et al., 1996; Earnest, 1999; Rosenfeld, 1999; Baehr, et al., 1999).

Handbook of Neurofeedback
© 2007 by The Haworth Press, Inc. All rights reserved.
doi:10.1300/5889_14

TABLE 14.1. Depressive subtypes and anxiety clinical/QEEG correlations and neurofeedback protocols.

	Genetic	Acquired	Response to psychotherapy	Associated with QEEG abnormality	Symptom-based NF training protocols
1. Endogenous depression (unipolar)	✓		Poor	Slowing F8 (trait marker)	↓ 2-7/↑ 15-18 F8
2. Cognitive depression (unipolar)	✓		Yes	Slowing F7 (trait marker)	↓ 2-7/↑ 15-18 F7
3. Manic/ depressive (bipolar)	✓		Poor	Slowing F3 (trait marker for depression) Excess frontal beta (trait marker for mania)	Combined training → stabilize
4. Reactive depression		✓	Yes	No trait markers Alpha asymmetry, L > R (CZ reference) (state marker)	Normalize alpha power or coherence asymmetry
5. Anxiety	✓	✓	Poor	Excess of high beta (20-30 Hz) Any brain area (may be trait or state marker)	Decrease high-frequency beta (whatever location)

THE NEUROBIOLOGY OF DEPRESSION

Adolphs and Tranel (2004) reviewed the neurobiology of emotions generally and in depression and mania, specifically. Neural structures that process emotions in humans include the left and right hemispheres, amygdala, orbitofrontal cortex, basal ganglia, cingulate gyrus, and hippocampus. The left cerebral hemisphere is more involved in positive emotions, and the right hemisphere is more involved in negative emotions. Davidson and Irwin (1999) posited an approach/withdrawal dimension, correlating increased right hemisphere activation with increases in withdrawal behavior (including emotions such as fear or sadness, as well as depressive tendencies), and increased left hemisphere activity with increase in approach behaviors (including emotions such as happiness). An important key issue for neurofeedback therapists is what exactly constitutes "activation." We will address this in the QEEG section of this chapter. Major depression has been associated with damage to the frontal lobes, especially the left frontal pole (Starkstein & Robinson, 1991). Positron Emission Tomography (PET) studies have shown that a region under the genu of the corpus callosum, the subcallosal gyrus, is consistently underactivated in patients with depression (Ongur, Drevets, & Price, 1998). As reviewed by Liotti and Mayberg (2001) depression also is associated with hypometabolism in the cingulate cortex and occasionally in other areas such as the orbitofrontal, insular, and anterior temporal cortices, amygdala, basal ganglia, and thalamus.

Reports on increased activation of any particular area have not consistently been associated with depression. Liotti and Mayberg (2001) found that induced sadness was associated with metabolic activation of limbic and paralimbic regions, ventral anterior cingulate, insula, and cerebellar vermis. Furthermore, Mayberg, Brannon, Tekell, Silva, and McGinnis (2000) found that recovery from depression was associated with activation in dorsal cortical, inferior parietal, dorsal anterior cingulate, and posterior cingulate areas. There were concomitant decreases in ventral limbic and paralimbic areas, including the subgenual cingulate and ventral, mid– and posterior insula, hippocampus, and hypothalamus.

Anxiety, on the other hand, correlates with increased regional cerebral blood flow (rCBF) in posterior cingulate and bilateral inferior parietal lobules. Since comorbid depression and anxiety are common, it is important to recognize the different areas that are activated or inhibited by both depression and anxiety. These relationships are depicted in Table 14.1, illustrating the presumed role of these areas in producing or inhibiting depression and anxiety or their opposites, happiness/calmness. While this model is admittedly oversimplified and all details not proven, it does serve a heuristic purpose for approaching depression and anxiety using neurofeedback. This approach will be discussed in the neurofeedback section.

QEEG AND DEPRESSION

EEG and QEEG are excellent approaches to measuring activation of cerebral cortical areas, but do not access all cortical areas (when the 10/20 system is used). Available databases do not reliably indicate activation or inhibition of subcortical structures, unless low-resolution electromagnetic tomography (LORETA) is used. There are few studies of depression using LORETA, and a coherent description of subcortical structures activated or inhibited in depression does not exist.

What exactly constitutes an activated EEG for a given brain area? Most people would agree that delta and theta rhythms indicate a hypoactive state. Alpha rhythms are associated with more activation, and increasing levels of beta are generally associated with further activation. Table 14.2 indicates the clinical states typically associated with frontal rhythms as seen in the clinical setting. A QEEG, involving a normative database, is necessary to determine whether the rhythms seen are normal, low, or high compared to the normal population. Generally, in neurofeedback, the goal is to normalize the activity by

TABLE 14.2. Frontal rhythms and commonly associated behavioral states.

Frontal rhythm	Behavioral state
Delta (R or L)	Sleepy
Theta (R or L)	Drowsiness
Alpha (R or L)	Awake, calm, unfocused
Beta 1 (12-15 Hz) (R)	Calm, observant
Beta 2 (15-18 Hz) (L)	Fully focused, attentive, less depressed
Beta 3 (19-30 Hz) (R or L)	Anxious, irritable

uptraining low frequency power values, downtraining high values, and leaving normal values alone.

Commercially available databases usually use a linked ears reference, as it approximates a neutral reference in most cases. As mentioned earlier, it is important to recognize that CZ is not a neutral reference, that is, it is an active reference. For this reason, no available databases use a CZ reference.

A second technical point is also important with reference to using neurofeedback to treat depression (or other disorders) and to measure EEG changes resulting from treatment. Push-pull amplifiers measure the difference in potential between two electrodes. If one of the electrodes is nonactive (a reference electrode), then one can measure the potential at the active electrode. If both references are active, it is not possible to know which electrode has the higher or lower value, or whether both electrodes have a higher or lower potential than a true reference electrode. Monopolar training utilizes a nonactive (reference) electrode; therefore, it gives one a certain measure of the effectiveness of training at the active electrode. Bipolar training, where both references are active, does not give a reliable measure of what is happening at either electrode. An increase in potential difference caused by bipolar training could represent one of the six possibilities:

	A	B
1. No change at electrode A, increase at electrode B	–	↑
2. No change at electrode B, increase at electrode A	↑	–
3. Increase at both electrodes, but more at B than A	↑ (+)	↑ (++)
4. Increase at both electrodes, but more at A than B	↑ (++)	↑ (+)
5. Decrease at both electrodes, but more at B than A	↓ (+)	↓ (++)
6. Decrease at both electrodes, but more at A than B	↓ (++)	↓ (+)

Similarly, a decrease in potential caused by bipolar training could also represent one of six possibilities. It is even more difficult to measure the result of asymmetry training, since it involves a ratio of increases or decreases.

A third technical point has to do with the choice of what to uptrain or downtrain. Since the neurobiological studies of depression indicate that left frontal activation is important in being happy rather than depressed, it would seem that training beta-2 (15-18 Hz) activity would be a more direct way to train the relevant area than would training to normalize symmetry between right and left frontal alpha, which might or might not be associated with an increase in left frontal activation in the 15-18 Hz range. This might account for failures in alpha asymmetry training for long-term prevention of depression in some cases.

John and his colleagues (Prichep, Lieber, & John, 1986) were the first to describe QEEG abnormalities associated with depression and depression subtypes. No one variable could identify a depressive disorder, but using 23 variables, in a multivariate analysis, they were able to correctly identify patients suffering with depression with 84 percent accuracy. The largest variances from normal included absolute power in the frontal-temporal regions (especially on the left), power symmetry in the temporal and frontotemporal regions, and the combined features for coherence in the anterior regions. Bipolar patients could be discriminated from unipolar patients using seven input variables. The variables that accounted for the most variance were left parietal-occipital beta power (deficient in unipolar, excess in bipolar), left hemisphere alpha power (deficient in bipolar), and anterior coherence (decreased in theta band in unipolar and decreased in beta band in bipolar patients). Accuracy was 87 percent for identifying unipolar individuals and 90 percent for identifying bipolar individuals. Lieber and Newbury (1988) also have delineated several subtypes of unipolar depression.

Lawson, Rogers, Barnes, Bodenhamer-Davis, and Reed (2000) have developed a new asymmetry metric that emphasizes coherence asymmetry rather than power asymmetry. Alpha coherence asymmetry is calculated as:

$$\frac{(\text{F3}/\text{CZ alpha coherence} - \text{F4}/\text{CZ alpha coherence})}{(\text{F3}/\text{CZ alpha coherence} + \text{F4}/\text{CZ alpha coherence})}$$

This alpha coherence asymmetry measure shows the differences between the amount of shared alpha activity between the central region (CZ) and the left frontal (F3) and right frontal (F4) areas. This metric helps to explain why frontal EEG alpha power asymmetry is more often significantly related to depression when analyzed with a vertex reference (CZ) than with a linked ears reference (A1/A2). The problem with using a vertex reference is that it is an active reference.

If alpha power over the right frontal lobe is similar to that at the vertex, little net alpha activity will be recorded. Conversely, if left frontal alpha power is very different from that at CZ, then a large differential amount of alpha power will be recorded. Frontal alpha power asymmetry using the CZ reference is therefore, a measure of the relationship between frontal and central brain alpha on the left and right. Coherence, as defined here, is a measure of the similarity of frequency activity between two brain sites with a constant phase relationship. There was a high correlation between depression severity and alpha coherence asymmetry ($r = 0.56$). The correlation with CZ alpha power asymmetry was lower ($r = 0.34$). It may well be that coherence training to normalize frontal alpha coherence asymmetry will prove to be more effective than alpha power asymmetry training for remediation of depression. However, no studies have yet been reported. Although alpha coherence asymmetry and alpha power asymmetry have a fairly high correlation ($r = 0.70$), they are measuring somewhat different parameters. Alpha coherence asymmetry may be a better metric for biofeedback training.

A second problem, addressed by Lawson (2001), is the role of comorbid anxiety on QEEG metrics. Anxiety tends to be associated with reduced alpha power in the right frontal lobe in the majority of cases (Sackheim, Greenberg, Weiman, & Gur, 1982; Gurnee, 2000). Clients who are both anxious and depressed may have coherence or power abnormalities with left or right preponderance. One, therefore, cannot reliably predict the direction of change produced by asymmetry training in this common type of patient. It is likely that additional specific training to decrease anxiety will be necessary to optimally help this group of patients.

Leuchter, Uijtdehaage, O'Hara, Cook, and Mandelkern (1999) have described a refined QEEG measure (cordance), which integrates information from absolute and relative power measures. This measure is highly correlated with rCBF. This measure may be used in the future for predicting outcomes of treatment for depression.

TREATMENT OF DEPRESSION WITH NEUROTHERAPY

There are no controlled studies of neurofeedback therapy for depression, and there also are no published references in which QEEG was used to guide neurofeedback training of depression. The first clinical neurofeedback approach was that of the Othmers (1994), based on the studies showing underactivation of the left hemisphere in depression. Decreasing theta (4-7 Hz) and simultaneously increasing beta-2 (15-18 Hz) at C3 was found to reduce depression in most patients (Othmer, 1994). For overaroused patients (anxiety, mania), right hemisphere training was done by decreasing 4-7 Hz and increasing 12-15 Hz activity at C4. Later, inhibition of 8-11 Hz activity was used by the Othmers (1997) to deal with underactivation states. In unstable states (such as manic-depressive or bipolar disorder), bipolar training often was found to be effective (increasing beta-2 [15-18 Hz] at T3/ FPI and increasing SMR [12-15 Hz] at T4/FP2). They note that excessive beta training may cause agitation, anxiety, mania, obsessive thoughts, compulsive behaviors, anger, aggressiveness, pressure in the chest, or a sensation of "crawling skin." Excessive SMR training may cause depression, irritability, or loss of emotional control. The Othmers report that left-sided beta-2 training increases ego strength and sense of well-being, whereas right-sided SMR training increases awareness of internal body state and social-emotional awareness of others (Othmer, 1997). Our results have been similar when using their approach.

Baehr and Baehr (1997) have used alpha asymmetry reduction to treat depression. In one clinical study, three of six patients improved on the Chambers and Beck Depression Inventory measures both immediately after training and at one and five years after neurofeedback training. Hammond (2001) had similar results in an independent study of frontal asymmetry training using the ROSHI procedure. Eight medication-resistant patients were trained for an average of 10.4 hours, with no other therapy. Mean improvement in MMPI depression scale scores of 28.75 T score points was found. All but one patient improved, and at one-year follow-up, improvement was maintained in all of those who improved. Putnam (2001) reported successful treatment with neurofeedback of depression associated with a stroke. Schneider, Heimann, and Mattes (2003) reported successful treatment of depression by down-regulating slow cortical potentials.

We report here our results using QEEG to guide neurofeedback in treating depressed patients, using two case histories to illustrate its utility. Our approach has been to identify the most significant abnormalities on QEEG and treat them with a series of protocols intended to normalize the specific abnormalities. If an abnormality is increased compared to normal, we downtrain it and if an abnormality is decreased compared to normal, we uptrain it. Usually five to ten sessions are done for each abnormality.

Recently, we have been using FP02 training to decrease theta (2-7 Hz) and increase beta (15-18 Hz) with depressed patients. They usually report feeling less depressed. This site is just medial to the right eyebrow. Although not proven, FP02 beta training appears to be a promising addition to depression protocols. Fisher (2003a,b) used this site, inhibiting delta and theta and rewarding alpha, to decrease fear, but she has not tried rewarding beta to decrease depression (personal communication).

CASE HISTORIES

Case 1 (Unipolar Disorder)

This 41-year-old woman had a long history of chronic depression. Treatment with a variety of antidepressant drugs did not help her depression. Training was begun with a classic Othmer protocol: C3 beta (reward decrease of 2-7 Hz and increase of 15 Hz at C3-monopolar training). She noted some improvement in her depression by the second session. By the tenth session, her depression was gone. A total of 16 sessions were done. She has been depression-free for over two years.

This type of blind (non-QEEG guided) training ("C3 beta") has been effective in our clinic about 80 percent of the times in remediating long-standing, drug-resistant unipolar depression.

Case 2 (Bipolar Disorder) (QEEG-Guided)

The client was a 61-year-old man with lifelong severe mood swings and intermittent bouts of severe depression. Lithium therapy was ineffective. Several antidepressants were tried without lasting benefit. Treatment with Topamax helped the depression, but triggered a sustained manic episode, during which the client got into trouble at work and was discharged. He again became severely depressed and took an overdose of medications in an attempt to commit suicide. The initial QEEG showed an increase in relative power of 7-9 Hz activity over the frontal and central regions bilaterally, and an increase in 8-9 Hz activity in both occipital regions. There was an increase in the relative power of 22-30 Hz activity in the left frontal/temporal regions. Decreased coherence was noted in alpha at O1/F7, in beta at F4/F8, in theta at F7/F8, and in delta at F7/F8.

He first completed 10 sessions to decrease 19-30 Hz at FP1 and noted marked improvement, with less anxiety, irritability, anger, and depression. Four sessions were done to decrease 7-9 Hz and increase 15-18 Hz. Five sessions were done to decrease 2-7 Hz and to increase 15-18 Hz at O2.

Upon completion of training, the client was no longer having either severe depression or manic episodes. He still had some anger related to his employment. He is in counseling to resolve these issues. He has stopped treatment with Cymbalta (antidepressant) but continues on Depakote (mood stabilizer). The follow-up QEEG revealed resolution of the slow abnormalities. The excessive high frequency beta activity had resolved in the left frontal and temporal areas, although there was still some excess 27-30 Hz activity in the parietal, central, and midfrontal areas. The decreases in coherence on the first study had normalized, with the development of increased coherence in several connections in left hemisphere delta and right hemisphere beta. These new hypercoherent abnormalities may represent a strategy used by the brain to ameliorate the original hypocoherent abnormalities. They were not accompanied by the development of any new symptoms.

CONCLUSIONS

Recent advances in the neurobiology of depression and anxiety have led to a better understanding of the roles of different brain areas in triggering depression, happiness, anxiety, or calmness. Activation (increasing 15-18 Hz) of the left frontal lobe generally triggers mood elevation, while hypoactivation (excess theta or alpha) of the left frontal lobe appears to cause failure of suppression of the subcortical structures that mediate the depressed state. Activation of the right orbital frontal lobe at 15-18 Hz can produce mood elevation. Higher frequency activation (21-30 Hz) of the right orbital frontal area, the posterior cingulate, or the inferior parietal lobules can trigger anxiety or mania, while calmness is usually associated with deactivation of these areas. Neurofeedback can be used to capitalize on these findings to remediate depression and anxiety, and promote happiness and calmness. QEEG and LORETA can be used to characterize the particular areas that need to be addressed in an individual patient, thereby producing the desired effects more quickly and persistently.

Recently, we have been using FP02 training to decrease theta (2-7 Hz) and increase beta (15-18 Hz) with depressed patients and they report feeling less depressed. Although not proven, FP02 beta training appears to be a promising addition to depression protocols.

REFERENCES

Adolphs, R. J., & Tranel, D. (2004). Emotion. In *Principles and practice of behavioral neurology and neuropsychology* (pp. 451-474). Philadelphia: Saunders.

Baehr, E., & Baehr, R. (1997). The use of neurofeedback as adjunctive therapeutic treatment for depression: Three case studies. *Biofeedback, 25*, 10-11.

Baehr, E., Rosenfeld, J. P., & Baehr, R. (1997). The clinical use of an alpha asymmetry protocol in the neurofeedback treatment of depression: Two case studies. *Journal of Neurotherapy, 2*, 10-23.

Baehr, E., Rosenfeld, P., Baehr, R., & Earnest, C. (1999). Clinical use of an alpha asymmetry protocol in the treatment of depressive disorders. In Evans, J., & Arbanel, A. (Eds.). *Introduction to QEEG and neurofeedback* (pp. 181-188). New York: Academic Press.

Davidson, R. J., & Irwin, W. (1999). The functional neuroanatomy of emotion and affective style. *Trends in Cognitive Sciences, 3*, 11-22.

Earnest, C. (1999). Single case study of EEG asymmetry biofeedback for depression: An independent replication in an adolescent. *Journal of Neurotherapy, 3*, 28-35.

Fisher, S. (2003a). *The fear protocol: The theory of FP02 and the implications of new clinical data.* Winter Brain Abstracts.

Fisher, S. (2003b). *Fear and FP02: The implication of a new protocol.* ISNR proceedings. 11th Annual Conference.

Gurnee, R. (2000). *QEEG subtypes of anxiety.* Abstract. Int. Soc. Neuronal Regulation.

Hammond, D. C. (2001). Neurofeedback treatment of depression with the ROSHI. *Journal of Neurotherapy, 4*, 45-56.

Lawson. R. (2001). *Anterior alpha asymmetry in anxiety and depression.* Abstract. Society for Neuronal Regulation.

Lawson, R., Rogers, R. Barnes, T., Bodenhamer-David, E., & Reed, S. (2000). *A comparison of exterior alpha asymmetry measures as predictors of depression severity.* Abstract. Society for Neuronal Regulation.

Leuchter, A. F., Uijtdehaage, S. A. J., Cook, I. A., O'Hara, R., & Mandelkern, N. (1999). Relationship between brain electrical activity and cortical perfusion in normal subjects. *Journal of Psychiatry Research, 90,* 125-140.

Lieber, A. L., & Newbury, N. D. (1988). Diagnosis and subtyping of depressive disorders by QEEG discriminates IV. Subtypes of unipolar depression. *The Hillside Journal of Clinical Psychiatry, 10,* 73-82.

Liotti, M., & Mayberg, H. S. (2001). The role of functional neuroimaging in the neoropsychology of depression. *Journal of Clinical and Experimental Neuropsychology, 23,* 121-136.

Mayberg, H. S., Brannan, S. K., Tekell, J. L., Silva, J. A., Makurvin, R. K., & McGinnis, S. (2000). Regional metabolic effects of fluoxetine in major depression: Serial changes and relationship to clinical depression. *Psychiatry, 48,* 830-843.

Ongur, D., Drevets., W. D., & Price, J. L. (1998). Glial reduction in the subgenual prefrontal cortex in mood disorders. *Proceedings of the National Academy of Sciences of the United States of America, 95,* 13290-13295.

Othmer, S. (1994). *Depression.* In Training Syllabus. Vol. II, EEG Spectrum, at a workshop conducted at Encino, CA.

Othmer, S. (1997). *Depression.* In Training Syllabus. Vol. II, EEG Spectrum, at a workshop conducted at Encino, CA.

Prichep, L. S., Lieber, A. L., & John, E. R. (1986). Quantitative EEG in depressive disorders. In Shagass, C. (Ed.) *Electrical brain potentials and psychotherapy,* Amsterdam: Elesvier.

Putnam, J. A. (2001). EEG biofeedback in a female stroke patient with depression. *Journal of Neurotherapy, 5,* 27-38.

Rosenfeld, J. P., Baehr, E., Baehr, R., Gottlieb, I. H., & Rangarndth, C. (1996). Preliminary evidence that daily changes in frontal alpha asymmetry correlate with changes in affect in therapy sessions. *International Journal of Psychophysiology, 23,* 137-141.

Rosenfeld, P. J. (1999). An EEG biofeedback protocol for affective disorders. *Clin. EEG, 31,* 7-12.

Sackheim, H. A., Greenberg, Weiman, A. C., Gur, R. C., & Hungerbuhler, J. P. (1982). Hemispheric asymmetry in the expression of positive and negative emotions. *Archives of Neurology, 39,* 210-218.

Schneider, F., Heimann, H., & Mattes, R. (2003). Self-regulation of slow cortical potentials in psychiatric patients. *Biofeedback, 17,* 2003-2214.

Starkstein, S. E., & Robinson, R. G. (1991). The roles of the frontal lobes in affective disorder following stroke. In Levison, A. S., Eisenberg, S. M., & Burton, A. (Eds.) *Frontal lobe function and dysfunction,* (pp. 212-218), New York: Oxford University Press.

Chapter 15

A Neurologist's Experience with QEEG-Guided Neurofeedback Following Brain Injury

Jonathan E. Walker

INTRODUCTION

There is a head injury epidemic in the United States, and in other countries where motor vehicles are in common use (Lobosky, 1996). When there is severe injury to the brain, with development of hemorrhage or brain edema, it is easy to diagnose with CT scan or MRI or raw EEG. However, in the majority of cases (over 85 percent), those routine studies are normal even when the patient has severe postconcussive sequelae. The gold standard for determining brain injury is the quantitative EEG (QEEG) (Thatcher et al., 1998). The most common abnormalities on QEEG in "mild" closed head injury (MHI) (i.e., patients who are alert and have no focal neurological deficits) are increases in coherence of theta and beta, decreases in phase of beta and alpha, beta amplitude asymmetries, and decreases in relative power of alpha. The predominant mechanism of injury is most likely diffuse axonal injury caused by shearing forces engendered by concussion (Maythaler, McAvery, & Hadley, 2001). The areas most affected are the brain stem, parasagittal white matter of the cortex, the corpus callosum, and the gray/white matter junctions of the cerebral cortex. The most common symptoms are poor short-term memory,

Handbook of Neurofeedback
© 2007 by The Haworth Press, Inc. All rights reserved.
doi:10.1300/5889_15

attentional difficulty, concentration difficulty, headaches, dizziness, depression, vision difficulty, cognitive deficits, anxiety, fatigue, irritability, poor speech fluency, and sleep disturbance (Walker, Norman, & Weber, 2002). Such postconcussive symptoms tend to improve with time, but 79 percent of MHI cases report at least one persistent symptom after three months, and 34 percent exhibit some level of functional disability after one year (Rimel, Giordani, Barth, Boll, & Jane, 1995). If posttraumatic symptoms persist at three months, they are likely to persist at six months and one year (Hoffman, Stockdale, & van Egren, 1981). Neuropsychological and cognitive rehabilitation approaches have not demonstrated significant effects on persistent postconcussive symptoms or disability (Silver et al., 1994; Rattok & Ross, 1994). Neurofeedback, on the other hand, has become increasingly effective in helping these patients reduce their symptoms, resolve their disabilities, and return to work. This review will cover all studies the author found in the literature with regard to neurofeedback to treat mild closed head injury. I will then present a few recent case histories in which neurofeedback was guided by power and coherence abnormalities on QEEG, illustrating the power of this approach. Finally, I will make some observations on why this approach has been slow to take hold in the neurological community, with suggestions as to how it can become more accepted.

REVIEW OF LITERATURE

The first reports of neurofeedback for MHI were those by Ayers (Ayers, 1983, 1987). Bipolar training was carried out to reduce 4-7 Hz activity and increase 15-18 Hz at F8/T4 for right hemisphere injuries. Previous psychotherapy had been ineffective. Six patients involved in one study had been randomly assigned to neurofeedback training. They reported subsidence of their mood swings, anger outbursts, and anxiety attacks. The patients continuing on psychotherapy alone did not experience improvement in these symptoms. This is the only controlled trial of neurofeedback for MHI in the literature to date.

The first reports on QEEG-guided neurofeedback for closed head injury were those of Hoffman and colleagues (Hoffman, Stockdale, & van Egren, 1981). They reported that 60 percent improved in self-reported symptoms and/or cognitive performance (Micro-Cog[R] assessment) after 40 sessions of neurofeedback. Later studies indicated improvement within 5-10 sessions (Hoffman, Stockdale, & Hicks, 1995; Hoffman, Stockdale, van Egeren, et al., 1996a,b). Those patients who improved with neurofeedback also evidenced improvement of their QEEGs. Tinius and Tinius (1996) also reported improved QEEGs in patients treated with neurofeedback for traumatic brain injury. Packard and Ham (1994) treated patients with persistent posttraumatic headache (greater than 1 year); 53 percent of the patients reported moderate or better relief of their headaches, 80 percent reported significant improvement in their ability to relax and cope with their pain, and 95 percent reported EEG biofeedback was helpful to some degree. The author of this paper and his associates reported a series of 26 patients with persistent posttraumatic symptoms (Walker, Norman, & Weber, 2002). Eighty-eight percent of the patients reported significant (greater than 50 percent) improvement in their symptoms (mean = 73 percent). All patients, who had been employed prior to the head injury, but could not work because of their symptoms, returned to work after neurofeedback training. These results are promising, but a double-blind placebo controlled study will be required to determine the true efficacy of the procedure. Thatcher (2002) has proposed such a study and outlined the research methodology that will be required.

PERSONAL EXPERIENCES

The author's entry into this field was stimulated by the success of Lubar (1991) in remediating symptoms of ADHD with neurofeedback. My training was in neurology and clinical pharmacology, and I was frustrated by the failure of head injury patients to respond to drug and behavioral treatment. It was my hope that neurofeedback would be helpful in relieving their symptoms and returning them to work. The development of increasingly better QEEG databases has greatly improved the ability to do precise training to remediate brain dysfunctions, as opposed to symptom-based training. Our first experiences with brain-impaired patients was using beta training, as pioneered by the Othmers (1995), and recently verified by Laibow, Stubblebine, and Sandground (2001). Results were good, but typically, about sixty sessions were required to return the patient to work

(Walker, 1996). Based on Horvat's experience that coherence training worked faster than power training (Horvat, 2004), our clinic began to train coherence instead. Indeed, we found that training was accomplished in about thirty sessions, enabling return to work (Walker, Norman, & Weber, 2002). Good discussions of coherence can be found in a paper by Thatcher (1998) and in the chapter in this text by Horvat. Thatcher had earlier found that coherence abnormalities are prominent in the QEEGs of head injured patients (Thatcher, Walker, Gerson, & Geisler, 1989). It is thought that normalization of coherence improves communication between areas that have been "disconnected" or "hyperconnected" as a result of axonal injury caused by concussion of the brain. The mechanism of improvement associated with successful coherence training is not known, but most likely represents learning by the brain (operant conditioning), in which nondamaged connections are used to bypass injured axons. Alternatively, transmitter release may be increased or decreased to accomplish the normalization of coherence. New synapses or connections may be formed, although this seems unlikely in neocortex.

RECENT ADVANCES

Thornton (2000) reported that coherence training of two brain-injured patients improved auditory recall by 85 and 168 percent. He has recently found even more impressive improvements in head injury symptoms using a new QEEG database to guide his training (2005). This database includes normal values for higher frequencies (gamma), as well as normal values for EEG changes associated with activation (EEG obtained while the client is reading, listening, writing, doing math). He then does training during activation, using the appropriate task. With this approach, he has achieved excellent results in MHI patients, as well as in children with learning disabilities. His data indicate that neurotherapy interventions are more effective than standard cognitive behavioral therapies. Also, neurotherapy is significantly less expensive. Another indication of the power of neurofeedback training is that some medically intractable posttraumatic seizures can be remediated using QEEG-guided neurofeedback (Walker & Davidson, 2004).

CURRENT PRACTICE OF QEEG-GUIDED
NEUROFEEDBACK AS USED IN OUR CLINIC

MHI patients are evaluated with a clinical history, a neurological evaluation, psychological testing, the Test of Variables of Attention (TOVA), and a QEEG. The QEEG is then used to guide the training. Both, power and coherence abnormalities, are addressed. If power or coherence abnormalities are increased compared to normal, they are downtrained. If power or coherence abnormalities are decreased compared to normal, they are uptrained. If abnormalities are numerous, which is often the case, we will first train the most significantly abnormal power abnormality found during eyes open (the most abnormally increased slow and fast frequencies). Then, we will train the most aberrant abnormality found during reading activation (usually an excess of slow frequencies). Next, we treat the statistically most significant coherence abnormalities in the delta, theta, alpha, and beta bands. Each protocol is for five sessions. We choose five sessions for each, because there are possibilities to overtrain. This does not usually occur in five sessions. Usually the patient is significantly improved after 30 to 35 sessions. On those rare occasions when the patient still has disabling symptoms, we will remap via QEEG and repeat this process. Once the patient reports amelioration of his symptoms, the TOVA and psychological tests are repeated, to verify for patient, families, employers, and insurance companies that the training has been effective.

FAILURES USING THIS APPROACH

Failures are uncommon, as evidenced by improvement in patients' symptoms, and the patients' return to work or school (Walker, Norman, & Weber, 2002). Obviously, this approach does not work if the patient does not get the testing or complete the training. Too often, it is a matter of affordability. Many MHI patients are out of work, out of money, and cannot get insurance. We have been willing to take a letter of protection from an attorney, so they can get the training, but this is financially risky, since the case may take a long time to prosecute, and there is no guarantee that the case will be won. We are fortunate in the State of Texas to have the Texas Head Injury Biofeedback Initiative, which mandates that if biofeedback is a covered benefit, then the patient's insurance company is to pay for the training. This statute should be a model for other states too. Unfortunately, not everyone has insurance. Medicare pays poorly for neurofeedback and Medicaid, not at all. It is incumbent on those of us in the field to become politically active and persuade our legislators what a powerful tool this is. We need to do the same with insurance companies, and show them how much money it saves them in the long run.

A second cause of failure is dropping out before training is completed. Having a MHI is a very stressful and confusing situation, and there are many reasons patients do not complete training—financial, social, and medical. One of the saddest reasons is that medical practitioners are often unfamiliar with neurofeedback and its effectiveness in MHI. They may advise the patient to try drugs, psychotherapy, or behavioral/cognitive therapy—which often results in less effective and more expensive and prolonged treatment.

Failure for the patient who completes training is rare in our experience; 95 percent of our patients experience some benefit, and greater than 50 percent improvement is the usual outcome. Almost everyone returns to work or school and is able to function relatively normally. Those who do fail with this approach may still use drugs, psychotherapy, and cognitive/behavioral therapy with some benefit.

APPROACHES TO GAINING ACCEPTANCE IN THE MEDICAL/NEUROLOGICAL COMMUNITY

It is the author's belief that a major problem is that the neurofeedback community has not been able to adequately educate physicians of the value of neurofeedback in MHI. Publications have been few, and rarely in mainstream medical publications. Most physicians are used to judging therapy according to the drug model (double-blind, placebo controlled trials). They do not understand that no two patients are trained the same way with neurofeedback. Some patients need to be pushed (e.g., to higher thresholds). Some need to be retrained (e.g., lowered thresholds). Some need to be left alone. Different sessions require different coaching. The difficulty is compounded when QEEG is used to guide training, since the abnormalities are different in each patient, and a unique set of protocols is required. We need to teach them that a better model for evaluating neurofeedback is a psychother-apeutic model, which allows modification of the protocol, depending on the patient's response to the training. Placebo training is easily de-tected by the patient, making blinding impossible; and noncontingent training may actually make the patient worse. QEEG-guided neuro-feedback is more analogous to neurosurgery than to drug treatment. A surgeon does not remove the same brain area in all of his brain tu-mor patients, but directs his attention to the area where the tumor is. Drugs, on the other hand, affect the brain in a diffuse, nonlocalized fashion.

In the final analysis, outcome studies, using historical or tradi-tional treatments and wait-listed participants as controls, will be nec-essary to persuade physicians and insurance companies that we have a better mousetrap. There are rigorous designs that are superior to the double-blind placebo control model (Armitage, 2002). Some of these are more appropriate for evaluating the efficacy of neurofeedback for MHI remediation.

FUTURE DIRECTIONS

Improvements in QEEG databases have been important in moving this field forward. However, there are still problems with the available databases (Lubar, 2004). Most do not separate out the various beta fre-quencies (12-15 Hz, 15-18 Hz, various gamma frequencies). Quite dif-ferent behavioral and cognitive effects are seen when different beta frequencies are trained. Also, traditional neurofeedback with scalp electrodes may not be addressing subcortical problems responsible for many of the symptoms of MHI. LORETA QEEG and neurofeedback may be able to address those problems better (Towler, 2004; Congedo & Joffe, this volume). Activation of the QEEG clearly changes power and coherence abnormalities, and activation training may be more effective than eyes closed or eyes open training (Thornton, 2005). Functional neuroimaging (e.g., fMRI, PET) promises to help under-stand the dynamics of neurofeedback, and may help us learn how to do better neurofeedback (Beauregard, 2004). QEEG-guided neurofeed-back is likely to be helpful in many neurologic disorders for which it has not yet been tried (Walker & Davidson, 2004).

SUMMARY

Neurofeedback, particularly QEEG-guided neurofeedback, is a powerful tool for remediating persistent posttraumatic symptoms of patients with mild or moderate head injury. It is a noninvasive, holistic, nontoxic, safe, rapid, and inexpensive way to remediate the symptoms in these patients. Our success in this area bodes well for future successful treatment of other psychological and neurological disorders.

REFERENCES

Armitage, P. (2002). *Statistical methods in medical research.* Blackwell: Oxford.

Ayers, M. E. (1983). Electroencephalographic feedback and head trauma. In *Head and neck trauma: The latest information and perspectives in patients with less than optimum recovery* (pp. 244-257). Los Angeles: UCLA Neuropsychiatric Institute.

Ayers, M. E. (1987). *Electroencephalographic neurofeedback and closed head injury of 250 individuals.* National Head Injury Conference.

Ayers, M. E. (1991). *A controlled study of EEG neurofeedback training and clinical psychotherapy for right hemisphere closed head injury.* National Head Injury Foundation Conference.

Beauregard, M. (Aug. 2004). *Effect of neurofeedback training on the neural substrate of executive deficits in ADHD children.* ISNR Conference. Abstract.

Hoffman, D. A., Stockdale, S., & Hicks, L. (1995). Diagnosis and treatment of head injury. *Journal of Neurotherapy, 1,* 14-21.

Hoffman, D.A., Stockdale, S., & van Egeren, L. (1981). Diagnosis and treatment of head injury. *Neurosurgery, 9,* 221-228.

Hoffman D. A., Stockdale, S., van Egeren, L. et al. (1996a). EEG neurofeedback in the treatment of mild traumatic brain injury. *Clinical EEG, 27,* 6.

Hoffman, D. A., Stockdale, S., van Egeren, L. et al. (1996b). Symptom changes in the treatment of mild traumatic brain injury using EEG neurofeedback. Abstract. *Clinical EEG, 27,* 164.

Horvat, J. (2004). *Management of closed head injury.* SNR Workshop.

Laibow, R. E., Stubblebine, A. N., & Sandground, H.(2001). EEG-neurofeedback treatment of patients with brain injury: Part 2, EEG parameters versus rehabilitation. *Journal of Neurotherapy, 5,* 45.

Lobosky, J. F. (1996). Epidemiology of head injury. In Naranya, K. (Ed.), *Neurotrauma,* New York: McGraw-Hill.

Lubar, J. F. (1991). Discourse on the development of EEG diagnostics and biofeedback for attention-deficit/hyperactivity disorders. *Biofeedback and Self-Regulation, 16,* 210-225.

Lubar, J. F. (2004). Quantitative Electroencephalographic Analysis Databases for Neurotherapy. *Journal of Neurotherapy, 7,* 1-169.

Maythaler, J. M., McCray, A., & Hadley, M. N. (2001). Current concepts: Diffuse axonal injury-associated traumatic brain injury. *Archives of Physical Medicine and Rehabilitation, 82,* 1461-1471.

Othmer, S. F., & Othmer, S. (1995). *Professional training syllabus,* EEG Spectrum, Encino, CA.

Packard, R. C., & Ham, L. P. (1994). Post-traumatic headache. *The Journal of Neuropsychiatry and Clinical Neurosciences,* Summer, 229-236.

Rattok, J., & Ross, B. (1994). Cognitive rehabilitation. In Silver, J., Ashman, T., Spielman, L., & Hibbard, M. (Eds.) *The Neuropsychiatry of traumatic brain injury* (pp. 703-729). Washington: American Psychiatric Press.

Rimel, R. W., Giordani. B., Barth, J. T., Boll, T. J., & Jane, J. A. (1995). Disability caused by mild closed head injury. *Journal of Neurotherapy, 1,* 14-21.

Silver, J., Ashman, T., Spielman, L., & Hibbard, M. (1994). *The neuropsychiartry of traumatic brain injury.* Washington: American Psychiatric Press.

Thatcher, R. W. (1998). Biophysical linkage between MRI and EEG coherence in closed head injury. *Neuroimaging, 8,* 307-326.

Thatcher, R. W. (2000). EEG-operant conditioning and traumatic brain injury. *Clinical EEG, 31,* 38-44.

Thatcher, R. W., Walker, R.A., Gerson, I., & Geisler, F. (1998). EEG discriminant analyses of mild head trauma. *Electroencephalography and Clinical Neurophysiology, 73,* 94-106.

Thornton, K. (2000). Improvement/rehabilitation of memory functioning with Neurotherapy/QEEG biofeedback. *The Journal of Head Trauma Rehabilitation, 15,* 1285-1296.

Thornton, K. (Jan. 2005). *EEG biofeedback for reading disabilities and traumatic brain Injury* (pp. 137-162). Psychiatric Clinics of North America.

Tinius T., & Tinius, C. (Sept. 20, 1996). *Neurotherapy for TBI.* Abstract. 4th Annual SSNR Conference.

Towler, K. (August 2004). *LORETA neurofeedback and automaticity.* 12th ISNR Conference.

Walker, J. E. (February 1996). *Rehabilitation of the patient with mild closed head injury.* Proceedings of the Future Health Conference.

Walker, J. E. (Jan. 2005). *Neurofeedback training for epilepsy* (pp. 163-176). Child and Adolescent Psychiatric Clinics of North America.

Walker, J. E., & Davidson, D. (August 2004). *QEEG-guided power and coherence training remediates tic disorder.* Abstract. 12th ISNR Conference.

Walker, J. E., Norman, C. A., & Weber, R. (2002). Impact of QEEG-guided coherence training for patients with a mild closed head injury. *Journal of Neurotherapy, 6,* 31-43.

Index

Page numbers followed by the letter "i" indicate an illustration; those followed by the letter "t" indicate a table.